T0317582

The Spanish Influenza
Pandemic of 1918–1919

Rochester Studies in Medical History

Senior Editor: Theodore M. Brown
Professor of History and Preventive Medicine
University of Rochester

Additional Titles of Interest

The Neurological Patient in History
Edited by L. Stephen Jacyna and Stephen T. Casper

The Birth Control Clinic in a Marketplace World
Rose Holz

Bacteriology in British India: Laboratory Medicine and the Tropics
Pratik Chakrabarti

Barefoot Doctors and Western Medicine in China
Xiaoping Fang

Beriberi in Modern Japan: The Making of a National Disease
Alexander R. Bay

The Lobotomy Letters
Mical Raz

Plague and Public Health in Early Modern Seville
Kristy Wilson Bowers

Medicine and the Workhouse
Edited by Jonathan Reinarz and Leonard Schwarz

Stress, Shock, and Adaptation in the Twentieth Century
Edited by David Cantor and Edmund Ramsden

*Female Circumcision and Clitoridectomy in the United States:
A History of a Medical Treatment*
Sarah B. Rodriguez

A complete list of titles in the Rochester Studies in Medical History series
may be found on our website, www.urpress.com.

The Spanish
Influenza Pandemic
of 1918–1919

Perspectives from the
Iberian Peninsula and the Americas

EDITED BY MARÍA-ISABEL PORRAS-GALLO
AND RYAN A. DAVIS

UNIVERSITY OF ROCHESTER PRESS

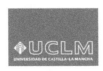

Copyright © 2014 by the Editors and Contributors

All rights reserved. Except as permitted under current legislation, no part of this work may be photocopied, stored in a retrieval system, published, performed in public, adapted, broadcast, transmitted, recorded, or reproduced in any form or by any means, without the prior permission of the copyright owner.

First published 2014

University of Rochester Press
668 Mt. Hope Avenue, Rochester, NY 14620, USA
www.urpress.com
and Boydell & Brewer Limited
PO Box 9, Woodbridge, Suffolk IP12 3DF, UK
www.boydellandbrewer.com

ISBN-13: 978-1-58046-496-3
ISSN: 1526-2715

Library of Congress Cataloging-in-Publication Data

The Spanish influenza pandemic of 1918–1919 : perspectives from the Iberian Peninsula and the Americas / edited by María-Isabel Porras-Gallo and Ryan A. Davis.
    p. ; cm. — (Rochester studies in medical history, ISSN 1526-2715 ; v. 30)
    Includes bibliographical references and index.
    ISBN 978-1-58046-496-3 (hardcover : alk. paper)
    I. Porras Gallo, M. Isabel (María Isabel), editor. II. Davis, Ryan A., editor.
III. Series: Rochester studies in medical history. 1526–2715
    [DNLM: 1. Influenza Pandemic, 1918–1919—history—Portugal. 2. Influenza Pandemic, 1918–1919—history—South America. 3. Influenza Pandemic, 1918–1919—history—Spain. 4. History, 20th Century—Portugal. 5. History, 20th Century–South America. 6. History, 20th Century—Spain. 7. Influenza A Virus, H1N1 Subtype—Portugal. 8. Influenza A Virus, H1N1 Subtype—South America. 9. Influenza A Virus, H1N1 Subtype—Spain. 10. Influenza, Human—history—Portugal. 11. Influenza, Human—history—South America. 12. Influenza, Human—history—Spain. WC 515]
    RA644.I6
    614.5ʼ1809041—dc23   2014029792

A catalogue record for this title is available from the British Library.

This publication is printed on acid-free paper.
Printed in the United States of America.

The editors would like to thank their respective universities—
the University of Castilla-La Mancha and Illinois State University—
for their monetary support of this project.

Contents

Introduction: Emerging Perspectives of the Spanish Influenza
Pandemic of 1918–19   1
  María-Isabel Porras-Gallo and Ryan A. Davis

Part One
Scientific Discourse: Now and Then

1 The Great Evolutionary Potential of Viruses: The 1918 Flu
   as a Paradigm of Disease Emergence   21
   Esteban Domingo

2 Spanish Flu in Brazil: Searching for Causes during the
   Epidemic Horror   39
   Liane Maria Bertucci

3 Ricardo Jorge and the Construction of a Medico-Sanitary Public
   Discourse: Portugal and International Scientific Networks   56
   Maria de Fátima Nunes

Part Two
Social Responses: Human and Institutional Actors

4 And to Make Things Worse, the Flu: The Spanish Influenza
   in a Revolutionary Portugal   75
   José Manuel Sobral, Maria Luísa Lima, and Paulo Silveira e Sousa

5 Between the Pandemic and World War I: The 1918–19 Influenza
   Pandemic in the Spanish Army, through the Eyes of the Press   93
   María-Isabel Porras-Gallo

6 The Reign of the Spanish Flu: Impact and Responses to the
   1918 Influenza Pandemic in Minas Gerais, Brazil   111
   Anny Jackeline Torres Silveira

7 The Spanish Flu in Bahia, Brazil: Prophylaxis and
   Healing Practices   130
   Christiane Maria Cruz de Souza

8   A Collaborative Experience: The Mutual Benefit Societies'
    Responses to the 1918–19 Influenza Pandemic in
    Pamplona, Spain   152
    Pilar León-Sanz

Part Three
Interpreting the Epidemic:
Sociocultural Dynamics and Perspectives

9   A Tale of Two Spains: Narrating the Nation during the
    1918–19 Influenza Epidemic   173
    Ryan A. Davis

10 The Spanish Flu in Argentina: An Alarming Hostage   194
    Hernán Feldman

11 Epidemic Disease, Local Government, and Social Control:
    The Example of the City of Alicante, Spain   215
    Josep Bernabeu-Mestre and Mercedes Pascual Artiaga

12 The Gendered Dimensions of Epidemic Disease: Influenza in
    Montreal, Canada, 1918–20   230
    Magda Fahrni

13 Remembering and Reconstructing: Fictions of the
    1918–19 Influenza Pandemic   248
    Catherine Belling

    Selected Bibliography   265

    List of Contributors   269

    Index   275

Introduction

Emerging Perspectives of the
Spanish Influenza Pandemic of 1918–19

María-Isabel Porras-Gallo
and Ryan A. Davis

Over the past decade the Spanish influenza pandemic of 1918–19 has commanded an increasing amount of attention from professionals and laypersons alike. In 1997 pathologist Jeffery Taubenberger and his team published the first partial genetic sequencing of the virus's RNA, bringing science one step closer to unlocking the mysteries of a disease that in 1918 dealt the first major blow to what Eugenia Tognotti has called the "scientific triumphalism" of the germ theory of disease.[1] The year 1918 was an era marked by the recent and astounding discoveries of the causative agents of diseases like cholera (1884), anthrax (1877), and tuberculosis (1882), and it was widely believed that laboratory trials would finally result in the isolation of the pathogenic agent of influenza. Moreover, a likely candidate already existed. On the heels of the nineteenth century's last large-scale flu epidemic in 1892, Richard Pfeiffer proposed that influenza was caused by *Haemophilus influenzae*, the bacillus later named after him. But his hypothesis was not universally accepted, and during the 1918–19 pandemic, the definitive case for Pfeiffer's bacillus failed to materialize, as laboratory studies produced no conclusive evidence that it was the microorganism responsible for causing the flu.[2] Not until 1933 were Patrick Laidlaw and his team able successfully to isolate a flu virus from humans.

Despite the importance of Laidlaw's discovery, it was merely the first step in addressing the many peculiarities of the Spanish flu. Although the pathogen responsible for causing influenza had been identified, numerous questions about the 1918 virus remained unanswered: why did it yield a W-shaped mortality curve, why was it extremely virulent, what was its etiology? By revealing the genetic code of the virus, Taubenberger and his colleagues' research held out the legitimate hope that these questions finally could be answered. The urgency to obtain answers and, more concretely, remedies (most notably in the form of a vaccine) escalated when it was discovered that the Spanish flu originated from an avian source and that it was basically the genetic "mother of all [influenza] pandemics."[3] In 2003, some years after the H5N1 "bird flu" had already jumped the species barrier and infected humans, Robert Webster and Elizabeth Walker warned in their article in *American Scientist* that "the world is teetering on the edge of a pandemic that could kill a large fraction of the human population."[4] Indeed, with the planet's population one genetic mutation away from a disaster—namely, one that would allow for human-to-human transmission of H5N1—is it any wonder the Spanish flu has been on the minds of so many people, whether professionals, politicians, or the general public?

Howard Phillips and David Killingray credit increased media attention for the recently renewed interest in the 1918–19 pandemic, though they see this coverage as sensationalist. For them, the "virological ventures of the 1990s caught a popular imagination already aroused by the drama of the 1997 Hong Kong chicken flu outbreak."[5] In many ways, the renewed interest in the pandemic coincides with a historical period marked by what Priscilla Wald refers to as the "outbreak narrative," which "in its scientific, journalistic, and fictional incarnations . . . follows a formulaic plot that begins with the identification of an emerging infection, includes discussion of the global networks through which it travels, and chronicles the epidemiological work that ends with its containment."[6] In 1918 it was precisely this last feature of the outbreak narrative of the Spanish flu (i.e., its containment) that failed to establish itself. Thus, unlocking the information of the specific microorganism responsible for causing the flu (identified since 1933 as a virus) and achieving the immunity of people by means of a specific vaccine was, and continues to be, seen as the key to ensuring the containment of future pandemics caused by the genetic progeny of the 1918 virus.

Moreover, since the urge to explain and control randomness—to say nothing of the desire to contain pathogens—is, as Charles Rosenberg eloquently reminds us, a central cognitive pressure exerted by epidemics, then we would do well to recognize in the buzz surrounding the genetic research on the virus a concomitant desire to bring psychological closure to the 1918–19 pandemic, which the WHO has described as "the single most devastating infectious disease outbreak ever recorded."[7] In other words, if closure is accomplished through the containment of epidemics, and containing future influenza pandemics is contingent on the genetic research on the 1918 virus, then if this research leads to the successful containment of future pandemics, it will also provide, as a concomitant, the psychological closure to the 1918–19 pandemic that has eluded us for the past ninety years.

It is perhaps not surprising, then, that at the same historical moment when the key of genetic sequencing seemed poised to unlock the mysteries of the 1918 virus and provide collective psychological closure to the pandemic experience, a wave of nonscientific narratives dealing explicitly and extensively with the Spanish flu also began to appear. We are thinking specifically of accounts like the CDC's *Pandemic Influenza Storybook*, the myriad works of literary fiction that have come onto the scene since 1997 (e.g., Thomas Mullen's *The Last Town on Earth*, Kevin Kerr's *Unity (1918)*, and Myla Goldberg's *Wickett's Remedy: A Novel*), documentaries and docudramas (e.g., *Black Dawn: The Next Pandemic*, *The American Experience: Influenza 1918*, *History Undercover: The Doomsday Flu*), juvenile graphic literature (e.g., Katherine Krohn's *The 1918 Flu Pandemic*), and historical scholarship. To be sure, interest in the 1918–19 pandemic has ebbed and flowed over time; however, never has there been such a concentrated focus on the pandemic from such varied perspectives at the same time, until the threat posed by the 1997 avian flu from Hong Kong.[8]

It was in this context of heightened anxiety and anticipation vis-à-vis pandemic influenza that Terrence Tumpey and his colleagues "resurrected" a genetically complete Spanish flu virus in 2005, in a sense showing that the line between media sensationalism and scientific reality is often quite thin. The authors justified their efforts in this fashion: "Because the emergence of another pandemic virus is considered likely, if not inevitable, characterization of the 1918 virus may enable us to recognize the potential threat posed by new influenza virus strains, and it will shed light on the prophylactic and therapeutic countermeasures that will be needed to control pandemic viruses."[9] Even as we were preparing this introduction, the world found itself in the midst of another pandemic—the H1N1 "swine flu." Since this novel virus essentially contained the genetic remains of the 1918 virus, the outcome of the pandemic could have had much of value to say about Tumpey and his colleagues' claim. Although similar to the 1918–19 pandemic in some respects, its severity has been much less, and, according to David Morens, Jeffery Taubenberger, and Anthony Fauci, "available evidence leads to the hope that the current pandemic virus will continue to cause low or moderate mortality rates if it does not become extinct."[10]

In any event, one factor that seems clear about the recent pandemic is that it has added yet another chapter to the perpetually unfolding story of the Spanish flu.[11] Moreover, it does so even as we struggle to answer some basic, nagging questions about the 1918–19 pandemic. In fact, Morens and Fauci's questions regarding the 1918–19 pandemic—Where did the 1918 virus originate? Why did so many young and healthy die? Why were there three waves?—remain just as pertinent in the aftermath of the 2009 pandemic since the answers continue to elude us.[12] Indeed, the Spanish flu seems destined to remain a difficult historical nut to crack.

Despite these lingering pathological and epidemiological questions, or perhaps because of them, the Spanish flu pandemic continues to be invoked frequently, both in professional and public spheres, as an important historical precedent that informs and shapes our understanding of, and response to, the current and future threats of pandemic influenza.[13] As a case in point, after combing through contemporary archives, Howard Markel and others were able to show that certain nonpharmaceutical interventions—such as school closings, the cancellation of public gatherings, isolation and quarantine—helped to mitigate the impact of the 1918–19 pandemic.[14] They argue that, in conjunction with the development of a vaccine and the use of medications, public health officials should consider similar measures in their planning for future pandemics. Similarly, in their examination of the Camp Brooks Open-Air Hospital of Boston during the 1918–19 pandemic, Richard Hobday and John Cason have recently echoed Markel and his colleagues' point of view.[15] In the context of HIV/AIDS, Elizabeth Fee and Daniel M. Fox have argued, "the rigorous application of historical methods can contribute to public understanding of the AIDS epidemic."[16] Markel and others' findings as well as those of Hobday and Cason would seem to corroborate their point in relation to the 1918–19 influenza pandemic.

Given the significance of the Spanish flu pandemic as an indispensable touchstone for grappling with more recent pandemic threats, it is encouraging that alongside the genetic work on the 1918 virus, and the epidemiological and pathological questions it raises, scholars from the social and human sciences have also engaged the pandemic. Epidemiological studies, which emerged after the isolation of the first flu virus in 1933 by Wilson Smith, Christopher Andrewes, and Patrick Laidlaw, paid particular attention to the 1918–19 pandemic, coinciding with the outbreaks of new pandemics in 1946, 1957, and 1968 and with new discoveries in the field of virology. Their frequency increased from the midseventies and, particularly, from the eighties, with notable contributions from Edwin Dennis Kilbourne, Gerald F. Pyle, K. David Patterson, Eugene P. Campbell, Andrew David Cliff, Peter Hagget, J. Keith Ord, W. Paul Gleezen, A. A. Payne, D. N. Snyder, T. D. Downs, R. E. Hope-Simpson, and Frank Macfarlane Burnet.[17] At the same time, another type of study appeared, analyzing the 1918–19 pandemic from a historical point of view, oriented toward demographic or medical history; these also became more common around the seventies. Together with local studies, other more general works were produced, such as those of Alfred W. Crosby in 1976 or E. Koenen in 1970.[18] While Crosby's study analyzed the development of the pandemic in the United States, Koenen's gave an overall picture of the pandemic worldwide and tracked the history of the flu over the centuries.[19] Historiographical interest in the Spanish flu in the midseventies was motivated by the alarm caused in the United States by the isolation in 1976 of a virus of swine flu, whose characteristics, according to researchers, appeared to be similar to those of the 1918 virus.[20] This event broadened the geographic scope of the research, although the majority of the work still corresponded to the United States.[21] In the 1980s, when the appearance of HIV/AIDS sparked new interest in infectious diseases generally, the geographic range of the research about the 1918–19 flu pandemic continued to increase, with studies analyzing what happened in different points of Africa, Indonesia, and India, as well as in Japan and Europe.[22]

The proximity of its eightieth anniversary, together with the Asian flu epidemic of 1997, once again brought the study of the great flu pandemic into prominence, and scientific journalists and academics produced a new wave of Spanish flu historiography.[23] Indeed, in 1998, some sixty scholars convened at the first academic conference dedicated entirely to the Spanish flu. Perhaps the most significant contribution of this gathering was the publication of Howard Phillips and David Killingray's *The Spanish Influenza Pandemic of 1918–1919: New Perspectives*. Offering a survey of both the historiography of the pandemic and the (then) current state of research into it, the volume helped establish not only a framework for comparative, interdisciplinary analysis of the pandemic experience but also a foundation on which subsequent scholarship could build. The six sections into which the various chapters are divided outline the parameters of this framework: "Virological and Pathological Perspectives," "Contemporary Medical and Nursing Perspectives," "Official Responses to the Pandemic," "The Demographic Impact," "Long-Term Consequences and Memories," and "Epidemiological Lessons of the Pandemic." As with any volume, important areas of analysis are omitted from their collection, many of which are directly addressed in the chapters to follow (e.g., the role of religion, literary fiction, mutual benefit societies, and regional studies of the pandemic experience).

In addition to offering new perspectives on the 1918–19 pandemic, Phillips and Killingray's volume marks off two distinct waves of Spanish flu scholarship. In his review of Esyllt W. Jones's *Influenza 1918: Disease, Death, and Struggle in Winnipeg*, Phillips describes the difference between the two waves in this fashion: "If what might be labeled the 'first wave' of scholarly histories of the 'Spanish' flu pandemic in the 1980s and 1990s paid particular attention to exploring the spread and deadly impact of the disease and getting it recognized as a topic worthy of serious study by historians, the 'second wave' of histories has been able to build on this foundation by putting particular aspects of the pandemic under lenses reflecting the authors' own fields of interest."[24] The chapters that follow correspond to both waves of flu scholarship since some geographic zones and certain questions have received more scholarly attention than others.[25] The group of cases that make up the chapters of this book have a dual aim: on the one hand, to analyze the role played by the Iberian Peninsula in the spread of the 1918–19 pandemic to the Americas; and, on the other, to deal with some of the areas omitted from Phillips and Killingray's volume and from the subsequent historiography.[26] The starting point of this book was the visit of Professor María-Isabel Porras-Gallo to Emory University in the spring of 2008, invited by Professor Ryan A. Davis. The opportunity was taken during her stay to sketch the outline of this monograph, originally conceived as the result of an international conference planned for the spring of 2009. After establishing initial contacts with the principal specialists collaborating in this volume, it was decided in view of the economic situation that it would be preferable to forego the conference and concentrate on the coordination of this book.

Specifically, the present volume targets three major gaps in Spanish flu scholarship. First, numerous chapters deal with geographic regions that do not figure prominently, if at all, in English-language publications about the pandemic. In addressing this issue, the chapters on Brazil (Bertucci, Silveira, Souza), Portugal (Nunes and Sobral, Lima, and Silveira e Sousa), and Argentina (Feldman) provide a representative sampling of the most updated research being done on the pandemic in these areas.[27] In a related fashion, with the chapters on Portugal we have included various ones on Spain (Porras-Gallo, León-Sanz, Davis, and Bernabeu-Mestre and Pascual Artiaga) to address the importance of the Iberian Peninsula as the point of connection, both epidemiologically and discursively, between Europe and the Americas in a context dominated by World War I. The war increased the traffic of the virus due to international travel and migration, but also included widespread problems of poverty, famine, and inadequate conditions of public hygiene.[28] Epidemiologically, soldiers and workers returning from central Europe to Portugal (which was involved in World War I) and Spain (which remained neutral) served as vectors for introducing the pandemic into these countries.[29] Both countries were in a critical economic, political, and social situation and were trying to implement an important process of transformation, including the need to modernize their health systems.[30] From there the pandemic spread to Latin America, or at least was often perceived to do so.[31] This leads us to select the cases of Brazil and Argentina, both such important and prominent gateways for the passage of civilian and military traffic of people and goods between Europe and America (as chapter 7 shows), to shed light on the relationship between this perception and the history of the 1918–19 pandemic. Yet, despite this, the case of Portugal is nearly absent from existing anthologies about the pandemic and only four recent essays in English have dealt with Spain's experience of the pandemic.[32]

Brazil, under its First Republic during the pandemic, took part in World War I and was in a state of political, social, and financial instability. As Liane Maria Bertucci explains in chapter 2, Rio de Janeiro and São Paulo, the two largest cities in Brazil, housed the Oswaldo Cruz Institute and the Butantã Institute, respectively, both of which had a very good relationship with the principal international scientific institutes and played an important role in the identification of the influenza "germ" during the Spanish flu. Argentina, unlike Brazil, maintained its neutrality in World War I and, after three decades of presidents close to aristocratic circles, the first relatively transparent election in 1916 brought Hipólito Yrigoyen, the leader of the Radical Party, to power. The experience of the pandemic there revealed the lack of verifiable statistics and the need to undertake major reforms and modernization in health terms.[33]

The discursive import of the peninsula is reflected in the nickname of the disease. Although it is now commonplace for critics to note that the Spanish flu did not originate in Spain, this move obscures the discursive opportunism whereby Spain was associated with the pandemic, leading some to mistakenly assume it originated there.[34] The fact that the disease was called the Spanish flu stems from the open and public nature with which the country, which was not involved in World War I, confronted the pandemic, as compared to the censorship dominant in belligerent countries that suffered from the flu at the beginning of the spring of 1918. For a disease that was only begrudgingly acknowledged by the major world powers—a phenomenon that contributed to it being "forgotten"—it is striking that Spain, which boasts such a rich trove of primary sources, has received such little attention in English-language historical criticism.

The second gap the present study fills involves the expanding theoretical and critical frameworks implemented to study the 1918–19 pandemic. Whereas the virus itself and certain major figures (like scientists) have been included in the history of the 1918–19 pandemic since it first occurred, only more recently have specific sociocultural dynamics been studied. In this vein, various chapters in this volume analyze such phenomena as social control (Bernabeu-Mestre and Pascual Artiaga), gender (Fahrni), class (Souza, Bernabeu-Mestre and Pascual Artiaga), religion (Sobral, Lima, and Silveira e Sousa; Souza), national identity (Davis), urban development (Silveira), and military medicine's reactions to the pandemic and its relationship with civilian medicine (Porras-Gallo). Other contributions to this volume offer innovative perspectives on common themes. For example, Maria de Fátima Nunes focuses on the renowned Portuguese doctor, Ricardo Jorge, to show how entwined sociosanitary policy from the period was with the persona of prominent figures. For her part, Pilar León-Sanz analyzes the role of mutual benefit societies, paragovernmental institutions that provided health care to members during the pandemic. In each case, the authors broaden our understanding of social and scientific dynamics by expanding the critical frame with which we have perceived the 1918–19 pandemic.

The third contribution this volume makes involves the particular relation between the 1918–19 pandemic and bacteriology qua explanatory framework.[35] The inability to identify the pathogen that caused the influenza had two related consequences that have not been fully appreciated by scholars of the pandemic. First, it called into question the epistemological validity of bacteriology as the principal explanatory framework for making sense of the pandemic. Although Eugenia Tognotti has recognized the challenge posed by the pandemic to bacteriology, most scholars seem to see the inconclusive laboratory results as simply a function of the historical moment.[36] In other words, scientists were unable to isolate the pathogen only because they lacked electron microscopes powerful enough to see it. But such a view minimizes the cognitive force that inheres in explanatory frameworks generally, and it specifically passes over the difficulty in some areas of achieving medical consensus because of this technological limitation.[37] Humans naturally seek to make sense of the world; thus, the failure of bacteriology to provide a definitive diagnosis of the pandemic disease—especially considering the weight of the germ theory—must have created a cognitive vacuum that left professionals and laypersons alike searching for answers all the more earnestly.[38] The second consequence, then, and the one explored by the chapters in part 3 of this volume, is that this cognitive vacuum was filled (at least in part) by narrative as opposed to laboratory means.

The Spanish Influenza Pandemic of 1918–1919: Perspectives from the Iberian Peninsula and the Americas is divided into three sections, the organizational logic of which resembles what in cinema is called a zoom-out shot. Section 1 focuses specifically on the flu pathogen and scientific attempts to understand it. Section 2 sheds light on the social context in which these attempts took place and the human and institutional reactions provoked by the pandemic. Finally, the chapters in section 3 explore the sociocultural resonances of these reactions and the pandemic experience in general. The first part—"Scientific Discourse: Now and Then"—begins with Esteban Domingo's exploration of the immense evolutionary potential of viruses, specifically the human influenza virus type A, the virus group to which the causative agent of the 1918 influenza belongs. From current viral knowledge, he shows how this virus "exploits all known types of genetic variation—mutation, recombination, and ressortment—to survive in the face of the host immune response and to produce potentially highly virulent strains." In chapter 2 Liane Maria Bertucci studies both the opinions and debates circulating in Rio de Janeiro and São Paulo during the pandemic and their subsequent developments in the postpandemic period. She shows how a team of Brazilian scientists produced findings supporting the "filterable virus" hypothesis independently of Charles Nicolle and Charles Lebailly in France and T. Yamanouchi in Japan. Juxtaposing chapters 1 and 2 provides readers with a clear contrast between what we now know about Spanish influenza in the early twenty-first century and what was known about it in 1918. In chapter 3, Maria de Fátima Nunes explores the central role of Ricardo Jorge, Portugal's preeminent public health official at the time of the 1918–19 influenza. Her chapter seeks to fill a critical void by elucidating the construction of a medical-sanitary public discourse around the pandemic in Portugal. She pays particular attention to the role Jorge played in establishing scientific connections between Portugal and other countries, especially in his capacity as the nation's representative to the Council for Public Hygiene attached to the League of Nations. Given Jorge's unique role as both scientist and public figure, chapter 3 provides a natural segue into section 2.

In detailing the role of institutional and human actors during the pandemic, the chapters of part 2—"Social Responses: Human and Institutional Actors"—reflect the epidemiological spread of the Spanish influenza, which passed from Spain to Portugal to Latin America. (All of the chapters in this section deal with Spain, Portugal, or Brazil.) In this sense, section 2 provides an evolving chronicle of the social responses to the pandemic that parallels its spread. In chapter 4, José Manuel Sobral, Maria Luísa Lima, and Paulo Silveira e Sousa present "an overview of the way this pandemic was experienced in Portugal, focusing particularly on the response of state agencies and civil organizations and on the role of the Catholic Church and Christian beliefs" (p. 77). The climate of intense political strife that characterized Portugal at the time invariably led to the politicization of the pandemic. In chapter 5 Porras-Gallo studies the reactions of Spain's Military Medical Service to the 1918–19 influenza pandemic, detailing both the debates about its social impact and the tensions and conflicts that arose between different sectors of society. She analyzes the military doctors' scientific opinions and their degree of modernity compared to those of the Civilian Health Service, assessing whether any conflicts of interest existed between the measures they both took in response to the epidemic, especially as these related to soldiers. Anny Jackeline Torres Silveira discusses the pandemic experiences of residents of Belo Horizonte—the capital of Minas Gerais, Brazil—in chapter 6, showing how the influenza contaminated both the press and the city's population even prior to the disease outbreak. She traces the spread of the viewpoint that the damages caused by the pandemic were due in large part to the so-called contagion of fear and illustrates how the acclaimed salubrity of the capital was insufficient to prevent the devastation caused by the influenza. Finally, she explores how the city's population mobilized itself to tackle the consequences generated by the perplexing experience of Spanish flu and the shortcomings of public authorities. For her part, Christiane Maria Cruz de Souza explores the repercussions of the pandemic in the lives of citizens of two other Brazilian cities, Bahia and Salvador, in chapter 7. Cruz de Souza focuses on the inhabitants' attitudes and their pacific resistance to public health measures that went against cultural practices related to illness and death rites. She also analyzes the therapeutic approaches used not only in academic medicine but also in domestic medicine and healing practices based on religion. Finally, in chapter 8, León-Sanz examines the role of mutual benefit societies in Pamplona, Spain, to shed light on both the history of these societies and their relationship with the Spanish state. They were part of a patchwork of health-related institutions antecedent to the modern welfare state that provided vital medical attention to workers and their families. She looks specifically at the efforts during the pandemic of the societies' physicians, who, as a general rule, were linked to the social hygiene movement in the city.

The chapters in part 3—"Interpreting the Epidemic: Sociocultural Dynamics and Perspectives"—shift the focus from a preoccupation with social questions to an emphasis on cultural issues. Specifically, the various authors explore the cultural resonances of either particular social responses to the epidemic (chapters 9 through 12) or the epidemic experience more generally (chapters 9, 10, and 13). As noted earlier, narrative plays a key role in the way people sought to make sense of their experience with the pandemic. In this sense, part 3 evinces a discursive focus that contrasts the epidemiological focus of part 2 and thus highlights the unique contributions of both perspectives while resisting the problematic isolation of one type from the other. Indeed, we believe that ignoring either of these approaches—rather than considering them in conjunction one with the other—will ultimately limit understanding of the Spanish flu pandemic. In chapter 9 Ryan A. Davis considers how the Spanish press represented epidemic events in Spain. His discursive analysis of the daily news coverage of the epidemic reveals an implicit distinction between an "epidemic Spain" and a "sanitary Spain." He traces the discursive evolution through the second epidemic wave and the struggle of the latter against the former, ultimately showing how this conflict structures the news of the epidemic into what we might call an emerging narrative about it. In a similar vein, Hernán Feldman examines in chapter 10 the shifting discursive focus of the main Argentine press during the influenza pandemic. Initially treating the disease as a joke, the press soon began to suspect the government was suppressing information to minimize public panic. Rather than quelling fears, however, this suppression revealed the existence of another narrative, that of the fear of fear (rather than the fear of influenza). Although the concept of prophylaxis would replace fear as the discursive center of gravity, it too would fail to allay Argentines' sense of defenselessness. Feldman thus illustrates how prophylaxis without supporting information perpetuates a notion of social defense that is as pernicious as the most unwarranted alarm. In chapter 11 Josep Bernabeu-Mestre and Mercedes Pascual Artiaga compare the sociosanitary, cultural, and political control mechanisms the municipal authorities of Alicante, Spain, implemented during the 1918 influenza epidemic in

relation to the most underprivileged members of society with those implemented during the 1804 yellow fever epidemic and the various cholera epidemics of the nineteenth century. Their comparative analysis reveals the
continuity and similarity in the arguments upheld by the political and sanitary discourses that justified the measures applied, despite the changes that
had occurred in scientific and medical knowledge and the developments
in hygiene and public health. Examining the 1918–20 influenza pandemic
through a gendered lens, Magda Fahrni shows in chapter 12 how the pandemic reaffirmed (and, very occasionally, altered) the respective roles and
responsibilities assigned to men and women in Montreal, Canada. Perhaps
not surprisingly, her analysis reveals that women were the primary caregivers during the pandemic. The obituaries of caregivers of both genders—who
include doctors, priests, and nuns—reflect the gendered traits of caregiving
during the 1918–20 influenza pandemic. Fahrni also explores how female
middle-class reformers drew on women's experiences during the pandemic in
their proposals regarding public health responses to the flu. Finally, in chapter 13 Catherine Belling surveys key texts in the growing body of literary representations of the Spanish flu pandemic, showing how fiction can in some
ways enhance our ability to imagine the pandemic as the sum of multiple,
richly felt experiences of particular individuals. Paradoxically, she does this
by illustrating how these texts tend to replicate, albeit in microcosm, the pandemic's resistance to subjective articulation by those who lived through it.

In sum, the collected essays of *The Spanish Influenza Pandemic of 1918–
1919: Perspectives from the Iberian Peninsula and the Americas* are designed to
enhance our understanding of the 1918–19 influenza pandemic by elucidating specific aspects that have received minimal attention until now
(such as social control, gender, class, religion, national identity, and military medicine's reactions to the pandemic and its relationship with civilian medicine); by showing the importance of the Iberian Peninsula as the
key point of connection, both epidemiologically and discursively, between
Europe and the Americas in the context of World War I; and, above all, by
raising more questions. The continued need for scholarship on the pandemic stems not just from the fact that pandemics are global in nature,
nor even that the 1918–19 pandemic occupies a singular role in world
history, but because the experiences of 1918–19 remain persistently relevant to contemporary life, as evidenced by the recent events of the 2009
pandemic. Our hope is that the following chapters both contribute to the
growing body of knowledge about the terrible Spanish flu—with a total
death toll of between forty or fifty million and one hundred million people, predominantly among young people (twenty to forty years old), during its three waves (spring and fall 1918 and spring 1919)—and encourage
further research into this most enigmatic of diseases, especially in the context of emerging and reemerging infectious diseases.[39]

Notes

1. Eugenia Tognotti, "Scientific Triumphalism and Learning from Facts: Bacteriology and the 'Spanish Flu' Challenge of 1918," *Social History of Medicine*, 16, no. 1 (2003): 97–110.

2. In chapter 2 Liane Maria Bertucci analyzes in depth both the opinions and debates circulating in Brazil about the influenza agent during the pandemic and the postpandemic period. This topic also appears in chapters 4 and 5 in connection with Portugal and Spain.

3. Jeffery K. Taubenberger and David M. Morens, "1918 Influenza: The Mother of All Pandemics," *Emerging Infectious Diseases* 12, no. 1 (2006): 15–22.

4. Robert G. Webster and Elizabeth Walker, "Influenza," *American Scientist* 91, no. 2 (2003): 122.

5. Howard Phillips and David Killingray, *The Spanish Influenza Pandemic of 1918–1919: New Perspectives* (London: Routledge, 2003), 21.

6. Priscilla Wald, *Contagious: Cultures, Carriers, and the Outbreak Narrative* (Durham, NC: Duke University Press, 2008), 2.

7. Charles E. Rosenberg, *Explaining Epidemics and Other Studies in the History of Medicine* (Cambridge: Cambridge University Press, 1992); World Health Organization, *Handbook for Journalists: Influenza Pandemic* (Geneva: WHO, 2005), 5. Total mortality estimates range from forty or fifty million to one hundred million, more than died in World War I, with the young and healthy being especially vulnerable. K. David Patterson, *Pandemic Influenza, 1700–1900: A Study in Historical Epidemiology* (Totowa: Rowman and Littlefield, 1986).

8. On the historical ebb and flow of scholarly interest in Spanish influenza, see Phillips and Killingray, *Spanish Influenza Pandemic*, 12.

9. Terrence M. Tumpey, Christopher F. Basler, Patricia V. Aguilar, Hui Zeng, Alicia Solórzano, David E. Swayne, Nancy J. Cox et al., "Characterization of the Reconstructed 1918 Spanish Influenza Pandemic Virus," *Science* 310, no. 5745 (2005): 79. See also Jacqueline M. Katz, "Preparing for the Next Influenza Pandemic," *American Society for Microbiology (ASM) News* 70, no. 9 (2004): 412–19; and Joshua Lederberg, "Infectious Disease as an Evolutionary Paradigm," *Emerging Infectious Diseases* 3 (1997): 417–23. Concern over another outbreak had already begun to register in certain circles, as reflected in the title of the conference "Pandemic Influenza: Confronting a Reemergent Threat," held in Bethesda, Maryland, from December 11 to 13, 1995. (Conference sponsors included the National Institutes of Health, the University of Michigan, the Centers for Disease Control and Prevention, the Food and Drug Administration, the US-Japan Cooperative Medical Science Program, and the World Health Organization.)

10. David M. Morens, Jeffery K. Taubenberger, and Anthony S. Fauci, "The 2009 H1N1 Pandemic Influenza Virus: What Next?" *mBio* 1, no. 4 (2010): 1, doi:10.1128/mBio.00211-10.

11. Esteban Domingo gives some illustrative information in chapter 1.

12. David M. Morens and Anthony S. Fauci, "The 1918 Influenza Pandemic: Insights for the 21st Century," *Journal of Infectious Diseases* 195 (2007): 1019.

13. For academic sources that treat the 1918–19 pandemic as a precedent, see Taubenberger and Morens, "1918 Influenza"; Adolfo García-Sastre and Richard J.

Whitley, "Lessons Learned from Reconstructing the 1918 Influenza Pandemic," supplement, *Journal of Infectious Diseases* 194, no. S2 (2006): S127–32; and Stacey Knobler, Alison Mack, Adel Mahmoud, and Stanley M. Lemon, *The Threat of Pandemic Influenza: Are We Ready? Workshop Summary* (Washington, DC: National Academies Press, 2005), www.nap.edu/catalog/11150.html, especially section 1 with perspectives by Barry, Taubenberger, Simonsen, and others. Consider also the following titles from articles in the popular press: Aaron Derfel, "Spanish Flu Pandemic a Stark Precedent," *Gazette* (Montreal) September 26, 2009; and Mark Humphries, "Lessons from the 1918 Pandemic: Focus on Treatment, Not Prevention," *Globe and Mail,* July 24, 2009.

14. Howard Markel, Harvey B. Lipman, J. Alexander Navarro, Alexandra Sloan, Joseph R. Michalsen, Alexandra Minna Stern, and Martin S. Cetron, "Nonpharmaceutical Interventions Implemented by US Cities during the 1918–1919 Influenza Pandemic," *Journal of the American Medical Association* 298, no. 6 (2007): 644–54.

15. Richard A. Hobday and John W. Cason "The Open-Air Treatment of Pandemic Influenza," supplement, *American Journal of Public Health* 99, no. S2 (2009): S236–42.

16. Elizabeth Fee and Daniel M. Fox, "Introduction: AIDS, Public Policy and Historical Inquiry," in *AIDS: The Burdens of History,* ed. Elizabeth Fee and Daniel M. Fox (Berkeley: University of California Press, 1988), 3.

17. Edwin Dennis Kilbourne, ed., *The Influenza Viruses and Influenza* (New York: Academic Press, 1975); Kilbourne, *Influenza* (New York: Plenum Medical Book, 1987); Gerald F. Pyle and K. David Patterson, "Influenza Diffusion in European History: Patterns and Paradigms," *Ecology of Disease* 2, no. 3 (1984): 173–84; Patterson, *Pandemic Influenza*; Eugene P. Campbell, "The Epidemiology of Influenza," *Bulletin of the History of Medicine* 13, no. 3 (1943): 389–403; Andrew David Cliff, Peter Haggett, and J. Keith Ord, *Spatial Aspects of Influenza Epidemics* (London: Pion, 1986); W. Paul Glezen, A. A. Payne, D. N. Snyder, and T. D. Downs, "Mortality and Influenza," *Journal of Infectious Diseases* 146, no. 3 (1982): 313–21; R. Edgar Hope-Simpson, "Recognition of Historic Influenza Epidemics from Parish Burial Records: A Test of Prediction from a New Hypothesis of Influenzal Epidemiology," *Journal of Hygiene, Cambridge* 91, no. 2 (1983): 293–308; Hope-Simpson, "The Method of Transmission of Epidemic Influenza: Further Evidence from Archival Mortality Data," *Journal of Hygiene, Cambridge* 96, no. 2 (1986): 353–75; Frank Macfarlane Burnet, "Influenza Virus A," in *Portraits of Viruses: A History of Virology,* ed. Frank Fenner and Adrian J. Gibbs (Basel, Karger, 1988), 24–37.

18. Local studies include Fred B. Rogers, "The Influenza Pandemic of 1918–1919 in the Perspective of a Half Century," *American Journal Public Health* 58, no. 12 (1968): 2192–94; Stuart Galishoff, "Newark and the Great Influenza Pandemic of 1918," *Bulletin of the History of Medicine* 43 (1969): 246–58; and D. I. Pool, "The Effects of the 1918 Pandemic of Influenza on the Maori Population of New Zealand," *Bulletin of the History of Medicine* 47, no. 3 (1973): 273–81.

19. Alfred W. Crosby, *Epidemic and Peace, 1918* (Westport, CT: Greenwood, 1976); E. Koenen, "Die Grippenpandemie 1918/19" (PhD diss., University of Cologne, 1970); Robert S. Katz, "Influenza 1918–19: A Study in Mortality," *Bulletin of the History of Medicine* 48, no. 3 (1974): 416–22.

20. The 1976 swine flu scare gave rise to special meetings and to the design and implementation of a controversial prophylactic plan against the illness, with the aim

of avoiding a disaster of the proportions of the 1918–19 pandemic. It also led to a series of publications, including the record of the various meetings held and different monographic studies on the 1918–19 pandemic, both local and general. Among them we should mention Alfred W. Crosby's monograph, *Epidemic and Peace*, and his contribution to the collective work edited by June E. Osborn: Crosby, "The Pandemic of 1918," in *History, Science, and Politics: Influenza in America, 1918–1976*, ed. June E. Osborn (New York: Prodist, 1977).

21. Philip C. Ensley, "Indiana and the Influenza Pandemic of 1918," *Indiana Medical History Quarterly* 9, no. 4 (1983): 3–15; Eileen Pettigrew, *The Silent Enemy: Canada and the Deadly Flu of 1918* (Saskatoon, Canada: Western Producer Prairie Books, 1983); G. M. Emerson, "The 'Spanish Lady' in Alabama," *Alabama Journal of Medical Sciences* 23, no. 2 (1986): 217–21; Judy M. Katzenellnbogen, "The Influenza Epidemic in Mamre," *South African Medical Journal* 74 (1988): 323–28.

22. Sources for Africa, Indonesia, and India include Don C. Ohadike, "Diffusion and Physiological Responses to the Influenza Pandemic of 1918–19 in Nigeria," *Social Science and Medicine* 32, no. 12 (1991): 1393–99. The extension of the geographic range of the historiography on the 1918–19 pandemic was pointed out in K. David Patterson and Gerald F. Pyle, "The Geography and Mortality of the 1918 Influenza Pandemic," *Bulletin of the History of Medicine* 65, no. 1 (1991): 4–21. On Japan, see Edwina Palmer and Geoffrey W. Rice, "A Japanese Physician's Response to Pandemic Influenza: Ijirō Gomibuchi and the 'Spanish Flu' in Yaita-Chō, 1918–1919," *Bulletin of the History of Medicine* 66, no. 4 (1992): 560–77. For studies of the pandemic in Europe, see Martha L. Hildreth, "The Influenza Epidemic of 1918–1919 in France: Contemporary Concepts of Aetiology, Therapy and Prevention," *Social History of Medicine* 4, no. 2 (1991): 277–94; William Ian B. Beveridge, "The Chronicle of Influenza Epidemics," *History and Philosophy of the Life Sciences* 13 (1991): 223–34; and Sandra M. Tomkins, "The Failure of Expertise: Public Health Policy in Britain during 1918–19 Influenza Epidemic," *Social History of Medicine* 5, no. 3 (1992): 435–54. Centered on the urban impact in several major European and American cities is Fred R. Van Hartesveldt, ed., *1918–19 Pandemic of Influenza: The Urban Impact in the Western World* (Lewiston: Mellen, 1993). A list of Spanish publications about the development of the 1918–19 influenza pandemic in Spain and its main cities can be found in María-Isabel Porras-Gallo, "Sueros y vacunas en la lucha contra la pandemia de gripe de 1918–1919 en España," *Asclepio* 60, no. 2 (2008): 261–88. The renewed relevance of the studies on the 1918–19 pandemic also led Alfred Crosby to publish a new version of his work from the seventies: *America's Forgotten Pandemic: The Influenza of 1918* (Cambridge: Cambridge University Press, 1989).

23. Among the main titles by scientific journalists, we would include the following: Lynette Iezzoni, *Influenza 1918: The Worst Epidemic in American History* (New York: TV Books, 1999); Gina Kolata, *Flu: The Story of the Great Influenza Pandemic of 1918 and the Search for the Virus That Caused It* (New York: Touchstone, 1999); David Getz, *Purple Death: The Mysterious Flu of 1918* (New York: Holt, 2000); and Peter Davies, *Catching Cold: 1918's Forgotten Tragedy and the Scientific Hunt for the Virus That Caused It* (London: Joseph, 1999). In 2000 a second edition was published, titled *The Devil's Flu: The World's Deadliest Influenza Epidemic and the Scientific Hunt for the Virus That Caused It* (New York: Holt, 2000). In a similar vein, but with more documentary support, is John M. Barry's *The Great Influenza: The Epic Story of the Deadliest Plague in History* (New

York: Viking Penguin, 2004). (In 2005 a new edition was published including a new afterword on avian flu). Among these more academic studies are those that take a demographic approach: Christopher Langford, "The Age Pattern of Mortality in the 1918–19 Influenza Pandemic: An Attempted Explanation Based on Data for England and Wales," *Medical History* 46, no. 1 (2002): 1–20; and Niall Johnson and Juergen Mueller, "Updating the Accounts: Global Mortality of the 1918–1920 'Spanish' Influenza Pandemic," *Bulletin of the History of Medicine* 76 (2002): 105–15.

24. Howard Phillips, review of *Influenza 1918: Disease, Death, and Struggle in Winnipeg*, by Esyllt W. Jones, *Bulletin of the History of Medicine* 83, no. 1 (2009): 226.

25. Phillips and Killingray, *Spanish Influenza Pandemic*, 23.

26. Among these are Amir Afkhami, "Compromised Constitutions: The Iranian Experience with the 1918 Influenza Pandemic," *Bulletin of the History of Medicine* 77, no. 2 (2003): 367–92; Tognotti, "Scientific Triumphalism"; Magda Fahrni, "'Elles sont partout . . .': Les femmes et la ville en temps d'épidémie, Montréal, 1918–1920," *Revue d'Histoire de l'Amérique Française* 58, no. 1 (2004): 67–85; Jean Guénel, "La grippe 'espagnole' en France en 1918–1919," *Histoire des Sciences médicales* 38, no. 2 (2004): 165–75; Lori Loeb, "Beating the Flu: Orthodox and Commercial Responses to Influenza in Britain, 1889–1919," *Social History of Medicine* 18, no. 2 (2005): 203–24; Geoffrey W. Rice, *Black November: The 1918 Influenza Pandemic in New Zealand*, 2nd ed. (1988; repr., Christchurch, Canterbury University Press, 2005); Stacey L. Knobler, Alison Mack, Adel Mahmoud, and Stanley M. Lemon, *Threat of Pandemic Influenza*; Niall Johnson, *Britain and the 1918–19 Influenza Pandemic: A Dark Epilogue* (New York: Routledge, 2006): 237–64; John M. Eyler, "De Kruif's Boast: Vaccine Trials and the Construction of a Virus," *Bulletin of the History of Medicine* 80 (2006): 409–38; and Heather MacDougall, "Toronto's Health Department in Action: Influenza in 1918 and SARS in 2003," *Journal of the History of Medicine and Allied Sciences* 62, no. 1 2007): 56–89. These works arose as a consequence of the new prominence reached by the Spanish flu following the epidemic of SARS in 2003, the news of the reconstruction in fall 2005 of the virus responsible for the Spanish flu, and the alarms that were sounded about a possible new pandemic similar to that of 1918. On the reconstruction of the Spanish flu virus, see Tumpey, Basler, Aguilar et al., "Characterization," 77–80. The 2009 flu pandemic has generated an abundant medical, virological, and epidemiological historiography, as well as medical history. Of particular note among the latter are the recent works of Michael Bresalier, including "Fighting Flu: Military Pathology, Vaccines, and the Conflicted Identity of the 1918–19 Pandemic in Britain," *Journal of the History of Medicine and Allied Sciences* 61, no. 3 (2011): 87–128, doi:10.1093/jhmas/jrr041; and "Uses of a Pandemic: Forging the Identities of Influenza and Virus Research in Interwar Britain," *Social History of Medicine* 25, no. 2 (2011): 400–24, doi:10.1093/shm/hkr162.

27. For additional English-language sources on Latin America, see Christiane M. Cruz de Souza, "The Spanish Flu Epidemic: A Challenge to Bahian Medicine," *História, Ciências, Saúde: Manguinhos* 15, no. 4 (2008): 945–72; and Adriana Da Costa Goulart, "Revisiting the Spanish Flu: The 1918 Influenza Pandemic in Rio de Janeiro," *História, Ciências, Saúde: Manguinhos* 12, no. 1 (2005): 1–41. Recent studies in other languages include Liane Maria Bertucci, "Entre doutores e para os leigos: Fragmentos do discurso medico na influenza de 1918," *História, Ciências, Saúde: Manguinhos* 12, no. 1 (2005): 143–57; Christiane Maria Cruz de Souza, "A gripe

espanhola em Salvador, 1918: Cidade de becos e cortiços," *História, Ciências, Saúde: Manguinhos* 12, no. 1 (2005): 71–99; Souza, "A gripe espanhola na Bahia: Saúde, política e medicina em tempos de epidemia" (PhD diss., Casa de Oswaldo Cruz/ Fundação Oswaldo Cruz, 2007); Souza, "As dimensões político-sociais de uma epidemia: A paulicéia desvairada pela gripe espanhola," *História, Ciências, Saúde: Manguinhos* 12, no. 1 (2005): 567–73; Cláudio Bertolli Filho, *A gripe espanhola em São Paulo, 1918: Epidemia e sociedade* (São Paulo: Paz e Terra, 2003); Ricardo Augusto Dos Santos, "O Carnaval, a peste e a 'espanhola,'" *História, Ciências, Saúde: Manguinhos* 13, no. 1 (2006): 129–58; Dora Dávila M. *Caracas y la gripe española de 1918: Epidemias y política sanitaria* (Caracas: Universidad Católica Andrés Bello, 2000); and Anny Jackeline Torres Silveira, *A influenza espanhola e a cidade planejada: Belo Horizonte, 1918* (Belo Horizonte: Argumentum Editora, 2007).

28. In chapter 1 Esteban Domingo shows the huge importance of these factors in the reemergence of the influenza.

29. More details concerning the role played by soldiers and workers as vectors of the pandemic in Spain and Portugal are available in chapters 3, 4, and 9.

30. More information about the Portuguese case can be found in chapter 3 and, especially, chapter 4. For the Spanish case, see María-Isabel Porras-Gallo, *Un reto para la sociedad madrileña: La epidemia de gripe de 1918–19* (Madrid: Complutense / Comunidad Autónoma de Madrid, 1997).

31. See chapters 6, 7, and 10 of this volume.

32. José Manuel Sobral, Maria Luísa Lima, Paula Castro, and Paulo Silveira e Sousa's volume gathers contributions to the first academic conference dedicated to the 1918–19 flu pandemic, held in Lisbon in 2007. See *A Pandemia Esquecida: Olhares comparados sobre a pneumónica, 1918–1919* (Lisbon: Imprensa de Ciências Sociais, 2009). English-language publications on Spain include Beatriz Echeverri Dávila, "Spanish Influenza Seen from Spain," in Phillips and Killingray, *Spanish Influenza Pandemic*, 173–90; Antoni Trilla, Guillem Trilla, and Carolyn Daer, "The 1918 'Spanish Flu' in Spain," *Clinical Infectious Diseases* 47, no. 5 (2008): 668–73; María-Isabel Porras-Gallo, "The Place of Serums and Antibiotics in the Influenza Pandemics of 1918–1919 and 1957–1958 Respectively" in *Circulation of Antibiotics: Journeys of Drug Standards*, eds. Ana Romero, Christoph Gradmann, and María Santesmases (Madrid: European Science Foundation, 2011), 141–60, ESF Networking Program DRUGS, Preprint no. 1 (2010), http://drughistory.eu/downloads/Madrid_Preprint.pdf; and Ryan A. Davis, "Don Juan versus Bacteriology: Competing Narrative Explanations of the 1918–19 Spanish Flu Epidemic in Spain," *Ometeca* 16 (2011): 171–89.

33. A more detailed description can be found in Hernán Feldman's chapter 10.

34. The historiography on the pandemic has located its origin in either China or the United States, with most scholars opining the latter. Crosby, *America's Forgotten Pandemic*, 25. Beatriz Echeverri Dávila, *La gripe española: La pandemia de 1918–19* (Madrid: Centro de Investigaciones Sociológicas / Siglo XXI, 1993), 20.

35. On explanatory frameworks, see Rosenberg, *Explaining Epidemics*.

36. Tognotti, "Scientific Triumphalism."

37. Porras-Gallo, "Sueros y vacunas."

38. Although one could argue that any number of diseases have exerted analogous cognitive pressure, the Spanish flu remains unique for a couple of reasons. Take, for instance, the plague. Unlike the Spanish flu, *yersinia pestis* came onto the

world stage long before the rise of bacteriology. During the black plague, then, it is reasonable to conclude that there were no expectations created by recent discoveries of the causative agent of other diseases. In a related fashion, if we consider AIDS, although no cure has been discovered yet, it is still the case that HIV was isolated relatively quickly. This was not the case with the Spanish flu. Also, we would add that although any number of emerging or reemerging diseases may portend a coming plague (see, e.g., Laurie Garrett, *The Coming Plague: Newly Emerging Diseases in a World Out of Balance* [New York: Penguin, 1995]), they do so at a time when, unlike the early twentieth century, medicine "has . . . drawn such intense doubts and disapproval." Roy Porter, introduction to *The Cambridge Illustrated History of Medicine*, ed. Roy Porter (New York: Cambridge University Press, 1996), 1. Finally, no other pandemic similar in magnitude to the Spanish flu has resulted from a disease so beset with assumptions about its benign nature.

39. Statistical information relating to the pandemic can be found in Patterson, *Pandemic Influenza*, and Patterson and Pyle, "Geography and Mortality."

Part One

Scientific Discourse

Now and Then

Chapter One

The Great Evolutionary Potential of Viruses

The 1918 Flu as a Paradigm of Disease Emergence

Esteban Domingo

RNA Viruses as a Paradigm of Rapid Evolution

The 1918 Spanish influenza is one of the most dramatic examples of the unpredictable threat that viral epidemics represent for the human population. In the words of Joshua Lederberg, "The survival of the human species is not a preordained evolutionary program. Abundant resources of genetic variation exist for viruses to learn new tricks, not necessarily confined to what happens routinely or even frequently."[1] Since 1918 we have learned about the nature of viruses, their structure, their replication in intimate relationship with their host cells and organisms, and their mechanisms of evolutionary change. Concerning the "tricks" mentioned by Lederberg, we have learned that influenza viruses can use a very large repertoire.

RNA viruses are replicated by RNA-dependent RNA (or DNA) polymerases (also termed "reverse transcriptases"), which tend to introduce incorrect nucleotides during template copying. The incorrect nucleotides are perpetuated in the genetic material of the viruses, unless the mistakes are corrected (by repair enzymes), or the genomes harboring them are eliminated by a process termed negative selection (as opposed to positive or Darwinian selection). The reason for this error-prone replication is that most viral polymerases lack an activity of error correction that is termed proofreading-repair activity. This is in contrast to cellular DNA polymerases (and some viral DNA polymerases) involved in DNA replication, which include such a correcting function. Other repair activities in the cell that can eliminate errors in DNA are not active on replicating RNA viruses. Mistakes during viral RNA replication average one misincorporation for every ten thousand nucleotides incorporated during template copying (fig. 1.1, pt. A).[2]

In addition to mutation, most RNA viruses can also undergo genetic recombination, a process by which a mosaic genome can be produced from two different parents. Mutation and recombination give rise to complex and dynamic mutant distributions termed "viral quasispecies" (fig. 1.1, pt. B).[3] Quasispecies dynamics provides a mechanism for the adaptability of RNA viruses. Fitness gains can be regarded as an optimization of mutant distributions. This view is supported by many experiments that have established that competitive replication in a given environment leads to fitness gain in that same environment, while the forced accumulation of mutations (naturally through population bottlenecks or artificially with mutagenic agents) leads to fitness loss. The quasispecies concept is an application to virology of a theory of the origin of life.[4] Some RNA viruses have a segmented genome, that is, their genetic information is split in two or more pieces of RNA. Segmented viruses can undergo genome segment reassortment, resulting in new combinations of RNA pieces (fig. 1.1, pt. C). Mutation, recombination, and reassortment are the mechanisms of genetic variation that RNA viruses use to generate diversity, the raw material for evolutionary change. Positive selection, together with statistical fluctuations in the frequency of genomes independent of selection (also termed random drift) contribute to the evolution of organisms, cells, and their parasites.

RNA viruses and other RNA genetic elements (satellite RNAs, viroids, etc.) coexist in our biosphere with the DNA-based life forms with which they coevolve. But the RNA genetic elements have the potential to evolve a million times faster than their host cells and organisms. As first stated by John J. Holland and his colleagues, "There are some disease implications for the DNA-based biosphere of this rapidly evolving RNA biosphere." One of these implications is that rapidly evolving RNA viruses can produce variant forms that may survive in the face of the immune response mounted by their host organisms or other interventions intended to stop their replication. The survival of mutant forms contributes to viral persistence within infected organisms, and, at the population level, to long-term persistence in nature. Some variants might be endowed with the capacity to recognize and penetrate new cell types, perhaps leading to a productive infection. Such modifications of host cell tropism may occasionally produce an altered host range, allowing the virus to multiply and infect a new host species. These factors are important disease implications of the rapidly evolving RNA biosphere in a DNA-based biosphere.[5]

Human influenza virus type A, the virus group to which the causative agent of the so-called Spanish influenza of 1918 belongs (according to sequencing data by Jeffery K. Taubenberger, Gina Kolata, Jeffrey R. Ryan and others), exploits all known types of genetic variation—mutation, recombination, and ressortment—to survive in the face of the host immune response and to produce potentially highly virulent strains (see fig. 1.2).[6]

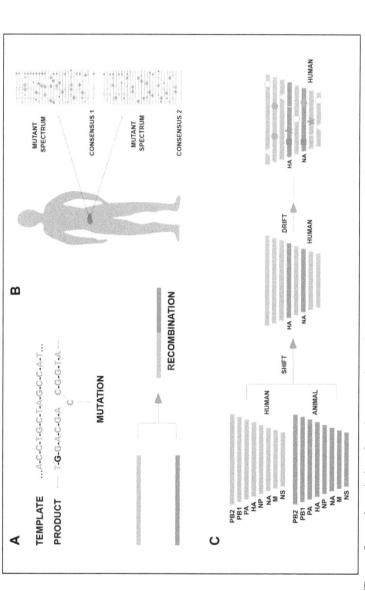

Figure 1.1. Types of genetic variation that viruses undergo during genome replication. (A) Incorporation of an incorrect nucleotide (C instead of T) during template copying. Below, formation of a recombinant genome. (B) RNA viruses rapidly become mutant spectra termed viral quasispecies (see text for further description). Viral genomes are depicted as horizontal lines, and mutations as various symbols on the lines. (C) Genome segment reassortment in the case of influenza virus type A. Reassortment between a human and an animal influenza virus may result in generation of a reassortant virus that includes the hemagglutinin (HA) and neuraminidase (NA) genes from animal origin. This process is termed antigenic shift, and has mediated the origin of several influenza pandemics. When mutations affect HA and NA the process is termed antigenic drift.

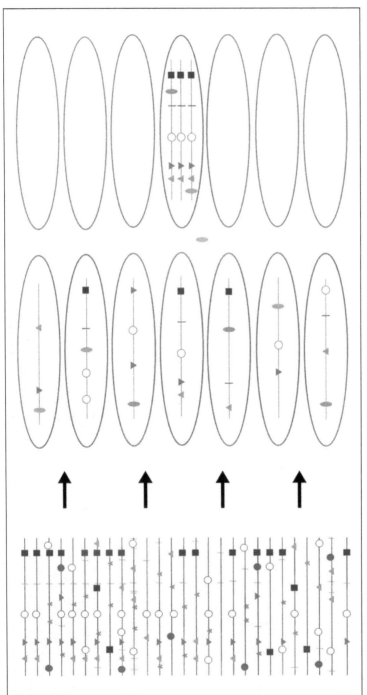

Figure 1.2. Virus genome heterogeneity in viral disease emergence and reemergence. When one or few variants reach a potential new host (depicted as ellipses in the middle) the probability of the genome being replication-competent is low, and only an adequate variant can be established in the new host (ellipses on the right). Contacts and establishment of new pathogens are unpredictable events (see text). Contact between swine and humans originated the 2009 human influenza pandemic.

Two Mechanisms of Antigenic Variation of Influenza Virus

The genome of influenza virus type A comprises about 13,500 nucleotides divided into eight RNA segments that encode one or more proteins: PB1 (polymerase basic 1), PB2 (polymerase basic 2), PA (polymerase acid)—PB1, PB2, and PA are components of the viral polymerase—HA (hemagglutinin), NP (nucleoprotein), NA (neuraminidase), M (matrix protein M1 and membrane protein M2), and NS (multifunctional protein NS1 and the nuclear export protein NEP/NS2) (fig. 1.1, pt. C). The major surface antigens of the virus (which determine the interaction of the virus with the cell and with the antibodies produced by the immune system) are the glycosylated proteins hemagglutinin (HA) and neuraminidase (NA), and these define the subtype composition of influenza virus type A. To the date of this writing, a total of sixteen H subtypes (H1–H16) and nine N subtypes (N1–N9) have been characterized, and they compose the majority of human and animal influenza viruses that have been identified.[7] Subtype composition is named by the letters H and N, followed by a number. For example, the 1918 influenza was caused by a virus of H1N1 subtype, while the so-called Hong Kong influenza of 1968 was associated with an H3N2 virus (fig. 1.2). But new HAs and NAs are likely to be discovered (the 1985 edition of *Fields Virology* listed thirteen H subtypes), either from additional viral reservoirs or because they arise by the recombination and mutation of the genes encoding extant HAs and NAs.

Human influenza viruses with a new subtype composition emerge usually through genome segment reassortment between a circulating human virus and an influenza virus of some animal reservoir. A new reassortant that incorporates antigenic determinants (HA and NA) from an avian virus but that maintains a number of genes that encode proteins adapted to replicate in human respiratory tissues has a good probability of being pathogenic for humans. The fact that the genes encoding the surface antigenic determinants HA and NA are from nonhuman origin implies that no (or weakly reacting) anti-HA or anti-NA antibodies for those specific antigens will be present in the human population, thus facilitating viral replication and circulation of the virus among humans. The generation of an influenza virus with a new antigenic protein due to reassortment is termed "antigenic shift" (fig. 1.1, pt. C).

Once a new subtype is established in the human population (or actually in any host) through a reassortment that has resulted in antigenic shift, variation through mutation continues at the genetic level, resulting in further antigenic variation. Thus, multiple sublineages of human, avian, and swine influenza viruses have been identified. Not only HA and NA but all viral genes continue to mutate in the absence of reassortment. Amino acid substitutions in HA and NA may modify the antigenic properties of the virus through a decrease of the affinity of the virus for antibodies. This is because antigen-antibody recognition (an important element of protection against viral infections) is based on precise amino-acid interactions. This gradual antigenic variation due to amino acid substitutions is termed "antigenic drift," and it is thought to contribute to the adaptation of influenza virus in the face of the host immune response (fig. 1.1, pt. C).

In addition to mutation and reassortment, genomic RNA segments of influenza virus can undergo molecular recombination, or the formation of a segment that includes part of the segment from a parental influenza virus and part from another influenza virus (fig. 1.1, pt. A).[8] Recombination can also involve influenza RNA and an unrelated RNA, although in this case virus viability is likely to be compromised. An increase in pathogenicity was observed in an influenza virus that included an insertion of a ribosomal RNA sequence in its HA gene.[9]

Dissecting the Steps in Disease Emergence

The term "emergence" of a human viral disease refers generally to a disease in the human population that had not been described previously and some-times also to the first occurrence of a viral disease in a given geographic area. AIDS is a human disease that emerged in the second half of the twentieth century, associated with infection by human immunodeficiency virus type 1, not known to have afflicted humans prior to its emergence. West Nile encephalitis emerged in the United States in New York in 1999 and spread rapidly throughout the country. The virus was endemic in eastern Africa, the Middle East, and eastern Europe. The term "reemergence" is often used to refer to the advent of a viral disease that had not occurred for a long time in the same geographic area. Following this nomenclature, influenza pandemics must be considered "reemergences." Three steps have been distinguished in the process of disease emergence and reemergence: the introduction, establishment, and dissemination of the pathogenic agent among individuals of a host species.

The introduction of a potential viral pathogen in a new host is highly unpredictable and dependent on the genetic makeup of the potential new host and of the virus, as well as on several sociological, ecological, and political influences.[10] The main factors contributing to the emergence of a viral disease are the following:

- Virus variation (mutation, recombination, reassortment) and adaptability
- The presence of virus reservoirs (in apparently infected animals) and vectors (mosquitoes, ticks)

- Susceptibility to infection by components of mutant spectra present in reservoirs and vectors
- Climatic conditions that may affect virus stability and proliferation and movements of viral vectors
- Changing ecosystems due to climate change (global warming) or economic development (construction of dams, deforestation)
- Human demographics and behavior, including large megacities that increase human-to-human contacts or drug use due to economic or psychological conditions
- Technology and industry (blood transfusion, organ transplantation, use of antiviral agents that promote selection of resistant viral mutants, thus limiting the therapeutic possibilities)
- International travel and commerce, which increases contact between humans, animals, and viral vectors
- Poverty, famine, and absence of public health measures
- Lack of political will, priority of economic interests over social needs, and late reporting of a disease outbreak
- Bioterrorism and agroterrorism[11]

These different influences are interconnected in such a way that they affect the probability that infected hosts or free viral particles come into contact with potentially new host species. Contact between viral pathogens and hosts is a highly stochastic and unpredictable event. Increase of virus traffic, that is, the amount of virus and the number of disseminating vectors (humans, animal, insects, objects, etc.), is one of the major influences in the introduction step.[12] For example, water surfaces as a result of elevated rainfall provide breeding habitats for mosquitos, and this results in an increase of mosquito-borne viral infections. Similarly, climatic change may modify the migration habits of birds, thereby exposing viruses carried by birds to new habitats.

Emergent human viruses are not generated de novo (at least in the vast majority of cases). They exist in natural, nonhuman reservoirs and must find their way to humans. The higher the number of natural reservoirs of a virus and the more frequent the contact between humans and these reservoirs, the higher the probability of introducing a new virus into the human population. Emergent and reemergent human viral diseases can be due either to ancestral human viruses that have acquired or enhanced their virulence or, more commonly, to viruses from some animal reservoir. In the latter case the virus is said to have a "zoonotic" origin. Since an infected animal produces and can shed a spectrum of viral mutants, the higher the number of infected animals, the higher the repertoire of virus variants exposed to the environment. The probability that a potential new host (human or any individual of a species different from the one that sustains the infection) encounters a virus variant that can produce a productive infection is higher the higher the number of variants available. A lottery of contacts and consequences is created. A virus is established in a new host when it can replicate and produce infectious progeny in that host. It is suspected that many encounters between viruses and potential new hosts take place regularly but that only a tiny minority of them lead to the successful establishment of the virus in the new host (fig. 1.2).

Once a virus is established in a new host species, the capacity of the infection to spread depends on the efficiency of each infected individual to infect other individuals. In highly populated urban areas, the chances of pathogen transmission increase because any infected individual has a high probability of encountering a susceptible individual. Depending on the average number of infected contacts per each infected host (a basic parameter in epidemiology termed "Ro," or "basic reproductive ratio"), the virus will spread (Ro > 1) or decay (Ro < 1). An example of an infection dynamics with Ro > 1 is the current AIDS epidemic, and an example of infection episodes with Ro < 1 (or that evolved to have an average Ro < 1) is the severe acute respiratory syndrome (SARS) outbreak of 2003. This does not mean that as the SARS coronavirus replicates in some other host or animal reservoir (pteropid bats or civet cats) it will not acquire mutations that render it more efficient for human transmission, with Ro > 1.[13] The evolution of virulence is subject to typical indeterminations inherent to RNA virus evolution due to the random nature of genetic change. For example, there were three waves of the Spanish influenza pandemic of 1918, each displaying a different degree and level of virulence (fig. 1.3).[14]

Viral transmission often constitutes a bottleneck event (infection initiated by one or few virus particles) that results in fitness decrease in a process known as "Muller's ratchet" (small arrows in fig. 1.4).[15] It has been suggested that this effect may ensure that even the most virulent viruses could, as a result of the operation of Muller's ratchet, immunize rather than kill at least a fraction of the host population.[16] Fitness decrease, together with a gradual increase of immunized host individuals, may contribute to the (often mysterious) fading away of an epidemic.

The events involved in the introduction, establishment, and dissemination of a new pathogen can all be influenced by the quasispecies dynamics of viral populations, although the genetic requirements for the three processes need not be the same. The encounter of a virus with a potential new host is in reality the encounter of a mutant distribution with that host (fig. 1.1, pt. B; fig. 1.4). Such an encounter can involve only one genome of the distribution (which is the most extreme example of a bottleneck event) or a number of genomes from the distribution. Despite the hypothetical nature of figure 1.2, all RNA viruses examined to date are mutant distributions (quasispecies), not genomes with a repeated nucleotide sequence.

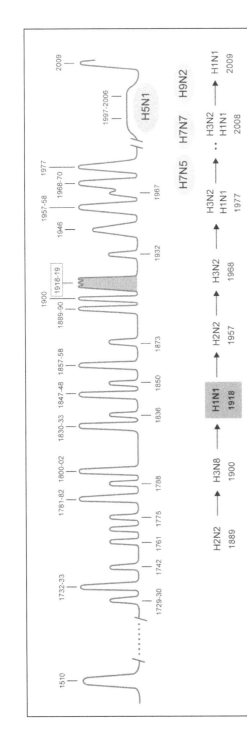

Figure 1.3. Representation of the major recorded influenza epidemics and pandemics. The size of the peaks is approximately proportional to the geographical extent of the epidemic, independently of its severity in terms of human deaths. Records and subtype assignments prior to 1918 are uncertain. Subtypes encircled correspond to avian viruses that have caused human infections (see text).

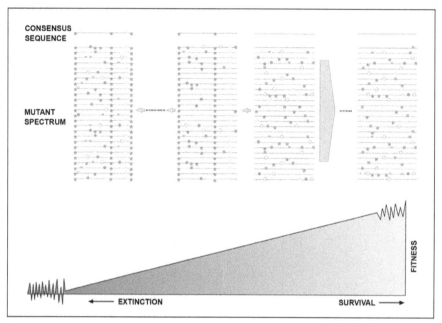

Figure 1.4. A viral mutant spectrum (similar to the ones depicted in figure 1.1B) is allowed to replicate in large populations (large arrow), and, as a consequence of competition among replicating genomes, the ones that replicate most efficiently dominate, and the virus gains fitness (tends to survive) in that particular environment. In contrast, the forced accumulation of mutations (small arrows) leads to fitness loss because mutations tend to be detrimental, and, as a consequence, the virus approaches extinction. This figure is modified, with permission, from Domingo, "Quasispecies."

Thus, despite indeterminations on how the introduction and establishment steps take place, the scenario conveyed in figure 1.2 is the most realistic one according to current knowledge of RNA virus genetics.[17]

Role of Viral Genome Variation in Disease Emergences and Reemergences

Emergences of human viral diseases have occurred at a rate of about one per year over the past four decades. Such emergences are usually (but not exclusively) associated with RNA viruses that can undergo frequent recombination and genome segment reassortment, suggesting that genome plasticity is important for emergence. But it is not easy to distinguish between variation required for the virus to be established in a new host from variation that provides just a nonessential replicative advantage in the new host or even variation that has no significant effect on virus replication. In one particular designed experiment, it was shown that an initial, ineffective replication of a swine foot-and-mouth disease virus in the guinea pig was soon followed by selection of virus mutants that improved replication and allowed the actual establishment of the virus as a pathogen for the guinea pig.[18] There might be a gradation of potentialities, ranging from viral pathogens that can replicate with sufficient efficiency to produce adaptive variation to viral pathogens that do not reach such minimal efficiency and cannot become productively adapted to the new host. The concept of genetic barrier refers to the extent of genetic variation (constellations of mutations, recombination or reassortment events, etc.) required for adaptation to a new environment. In the process of adaptation, the mutant spectrum complexity and the virus population size may play important roles.[19] As illustrated in figure 1.4, an adaptive variant may reach a target host if the virus population size attains a sufficient value (to provide multiple variants) and would have a low probability of encountering a target host when the number of variants is limited. There might be subtle random events (which affect the virus population size and numbers of variant genomes) that tilt a virus toward survival or extinction when exposed to new host candidates.

Factors in the Reemergence of Influenza

Influenza virus type A has all the ingredients to be prone to periodic readaptations and reemergences as a disease agent. Genetically it can undergo mutation, recombination, and reassortment (fig. 1.1). Ecologically, it has several animal reservoirs, notably wild waterfowl, swine, and horses. From wild aquatic birds, the virus can be transmitted to domestic poultry. Other hosts may also sustain the infection. For example, the H5N1 avian virus (fig. 1.3) that has caused about three hundred human deaths can infect and be transmitted among cats, and the virus has produced high mortality in tigers and leopards. The influenza virus can replicate in the digestive tract of waterbirds without causing disease, yet these animals shed the virus in large numbers, and viral particles can be found in lakes. Migratory birds can spread the influenza virus very efficiently, thereby increasing the probability of reassortment with viruses from mammalian species. The virus can be transmitted also from pigs to humans and poultry to humans, among other transmission pairs.[20] Human-to-human transmission through aerosols (favored by coughing and sneezing prompted by the infection) is facilitated by several of the sociological factors listed earlier (urbanization, rapid travel, migrations, late reporting of the onset of disease, the gathering of infected poultry or pigs with humans in farms or markets, etc.). Infection spread to ducks and chickens, and the virus evolved to be pathogenic for chickens. Then the virus reached domestic ducks and geese, where its genome underwent segment reassortment with other influenza viruses of aquatic birds. The new reassortant viruses were established in domestic chickens, swine, and humans. These infections were facilitated by mutations in several genes encoding different viral proteins. A boy died of infection from an H5N1 virus in Hong Kong in 1997. Additional human cases were reported that were associated with contacts between humans and infected poultry. In 2003 additional human infections occurred in several countries of Africa, Asia, the Pacific, and the Middle East.

Fortunately, the current H5N1 virus is not transmitted efficiently among humans. But the genetic material of the H5N1 virus continues to diversify through mutation, and more recent isolates appear to cause systemic (generalized) infections in humans, where they are resistant to anti-influenza virus drugs.[21] This account, and the presence of additional avian influenza viruses of subtypes H7N5, H7N7, H9N2, together with the presently cocirculating human H3N2 and H1N1 viruses, raises the possibility for and fear of additional reassortments and mutations that may result in a virus that can be efficiently transmitted among humans. A virus of subtype H1N1, most likely of swine origin, produced the influenza pandemic of 2009, with the first cases reported in Mexico, and tens of thousands of people were infected worldwide (fig. 1.3).

History of Influenza Epidemics and Pandemics

An examination of some of the influenza virus epidemics and pandemics recorded to date (fig. 1.3) indicates that they have occurred regularly during at least three centuries. Although it is generally accepted that sociological and ecological modifications accentuated in the course of the twentieth century favor disease emergences, history tells us that some influences were already in operation in the eighteenth century. There is considerable uncertainty as to the subtypes of the virus that caused the early 1889 epidemic, although some evidence suggests that viruses similar to H2N2 and H3N8 might have circulated.[22] The 1830–33 epidemic originated in China and then spread through Russia and Europe. From a properly epidemiological perspective, the Spanish influenza was not Spanish, as shown in the introduction to this volume.[23] The H1N1 virus associated with the severe 1918 pandemic was the first influenza to be well characterized biologically thanks to virus reconstruction from archival materials and genetic engineering.

The Asian influenza of 1957 originated in southern China, and successive waves reached Japan, Europe, and the United States, with one million deaths worldwide. Molecular and serological evidence suggests that the 1957 H2N2 virus originated from a virus derived from the 1918 H1N1 virus, in which segments PB1, HA, and NA were replaced by those of an avian H2N2 virus. In turn, the 1968 H3N2 virus originated from H2N2 virus, in which PB1 and HA were replaced by the corresponding segments of a virus, again of avian origin (fig. 1.1, pt. C).[24]

The H2N2 virus was replaced by the H3N2 virus in 1968 (fig. 1.3) and gave rise to the "Hong Kong influenza" that spread worldwide in 1969–70. The H3 and PB1 genes of this virus were of avian origin. An H1N1 influenza virus closely related to a virus that had circulated in the 1950s reemerged in 1977 in the so-called Russian influenza, with the first cases of disease recorded in China. H1N1 and H3N2 viruses have continued to cocirculate in the human population, undergoing continuous genetic and antigenic drift.

A new H1N1 variant recently caused an influenza outbreak in Mexico that has extended to other parts of the globe.[25] The initial analyses of the genomic segments of this new virus suggest that PB1 originated from a human virus, PB2 and PA from an avian virus, and HA, NP, NA, M, and NS from swine viruses (genome segments are described in a previous section and in fig. 1.1, pt. C), although the precise origin of the genome segments is still under study. This new genome constellation has resulted in efficient replication in humans and human-to-human transmission, which ensures its rapid spread in the human population. It appears that the new virus might have originated in swine and that HA and NA had undergone drift in swine prior to their incorporation in a virus able to be established in humans. Thus, despite the virus retaining the H1N1 subtype, vaccines administered in recent years (which include H1N1 and H3N2 viruses in their formulation) are unlikely to confer solid protection. Several factors included in the bulleted list (intensive farming, contact between humans and pigs, late reporting of the initial cases, etc.) have contributed to the onset of this new human pandemic. The new influenza illustrates once again the unpredictable nature of viral disease emergence, since surveillance efforts were concentrated on the avian influenza viruses circulating in Asia (mainly H7N5, H7N7, and H9N2; see fig. 1.3), while the introduction and establishment events in this case occurred in Central America and involved an H1N1 virus, the same subtype as the 1918 flu. Thus, successions of antigenic shifts with continued genetic and antigenic drift in multiple animal species have probably been at the basis of the major influenza epidemics recorded over the past centuries (compare figs. 1.1, pt. C, and 1.3).

Struggle to Reconstruct an Ancient Pathogen

The origin of the deadly H1N1 1918 influenza virus and the determinants of its extreme virulence are one of the major mysteries of virology. Samples of the

RNA from the virus were recovered from lung tissue specimens from US soldiers who died during the pandemic and who had been fixed in formalin and kept in paraffin wax. Lung tissue was also obtained from an Inuit woman who was a victim of the flu and whose body was kept in permanently frozen subsoil in the Seward Peninsula, Alaska.[26] This allowed for the reconstruction of the viral genes associated with the 1918 influenza virus and the engineering of the constellation of genes, which enabled their expression products to generate infectious viruses (a process termed "reverse genetics").[27] The main determinant of its high pathogenicity was probably HA, which induced cytokines and chemokines from macrophage (sometimes referred to as a "cytokine storm"). Such induction led to hemorrhage, one of the effects observed in infected humans during the pandemic. One of the amino acid substitutions in HA determined binding of the virus to human cell receptors, and other genetic signatures suggested that HA was of an avian origin. In addition, other genes contributed to pathogenicity, including PB2, in airborne transmission.[28]

It is not clear whether the virus that caused the 1918 pandemic was a reassortant, an avian virus that jumped into humans, that replicated first in some mammalian species before infecting humans, or that circulated in humans and then acquired high pathogenicity.[29] The reconstructed 1918 influenza virus can infect pigs, although the infection is not lethal as it is in the infection of mice, ferrets, and macaques. It is likely that during the 1918 epidemic, the virus infected pigs and originated a lineage of H1N1 influenza viruses.[30] Phylogenetic evidence has suggested that the HA gene of the 1918 virus was a true recombinant (fig. 1.1, pt. A) and that the recombination event probably coincided with the onset of the epidemic. One stretch of the HA gene was related to the corresponding region of swine influenza viruses, while the flanking regions were related to sequences of viruses from a human lineage. Two possible parental viruses cocirculated before 1918. The recombinant did not survive to be epidemiologically significant once the 1918 pandemic faded.[31] The molecular studies agree that, not surprisingly, at some point the ancestors of the 1918 H1N1 virus were avian viruses. But how the virus evolved prior to acquiring virulence for humans constitutes an example of the indetermination inherent to the establishment of a virus pathogen in a new host species.

Although several virulence determinants intrinsic to the 1918 influenza virus (hemagglutinin, polymerase complex, NS1) most likely influenced the severity of the pandemic, other factors might also have contributed to the elevated mortality.[32] Some of the social factors in the bulleted list are expected to accentuate disease severity during war times, in which nutritional limitations, stress, and suboptimal immune status must have been frequent among people involved. The gathering of soldiers at some specific locations, the transport of troops over long distances, and the disruption of surveillance and preventive measures during the war might have facilitated disease severity. It has been debated (several observations of the reconstruction of events in the 1918 influenza pandemic have proven to be especially prone to debate) whether bacterial infections contributed significantly to the mortality of individuals infected with the influenza virus, a phenomenon known as "copathogenesis." The opportunistic infections in AIDS patients, prompted by the deterioration of the immune system caused by human immunodeficiency virus type 1, constitute an extreme example of "copathogenesis." Despite the remarkable success in reconstructing the virus that caused the 1918 influenza, the origin of the virus and the factors that determined its virulence are likely to remain largely a mystery, as María-Isabel Porras-Gallo and Ryan A. Davis have pointed out in the introduction to this volume.

On Unexpected Evolutionary Events

Genetic variation is blind and the outcome uncertain. It is not possible to anticipate whether the virulence of a virus will increase, decrease, or remain the same as a pandemic progresses. It has been largely a matter of chance that we have the infectious diseases that we have, and we cannot predict those of subsequent generations of humans. Evolution renders virulence and the capacity of human-to-human transmission unpredictable. Evolution will select for viruses resistant to antiviral agents unless drug use is restricted to the patients who obviously need them. The challenge of a potentially devastating influenza pandemic demands surveillance approaches aimed not only at detecting influenza but also at penetrating molecular and biological features of the circulating, ever-evolving viruses, including avian viruses. These are not easy tasks, and the threat of influenza pandemics is likely to continue indefinitely.

Genetic change has constructed the biosphere of which we are a part. Diseases associated with genetic change (those resulting from chromosomal mutations or aberrations or cancer and those caused by dynamic pathogenic agents, etc.) are unavoidable by-products of the very same mechanisms that permitted life to appear and evolve. We live in a world increasingly recognized as complex, that is, run by multiple interacting agents, with outcomes that cannot be immediately explained as the sum of the individual actions of their participating parts. Emerging and reemerging infections are an illustration of biological complexity and thus a challenge for public health.

Acknowledgments

I am indebted to José Belio for the preparation of illustrations. Work in Madrid was supported by grants from BFU2008-02816/BMC and from FIPSE 36558/06. CIBERehd is funded by Instituto de Salud Carlos III.

Notes

I dedicate this article to the memory of Christof K. Biebricher for his friendship and unforgettable discussions on quasispecies.

1. Joshua Lederberg, "Viruses and Humankind: Intracellular Symbiosis and Evolutionary Competition," in *Emerging Viruses*, ed Stephen S. Morse (Oxford: Oxford University Press, 1993), 8.

2. Additional information is available from the sources on which figure 1.1 is based: Esteban Domingo, "Quasispecies: Concept and Implications for Virology," *Current Topics in Microbiology and Immunology* 299 (2006): 51–82; Esteban Domingo, "Virus Evolution," in *Fields Virology*, ed. David M. Knipe and Peter M. Howley, 5th ed. (Philadelphia: Lappincott Williams and Wilkins, 2007), 389–421; S. Jane Flint, Lynn William Enquist, Vincent R. Racaniello, and Anna Marie Skalka, *Principles of Virology, Molecular Biology, Pathogenesis and Control of Animal Viruses* (Washington DC: ASM Press, 2009); and Peter Palese and Megan L. Shaw, "Orthomyxoviridae: The Viruses and Their Replication," in *Fields Virology*, 1647–89.

3. Domingo, "Quasispecies"; Domingo, "Virus Evolution."

4. Esteban Domingo and Simon Wain-Hobson, "The 30th Anniversary of Quasispecies: Meeting on 'Quasispecies: Past, Present and Future,'" *EMBO Reports* 10, no. 5 (2009): 444–48; John J. Holland, "Transitions in Understanding of RNA Viruses: An Historical Perspective," *Current Topics in Microbiology and Immunology* 299 (2006): 371–401.

5. John J. Holland, Konrad Spindler, Frank Horodyski, Elizabeth A. Grabau, Scott VandePol, "Rapid Evolution of RNA Genomes," *Science* 215, no. 4540 (1982): 1577–85; Domingo, "Virus Evolution."

6. Jeffery K. Taubenberge, Ann H. Reid, Amy E. Krafft, Karen E. Bijwaard, Thomas G. Fanning, "Initial Genetic Characterization of the 1918 'Spanish' Influenza Virus," *Science* 275, no. 5307 (1997): 1793–96; Gina Kolata, *Flu: The Story of the Great Influenza Pandemic of 1918 and the Search for the Virus That Caused It* (New York: Farrar, 1999); Jeffrey R. Ryan, *Pandemic Influenza: Emergency Planning and Community Preparedness* (Boca Raton: CRC / Taylor and Francis Group, 2009).

7. See Palese and Shaw, "Orthomyxoviridae."

8. Mark J. Gibbs, John S. Armstrong and Adrian J. Gibbs, "The Haemagglutinin Gene, but Not the Neuraminidase Gene, of 'Spanish Flu' Was a Recombinant," *Philosophical Transactions of the Royal Society of London B: Biological Sciences* 356, no. 1416 (2001): 1845–55.

9. Detlev Khatchikian, Michaela Orlich, and R udolf Rott, "Increased Viral Pathogenicity after Insertion of a 28S Ribosomal RNA Sequence into the Haemagglutinin Gene of an Influenza Virus," *Nature* 340, no. 6229 (1989): 156–57.

10. Mark S. Smolinski, Margaret A. Hamburg, and Joshua Lederberg, *Microbial Threats to Health: Emergence, Detection and Response* (Washington, DC: National Academies Press, 2003). As pointed out in the introduction to this volume, several of these factors converged at the time of the Spanish influenza as a consequence of World War I and its effects.

11. This list is adapted from the following sources: Morse, *Emerging Viruses*; Stephen S. Morse, *The Evolutionary Biology of Viruses* (New York: Raven, 1994); Flint, Enquist, Racaniello, Skalka, *Principles of Virology*; Esteban Domingo and John J.

Holland, "Complications of RNA Heterogeneity for the Engineering of Virus Vaccines and Antiviral agents," *Genetic Engineering* 14 (1992): 13–31.

12. Stephen S. Morse "The Viruses of the Future? Emerging Viruses and Evolution," in Morse, *Evolutionary Biology of Viruses.*

13. Martin A. Nowak, *Evolutionary Dynamics* (Cambridge, MA: Belknap Press of Harvard University Press, 2006).

14. Data for figure 1.3 compiled from the following sources: William Ian Beardmore Beveridge, *Influenza: The Last Great Plague; An Unfinished Story of Discovery* (Heinemann: London, 1977); Palese and Shaw, "Orthomyxoviridae"; Robert G. Webster, William J. Bean, Owen T. Gorman, Thomas M. Chambers, and Yoshihiro Kawaoka, "Evolution and Ecology of Influenza A Viruses," *Microbiological Reviews* 56, no. 1 (1992); Flint, Enquist, Racaniello, and Skalka, *Principles of Virology*; Jeffrey R. Ryan, ed., *Pandemic Influenza: Emergency Planning and Community Preparedness* (Boca Ratón: CRC Press, 2009); Novel Swine-Origin Influenza A (H1N1) Virus Investigation Team, "Emergence of a Novel Swine-Origin Influenza A (H1N1) Virus in Humans," *New England Journal of Medicine* 360, no. 25 (2009).

15. Domingo, "Virus Evolution."

16. E. Duarte, D. Clarke, Andrés Moya, Esteban Domingo, "Rapid Fitness Losses in Mammalian RNA Virus Clones Due to Muller's Ratchet," *Proceedings of the National Academy of Sciences USA* 89, no. 13 (1992): 6015–19.

17. Domingo, "Quasispecies"; Domingo, "Virus Evolution"; Holland, "Transitions in Understanding"; Domingo and Wain-Hobson, "30th Anniversary of Quasispecies."

18. Eric Baranowski, Carmen M. Ruiz-Jarabo, Esteban Domingo, "Evolution of Cell Recognition by Viruses: A Source of Biological Novelty with Medical Implications," *Advances in Virus Research* 62 (2003): 19–111; José Ignacio Núñez, Eric Baranowski, Nicolas Molina, Carmen M. Ruiz-Jarabo, Carmen Sánchez, Esteban Domingo, and Francisco Sobrino, "A Single Amino Acid Substitution in Nonstructural Protein 3A Can Mediate Adaptation of Foot-and-Mouth Disease Virus to the Guinea Pig," *Journal of Virology* 75, no. 8 (2001): 3977–83.

19. Julie K. Pfeiffer and Karla Kirkegaard, "Increased Fidelity Reduces Poliovirus Fitness under Selective Pressure in Mice," *PLoS Pathogens* 1 (2005): 102–10; Marco Vignuzzi, Jeffrey K. Stone, Jamie J. Arnold, Craig E. Cameron, and Raul Andino, "Quasispecies Diversity Determines Pathogenesis through Cooperative Interactions in a Viral Population," *Nature* 439 (2006): 344–48.

20. Webster, Bean, Gorman, Chambers, and Kawaoka, "Evolution and Ecology of Influenza A Viruses"; P. F. Wright, G. Neumann, and Y. Kawaoka, "Orthomyxoviruses," in Knipe and Howley, *Fields Virology*, 1691–1740.

21. Wright, Neumann, and Kawaoka, "Orthomyxoviruses."

22. Beveridge, *Influenza: The Last Great Plague*; Wright, Neumann, and Kawaoka, "Orthomyxoviruses."

23. In the introduction Porras-Gallo and Davis provide basic information about the massive mortality produced by the pandemic.

24. Flint, Enquist, Racaniello, and Skalka, *Principles of Virology.*

25. Fatimah S. Dawood, Seema Jain, Lyn Finelli, Michael W. Shaw, Stephen Lindstrom, Rebecca J. Garten, Larisa V. Gubareva, Xiyan Xu, Carolyn B. Bridges, Timothy M. Uyeki, Novel Swine-Origin Influenza A (H1N1) Virus Investigation Team, "Emergence of a Novel Swine-Origin Influenza A (H1N1) Virus in Humans,"

New England Journal of Medicine 360 (2009): 2605–15; Sebastian U. Schnitzler and Paul Schnitzler, "An Update on Swine-Origin Influenza Virus A/H1N1: A Review," *Virus Genes* 39, no. 3 (2009): 279–92.

26. Kolata, *Flu;* Taubenberger, Ann H. Reid, Amy E. Krafft, Karen E. Bijwaard, Thomas G. Fanning, "Initial Genetic Characterization"; Ryan, *Pandemic Influenza.*

27. Jeffery K. Taubenberger Ann H. Reid, Raina M. Lourens, Ruixue Wang, Guozhong Jin, and Thomas G. Fanning, "Characterization of the 1918 Influenza Virus Polymerase Genes," *Nature* 437, no. 7060 (2005): 889–93.

28. Neal Van Hoeven, C. Pappas, J. A. Belser, T. R. Maines, H. Zeng, Adolfo García-Sastre, R. Sasisekharan, J. M. Kat zand Terence M. Tumpey, "Human HA and Polymerase Subunit PB2 Proteins Confer Transmission of an Avian Influenza Virus through the Air," *Proceedings of the National Academy of Sciences USA* 106, no. 9 (2009): 3366–71.

29. Mark J. Gibbs and Adrian J. Gibbs, "Molecular Virology: Was the 1918 Pandemic Caused by a Bird Flu?," *Nature* 440, no. 7088 (2006): E8, discussion E9–10; J. Antonovics, M. E. Hood, and C. H. Baker, "Molecular Virology: Was the 1918 Flu Avian in Origin?," *Nature* 440, no. 7088 (2006): E9, discussion E9–10; Jeffery K. Taubenberger, Ann H. Reid, Raina M. Lourens, Ruixue Wang, Guozhong Jin and Thomas G. Fanning, "Reply," *Nature* 440 (2006): E9–E10; Geoff Vana and Kristi M. Westover, "Origin of the 1918 Spanish Influenza Virus: A Comparative Genomic Analysis," *Molecular Phylogenetics and Evolution* 47, no. 3 (2008): 1100–10.

30. Hanna M. Weingartl, Randy A. Albrecht, Kelly M. Lager, Shawn Babiuk, Peter Marszal, James Neufeld, Carissa Embury-Hyatt et al, "Experimental Infection of Pigs with the Human 1918 Pandemic Influenza Virus," *Journal of Virology* 83, no. 9 (2009): 4287–96.

31. Gibbs, Armstrong, and Gibbs, "Haemagglutinin Gene."

32. Christopher F. Basler and Patricia V. Aguilar, "Progress in Identifying Virulence Determinants of the 1918 H1N1 and the Southeast Asian H5N1 Influenza A Viruses," *Antiviral Research* 79, no. 3 (2008): 166–78.

Chapter Two

Spanish Flu in Brazil

Searching for Causes during the Epidemic Horror

Liane Maria Bertucci

In Brazil the first systematic scientific discussions about the Spanish flu epidemic took place in September 1918, after members of the Brazilian Medical Mission and soldiers of the Brazilian army—whose ships had anchored in Dakar, Senegal (then a French colony)—contracted the disease, many of whom died.[1] Dakar was one of the main ports for the transit of international troops headed for the war in Europe.[2] While the Brazilian government was discussing how to send medicines to victims and whether to bring all their soldiers and doctors in Africa back to Brazil, the Brazilian newspapers published articles telling of the visit of the English ship *Demerara* to Brazil.[3] The ship departed England from Liverpool and docked at Rio de Janeiro on September 14, after stopping at Lisbon, Recife, and Salvador. During the trip various passengers took ill and five people died. In Rio de Janeiro the sick were taken to the Hospital de Isolamento (Hospital of Isolation), and the ship was disinfected by Brazilian sanitation authorities. Many passengers entered the city, some of whom became ill in the following days.[4] In late September information about patients in port towns began to be published nationwide, and within a few days victims of the Spanish flu were found in the interior of Brazil.

An illness that aroused little attention in the medical community in the 1910s, the flu was classified by most scientists as a microbial, endemic, and worldwide disease that caused nasal mucus, a mild fever, a cough, and body pains, generally without many complications or risk of death. In short, it was considered a benign disease. According to the "Bibliografia brasileira da grippe" published in 1919 in the *Archivos Brasileiros de Medicina*, thirteen works about the disease had been published in the country in the nineteenth century: two articles discussed the 1889–90 pandemic, four dealt with the epidemic of 1835, and seven dealt with flu or related illnesses in other years, whether epidemic or not. In contrast, between 1901 and 1917, twenty-eight studies were published in Brazil. The authors of these texts discussed flu epidemics of the late nineteenth and early twentieth centuries, giving clinical descriptions of patients, information about treatments, and their thoughts on Pfeiffer's bacillus.[5]

In 1892 German pathologist Richard Pfeiffer announced that a bacillus, *Haemophilus influenzae*, was the cause of flu. His thesis about what became known as Pfeiffer's bacillus resulted in increased interest in the disease on the part of the international scientific community, and myriad studies were carried out in an attempt to prove or debunk his findings.[6] While some scientists (such as August Wassermann) claimed there could be no flu without *Haemophilus influenzae*, others (like Heinrich Curschmann) claimed the bacillus was not always found in a patient who was clinically believed to have the flu.[7] Many doctors (among them G. Jochmann, Paul Clemens, Fernand Bezançon, and S. Israel De Jong) who examined bodily fluids collected from patients (mucus, blood, etc.) reported a low rate of Pfeiffer's bacillus.[8] In the second half of 1918, when these debates were still prevalent, interest in flu, its diagnosis, and its etiological agent grew tremendously in Brazil and the world due to the devastation caused by the so-called Spanish flu.[9]

My previous research on this pandemic has focused on the social, cultural, economic, demographic, and sanitary impact of this episode in Brazil, as well as on the more general social reactions from laypeople, politicians, and doctors. The present chapter focuses more on Brazilian scientists' scientific work during the epidemic as an expression of the development of Brazil. Specifically, it discusses the studies, opinions, and debates about the flu that were carried out in Rio de Janeiro and São Paulo (the two largest cities in Brazil) during the time of the Spanish flu and some of its developments in the following years. Between the late 1910s and the early 1920s part of the Brazilian scientific community, using studies from around the world, debated different theses and studied hypotheses about the flu. In 1918 the first great debate that Brazilian doctors had concerned the real nature of the disease: was it or was it not the flu? The diagnosis of the epidemic as flu (a relative consensus among doctors worldwide) led to another question: was there a difference between the Spanish flu epidemic and the flu beginning to affect Brazilians in September 1918? By October no one doubted the diseases were one and the same, and in light of the pressing epidemic circumstances, members of the Brazilian scientific community shifted the focus of their studies from identifying the disease to determining whether a bacillus or a filterable virus caused it. Establishing the cause of the flu was seen as the path to controlling it, discovering its cure, and ultimately preventing it.[10]

By examining the research reports of the Butantã Institute in São Paulo and the Oswaldo Cruz Institute in the Manguinhos district of Rio de Janeiro, especially the original experiments conducted by Drs. Aristides Marques da Cunha, Octavio de Magalhães, and Olympio da Fonseca, as well as reports from medical faculties and hospitals in the two cities, we can recreate doctors' initial discussions of the flu epidemic, including their doubts and differing opinions about the disease.[11]

Was It Really the Flu?

After the events in Dakar, medical and scientific discussion concerning the disease began to take place in Brazil's two most important metropolises, Rio de Janeiro and São Paulo.[12] With around 528,200 inhabitants, the city of São Paulo, capital of the richest state in the country and the largest producer of coffee, rivaled the national capital Rio de Janeiro in importance with its industries, banks, and prosperous commerce. Rio de Janeiro, with a population of approximately 914,200, also had a high concentration of important financial and economic activities in its urban region.[13] Both cities were political and administrative centers with research institutes and scientific academies, laboratories, and faculties that were respected overseas and that served as a model for the rest of the country. Among the most important were the Oswaldo Cruz Institute and the Butantã Institute, which, in addition to publishing original studies that enjoyed international circulation, engaged in bacteriological research and medical experiments dealing specifically with problems in Brazil.[14] Researchers at these institutes were in constant contact with the major scientific centers around the world, following the most recent developments in medicine and science and publishing the results of their own research. As a result, they acquired knowledge that fostered new research and studies.[15]

In September 1918 doctors in both cities, whether affiliated with the Oswaldo Cruz and Butantã Institutes or not, began discussing the Spanish flu epidemic. Two key questions arose in their discussions. First, was the illness affecting Africans and Europeans the flu or some other type of illness? Second, was the flu that was beginning to spread in Brazil in late September the same one affecting people in Africa and Europe?

Following the first outbreak in early 1918, which was characterized by low virulence, doctors from a number of countries debated which disease caused the Spanish flu epidemic. Medical opinion was divided among three possibilities, each one based on different nosological features: flu, dengue fever, or pappataci fever (also known as three-day fever).[16]

On September 25, at a meeting of the São Paulo Academy of Medicine, Dr. Ludgero da Cunha Motta suggested "investigating what morbid agent, known as Spanish flu, was actually causing the loss of so many precious lives of our poor and neglected colleagues who had left for Europe with the double duty of healing the sick and acting as patriots."[17] The first conclusion they reached was that there were not enough clinically detailed descriptions of the Brazilians who had fallen prey to the illness in Senegal to offer a proper diagnosis. Nevertheless, this did not prevent robust debate of the issue, even if this debate was based on contemporary medical literature rather than on clinical trials or experiments. Cunha Motta informed the members of the academy that the most widespread theory among Brazilian doctors was that the Brazilian soldiers and members of the Medical Mission had fallen victim to pappataci fever. But he disagreed.

Cunha Motta discarded this possibility because the number of deaths, and the fact that people in Dakar were dying so quickly, were not in keeping with the normal characteristics of three-day fever. In partial disagreement with his colleague, Dr. Octavio de Carvalho argued that although traditionally considered a benign disease in the scholarly literature, pappataci fever, as well as dengue fever and the flu, could become virulent under "special circumstances," such as those observed in a number of men (in barracks and ships and battlefields) at that time. Therefore, it was his understanding that under the name of Spanish flu, any one of the three diseases could become an epidemic.[18]

Dr. Eduardo Monteiro advanced a similar hypothesis to explain the epidemic in Europe, basing his conclusions on information published in France concerning discussions that took place on May 17 at the Société Médicale des Hôpitaux de Paris (Medical Society of the Hospitals of Paris). In the case of disease in Africa, however, he preferred to wait for clinical descriptions. At the meeting in Paris, Drs. Chauffard, Massary, and Netter claimed the disease spreading throughout Europe was the flu, whereas Dr. Brun claimed it was dengue fever. At the same time, military doctors in the Mediterranean basin had found it to be three-day fever. For Monteiro, such diverging diagnoses suggested the three diseases could be spreading over Europe at the same time. The similarity between some of the symptoms of the three illnesses made it difficult for the lay public and "not very learned physicians" to distinguish one from the other. In this sense, the Spanish flu became an umbrella term that referred to all three.[19]

Nevertheless, the characteristics of the disease changed dramatically between the May meeting in Paris and the meeting at the São Paulo Academy of Medicine in September. The early diagnoses of the disease as either dengue fever or three-day fever were gradually rejected because of the high level of virulence, which had never been seen before, and the fact that the disease was spreading so rapidly. The number of clinical descriptions of the disease multiplied in a matter of weeks and bacteriological and necroscopic analyses were carried out as the spread of the epidemic reached a global scale. Most medical researchers identified the disease as the flu.[20] In Brazil a telegram sent from Africa by Dr. José Thomaz Nabuco de Gouvêa, head of the Brazilian Medical Mission, to the federal government (picked up by newspapers on September 26) reported that the African disease was, in fact, the flu. Similarly, a report on the epidemic in Europe, obtained by Brazilian authorities in France, also described the disease as the flu. In other words, it was the same epidemic of Spanish flu that was raging on both African and European soil.

A number of Brazilian doctors, however, adopted the theory that the flu that had begun to spread in Brazil in late September was different from the one spreading in Europe and Africa. As mentioned in the introduction to this volume, the virulence of the Spanish flu was blamed on the conditions of the Great War; specifically, the battlefields in Europe and the ports in Africa where troops docked (such as Dakar) on their way to the battlefields. Such was the opinion of Dr. Carlos Seidl, head of the Diretoria Geral de Saúde Pública (Directorate General of Public Health), run by the federal government, who aired his opinion on this "contemporary matter of great interest" at a session of the Brazilian Academy of Medicine in Rio de Janeiro on October 10, 1918. For Seidl, although the epidemics spreading in Africa and Europe and Brazil were all flus, the type of flu in Europe and Africa was much more virulent than the one in Brazil. He stated that general prophylactic actions such as isolation had a minimal impact on the flu (whether Spanish or not), which was an extremely contagious disease, and that only individual prophylaxis would be in any way effective. He recommended taking quinine salts to prevent the flu and rigorous antisepsis of the mouth and nose.[21]

Dr. Garfield de Almeida agreed with Seidl, asserting that although it was the same flu affecting people in Europe, Africa, and Brazil, the difference was the lethality of the disease in Europe and Africa. According to Dr. Almeida, this difference, which contrasted the typical benign characteristics of the flu overseas, was due to the type of conditions that many men were submitted to in the military camps, navy ships, and battlefields. The conditions caused by World War I were a deciding factor in the form the disease took in Europe and Africa (where it would also be aggravated by the climate).[22]

The other members of the academy present at the meeting fully agreed with Seidl and Almeida, with one exception: Adm. João F. Lopes Rodrigues, head of the Serviço Sanitário da Armada Nacional (Sanitation Service of the National Fleet). The admiral, who reported that he had taken care of more than two hundred flu-stricken sailors in two days, believed it was some other disease that had killed the Brazilians in Africa. In the opinion of the Lopes Rodrigues, even considering that the flu could kill, it seemed impossible that this disease could kill so many young people so quickly. His words caused quite a stir among the academy's doctors and, in an attempt to reestablish a consensus among them, his colleagues reminded Lopes Rodrigues that their diagnosis of the disease was based on information gathered by Dr. José Thomaz Nabuco de Gouvêa in Dakar.[23] The admiral stuck to his opinion that it was not the flu but also stated that he did not know what illness had killed the soldiers in Africa.[24]

While doctors were discussing the epidemic, the number of victims in Brazil was rising. On October 10 Rio de Janeiro had 440 patients. Two days later the number had reached approximately 20,000. In São Paulo, on October 15, medical and government authorities confirmed the first case of the flu epidemic, a young man arriving from Rio de Janeiro who had been admitted to the Hospital of Isolation two days before.[25] Within two weeks some 30,000 people in the city had come down with the flu. As a result, the theory that the flu in Brazil was different from that of Europe and Africa was dismissed. In a matter of days authorities began to record the number of deaths occurring nationwide.[26]

Bacillus versus Filterable Virus: A Long-running Dispute

With the confirmation of the first cases of Spanish flu in Brazil, the government took measures to care for the sick and help the families of poorer victims. Not only did doctors, nurses, pharmacists, medical academics, and other health care professionals go to work across the nation, but the nation also witnessed increased solidarity among the lay public as the number of victims and deaths due to the illness grew.[27] Many people helped collect and distribute medicine and food, provide help to the victims and their families, and make donations to organizations, such as the Brazilian Red Cross, which were providing aid to the sick.[28]

On October 18, as this nationwide campaign was gaining momentum, Dr. Carlos Seidl was dismissed from the Directorate General of Public Health due to the numerous criticisms he received in the Rio de Janeiro press, which were published all over the country.[29] He was accused of "indifference," owing to the few steps he had taken to halt the spread of the disease.[30] Despite this criticism, however, there was in reality little he could have done to deal with such a virulent flu that had confused men of science and decimated the population. One key to dealing with the epidemic involved identifying the etiological agent of the disease, which would help determine what action to take to prevent and combat it. Therefore, while doctors were telling the general population that it was necessary to wait out the six weeks of the epidemic cycle and providing medication to alleviate the suffering of the sick and help their families (as there was no effective treatment, only palliative treatments), they were also carrying out research in Rio de Janeiro and São Paulo in an attempt to define the cause of the disease.

As the epidemic progressed, doubts that Pfeiffer's bacillus was the causative agent of the epidemic flu increased in medical communities throughout the world, which prompted a number of Brazilian doctors to examine the hypothesis that a filterable virus causes the flu (whether Spanish or not).[31] Many of these doctors were familiar with Walter Kruse's 1914 study (later developed by George Foster), which had succeeded in reproducing the symptoms of a common cold in four people from a filtrate (in a Berkefeld candle) of nasal secretion of an affected patient. Most of the experiments conducted in Brazil used blood or mucus filtrates from flu victims.

Dr. Carlos Chagas (who discovered Chagas disease), director of the Oswaldo Cruz Institute, performed initial bacteriological studies of throat secretions and blood samples collected from soldiers in the Quinquagésimo-Sexto Batalhão de Caçadores do Exército Brasileiro (Fifty-Sixth Hunters Battalion of the Brazilian Army). These men were among the first confirmed cases of the epidemic in Rio de Janeiro. Overloaded with work at the Directorate General of Public Health, whose command he had assumed after the dismissal of Dr. Carlos Seidl, Chagas was forced to abandon his experiments; however, Drs. Astrogildo Machado and Costa Cruz later completed his work. The doctors detected an abundance of a type of diplococcus (a round bacterium of pairs of two joined cells) in the samples collected from the patients, which led them to form the hypothesis that this diplococcus was the cause of the flu. After running tests, they reported that "the inoculations made in laboratory animals were negative and no secure conclusion can be made from the *in anima nobili* experiments carried out during the epidemic invasion."[32] Consequently, their hypothesis was discarded.

Necropsies were also conducted on deceased flu victims after the first deaths from the epidemic were reported in Rio de Janeiro on October 12 and, nine days later, in São Paulo. The American pathologist Bowman C. Crowell, who had recently arrived to organize and head the pathological anatomy division of the Oswaldo Cruz Institute, conducted the earliest post mortem research.[33] In December 1918 Crowell recorded the conclusions of his research: "There was a notable similarity in the cases [studied] and we believe we are justified in describing them as examples of a single entity. On the other hand, we are aware that more accurate knowledge of the etiology might show that we have been dealing with more than one entity. We know that in some of our cases there was a complication caused by lobar pneumonia."[34]

Dr. Arnaldo Vieira de Carvalho, director of the Faculdade de Medicina e Cirurgia de São Paulo (Faculty of Medicine and Surgery in São Paulo) and coordinator of the makeshift hospitals established to treat the victims in the city, conducted necroscopic examinations to determine why the disease was so lethal. His conclusions were similar to Crowell's: the pathological analyses justified a flu diagnosis, though there were also signs that pneumonia was responsible for the deaths. But while Crowell was cautious in his statements, explicitly advocating for the need to define the etiology of the disease, Dr. Vieira de Carvalho declared that it was likely that two diseases were spreading epidemically in São Paulo: flu and pneumonia.[35] Most doctors disagreed with Vieira de Carvalho's assertion, in spite of the pulmonary complications caused in organisms debilitated by the flu and cases of pneumonia. For instance, Dr. Deolindo Galvão, a member of the São Paulo Academy of Medicine, defended the theory of Pfeiffer's bacillus. For him, one of the characteristics of *Haemophilus influenzae* was its ability to predispose a person to secondary infections such as pneumonia by debilitating the victim's organism. This characteristic of the bacillus made it impossible to detect in the organism of some patients, namely, those in which the agents of opportunistic diseases prevailed. Accordingly, he stated, "I have never considered, in our current situation, pneumonia to be a separate, isolated [epidemic] disease."[36]

During the Spanish flu epidemic, Pfeiffer's bacillus was repeatedly identified—in greater or lesser quantity—in the blood and mucus samples from victims. In some cases, it was found in combination with other microorganisms such as pneumococcus and streptococcus. Finding *Haemophilus influenzae* in the samples collected from Spanish flu victims, even in small quantities, seemed to support those who believed in the bacillus theory. At the same time, reports from a number of pathologists who carried out research during this outbreak supported the theory of a filterable virus. These reports were based on clinical and epidemiological comparisons between the 1918 flu and other human illnesses (such as measles) as well as animal illnesses that were caused by a "filterable germ."[37] In short, doctors on both sides of the debate pointed to a number of studies in defense of their respective theories.

In this context, the director of the Serviço Sanitário do Estado de São Paulo (State Sanitation Service of São Paulo), Dr. Arthur Neiva, authorized the installation of a special ward at the makeshift hospital in the Escola de Farmácia de São Paulo (Pharmacy School of São Paulo) so that studies of the Spanish flu could be conducted.[38] At the Butantã Institute, in October and November, researchers prepared mucus cultures of patients with ether and physiological serum. After filtering the material, they injected it into a number of animals, though there was no apparent reaction.[39] In early October Dr. Arthur Moses, professor of microbiology at the Faculty of Medicine in Rio de Janeiro, began to conduct research in hospitals around the city. He first attempted to isolate and analyze Pfeiffer's bacillus. From both a bacteriological viewpoint and in cultures, he examined mucus from more than forty patients with varying degrees of the disease. The microscopic exams revealed the presence of *Haemophilus influenzae* in seven cases (in two of these cases at very low levels). He then prepared water-blood cultures of sheep, pigeons, and humans. Colonies of microorganisms similar to Pfeiffer's bacillus were found in larger quantity in the human water-blood mixture, but it was possible to isolate the bacillus only once. Although he collected samples from twenty-three patients, which he submitted to hemocultures, he was unable to isolate the bacillus. Similarly, the presence of *Haemophilus influenzae* was very small in material obtained from five necroscopic exams. Moses also conducted tests with cultures on a monkey, but the reactions of the animal were insignificant. His various experiments led him to conclude, "it cannot be confirmed that Pfeiffer's bacillus is indeed the determining factor of the flu." Rather, he believed his experiments had shown it was possible to conclude that the flu was caused by a filterable virus.[40]

When Moses published his results, he made specific mention of Dr. Henrique Beaurepaire de Aragão. Dr. Aragão carried out microscopic studies at the Oswaldo Cruz Institute, where he experimented with mucus cultures injected into animals.[41] Despite the inconclusive results of his research, he decided to publish his experiments in the November 9, 1918, volume of *Brazil-Médico*, convinced that a filterable virus was a more likely cause of the flu than a bacillus.[42]

On November 30, also in the *Brazil-Médico* journal, a "preliminary note" provided the initial results of three other doctors at the Oswaldo Cruz Institute: Drs. Aristides Marques da Cunha and Olympio da Fonseca, from the head office of the institute in Manguinhos, Rio de Janeiro; and Dr. Octavio de Magalhães at the branch in Belo Horizonte in Minas Gerais State.[43] Decades later Fonseca would claim that it was Cunha who expressed the "need to proceed with studies on the true etiology of the disease, since the role of Pfeiffer's bacillus, generally considered to be its producing agent, seems highly doubtful to us."[44] The detailed report of Cunha, Magalhães and Fonseca's research was published in late 1918 in the journal *Memórias do Instituto Oswaldo Cruz*. According to them, it was only when they were writing the report that they learned of the studies carried out in the second half of 1918 by the French doctors Charles Nicolle, Charles Lebailly and Henri Violle, whose procedures and results were similar to their own. They also stated they were aware of the work of H. Selter, "whose conclusions [about the filterable virus] are fully in agreement with the findings of our experiments."[45]

The stated purpose of Cunha, Magalhães, and Fonseca's research was to identify "[flu] germs existing randomly in the circulating blood." Accordingly, they made anaerobiotic hemocultures—in different media such as serum and glucose—of samples obtained from ten recent patients who were in their first day or two with the flu. The doctors paid special attention to the cultures in the "Noguchi medium," seeking to detect spirochetes or spherical corpuscles similar to those described by Simon Flexner when he was researching the agent that caused poliomyelitis.[46]

They also injected men, guinea pigs, and six species of monkeys with blood and mucus samples that had been prepared in cultures and duly filtered in Berkefeld and Chamberland candles.[47] The results of the experiments with injections of different doses and filtrates in monkey and guinea pigs ranged from no reaction to intense agitation and rising temperature in several of the animals. By rigorously monitoring the experiments, they were able to discard the possibility that the toxicity of the materials used had caused the reactions. In the case of the monkeys, the doctors compared the behavior of the animals selected for the experiments with that of other monkeys of the same species that had not been injected. In the tenth experiment, two monkeys (*Cebus*) were injected with the same mucus filtrate. One had had an intense reaction to the first injection days before, though there was no reaction at all to the second injection (this was the most interesting case of immunity observed by the doctors). The other monkey, which received its first filtrate injection, reacted violently, indicating the possible presence of a filterable virus.[48]

If the flu was indeed caused by a filterable virus in the blood of the patients, then it was believed that autohemotherapy would yield positive results in the acute, septicemic phase of the disease because it would act as an antigen. Cunha, Magalhães, and Fonseca tested this hypothesis even though it was difficult to determine the acute phase of the flu. Autohemotherapy was performed on forty-nine patients with results that were "favorable and, not rarely, excellent." But, as they stated, "Given the enormous accumulation of work during the acute phase of the epidemic, it was not possible to gather numerical data concerning the results of the autohemotherapy. . . . Since we do not know exactly what the septicemic stage of the infection is, the use of autohemotherapy may not provide constantly favorable results."[49]

Cunha, Magalhães, and Fonseca also conducted other studies involving humans, injecting mucus filtrates into six healthy men. Four were given a subcutaneous injection, with two of them receiving a single dose of 5 cc and two receiving injections of 5 cc and 10 cc. The other two men were injected with mucus filtrate through the pharynx. None of the six men, however, experienced a reaction. Nevertheless, they decided to test a "vaccine" from the virulent material collected from patients. They prepared a filtrate made of mucus treated with phenic acid and heated and tested it on the six patients. In five cases the patients' temperature, which averaged around thirty-nine degrees Celsius (102 degrees Fahrenheit), quickly fell to under thirty-seven degrees (98 degrees Fahrenheit) following the first dose, providing an encouraging result, at least initially.[50] But the low number of vaccinated patients did not convince the doctors of the effectiveness of the injection as a therapy for those affected by the disease. Moreover, because the epidemic was coming to an end, it was impossible to continue the experiments.

In reporting on their research, Cunha, Magalhães, and Fonseca put forward various hypotheses to account for the negative results of some experiments. One was that the candles used to obtain the filtrates could occasionally retain the filterable flu virus, which had occurred on some occasions during research involving filterable agents of other diseases. Another was that the filterable flu virus might disappear from the mucus or blood before the material was filtered. A third hypothesis held that the virus could have a "short period of existence in the circulating blood" and therefore disappear before the material could be collected or injected. Despite the negative results of some experiments, however, the doctors continued to affirm their belief that the flu was "an infection produced by a filterable virus."[51] At the same time, because their findings were preliminary and because the waning of the epidemic made it impossible to continue their research, they did not discard the need for further experiments to prove their theory definitely.

Flu Cause, the Theme after 1918

By the end of the epidemic, approximately 12,300 of the 600,000 cases of infection from the Spanish flu in Rio de Janeiro resulted in death. In São Paulo, of the 116,777 who contracted the disease, at least 5,331 died.[52] This great tragedy was repeated in other Brazilian cities (with a death toll reaching 180,000 in the country) and also around the world.[53] In the following years fear of an epidemic like that of 1918 haunted Brazil and the world and the number of scientific works published about flu multiplied.

In April 1919 those who attended the meeting in Milan to discuss the Spanish flu epidemic reported on the diversity of studies and opinions concerning the disease and spoke of the experiments that had been done at scientific institutes in a number of countries, including the experiments of Cunha, Magalhães and Fonseca at the Oswaldo Cruz Institute.[54] Dealing with persisting doubts about the etiology of the disease, an article published in 1919 in the Chicago journal *Archives of Internal Medicine* stated, "Pfeiffer's bacillus is the apparent cause of the epidemic disease, but its causal relationship has not been conclusively proved."[55] That same year the São Paulo journal *Archivos de Biologia* published a summary of the conclusions of Dr. Serafino Belfanti, director of the Istituto Sieroterapico Milanese (Milanese Sero-therapeutic Institute) in Milan. According to Belfanti, until science could shed more light on the etiology of the flu, it was possible to consider "the clinical and bacteriological duality of the flu and its complications."[56] In other words, he suggested the existence of two types of flu: one classic and benign and the other with serious symptoms. In Rio de Janeiro, also in 1919, Dr. Motta Rezende, the assistant to Dr. Antonio Austregésilo, one of the scientific directors of the journal *Archivos Brasileiros de Medicina*, concluded, "the latest works from overseas bring the news that a filterable virus was the efficient cause of the flu, and not the well-known Pfeiffer germ."[57] Similarly, two years later in São Paulo, Dr. Ulysses Paranhos, a member of the Brazilian Academy of Medicine, declared his opinion that the disease was "caused by a specific agent, probably a filterable virus."[58] Nevertheless, because Pfeiffer's bacillus was detected in people who had no symptoms of the flu, and not found in a number of people who were infected, it continued to divide scientific opinions all over the world.[59] In 1923 the *Archives of Internal Medicine* published the results of necroscopic studies carried out during the 1918 epidemic in Camp Devens (United States) by Drs. S. Burt Wolbach and Channing Frothingham, concluding, "The cause of the influenza epidemic has not been established."[60]

Among those who defended the Pfeiffer's bacillus theory was Professor James McIntosh, who conducted a number of bacteriological and pathological studies during the epidemic.[61] In 1922 a commentary on these studies published by the *British Medical Journal* stated, "Professor McIntosh severely criticizes the evidence that has been brought forward in support of the view that a filter-passing organism is concerned in the cause of the influenza, and he has no hesitation in rejecting it *in toto*."[62] The next year the *British Medical Journal* published a diagnosis of the Spanish flu epidemic prepared by the Pathological Section of the Sheffield Medical and Surgical Society: "one agent, and one only, was primarily responsible for the cases of the pandemic. This agent was the influenza bacillus."[63] In Rio de Janeiro, in 1924, the president of the Brazilian Academy of Medicine, Dr. Miguel Couto, when discussing the characteristics of the flu, declared that the gravity of the flu epidemic was due to the ability of Pfeiffer's bacillus to exacerbate the virulence of the agents of other diseases.[64]

As the foregoing examples demonstrate, the debate over the etiology of the Spanish flu raged on long after the epidemic had subsided, with articles in defense of both theories continuing to appear. Yet, despite their differences, all these researchers shared the common belief that, building on their hypotheses, experiments, and the discussions among peers, the etiology of the flu and the means of preventing and curing the disease would one day be definitively revealed. In 1933 this belief began to be confirmed when a London-based team comprising Drs. Christopher Andrewes, Wilson Smith, and Patrick Laidlaw identified a filterable and mutant virus, *Myxovirus influenzae*, as the cause of the disease. Moreover, since that time the experiments of Aristides Marques da Cunha, Octavio de Magalhães, and Olympio da Fonseca have gained recognition little by little in the international scientific community (along with other studies carried out in different parts of the world in 1918).[65] In 1950 Pierre Lépine, a virologist at the Pasteur Institute in Paris, declared that Cunha, Magalhães, and Fonseca's research with the monkeys had provided evidence of a filterable virus at the same time as and independently of Nicolle and Lebailly in France and T. Yamanouchi and his team in Japan.[66] But almost a hundred years later, as Porras-Gallo and Davis have indicated in the introduction to this volume, the so-called Spanish flu continues to challenge doctors.[67] Like their counterparts from the Spanish flu era, early twenty-first-century physicians and scientists hope that in the future the disease will finally be totally understood and controlled.

Notes

1. As Porras-Gallo and Davis have pointed out in the introduction to this volume, Brazil took part in World War I.

2. Liane Maria Bertucci, *Influenza, a medicina enferma* (Campinas: Universidade Estadual de Campinas, 2004), 92–96. The Brazilian soldiers first stopped at Freetown, Sierra Leone (a British protectorate and the main port in the west of Africa). According to Alfred W. Crosby, *Epidemic and Peace, 1918* (Westport, CT: Greenwood, 1976), and Beatriz Echeverri Dávila, *La gripe española: La pandemia de 1918–1919* (Madrid: Centro de Investigaciones Sociológicas / Siglo XXI, 1993), Boston (United States), Brest (France), and Freetown (Sierra Leone) were the main points from which the Spanish flu spread from August onward.

3. Medicines were sent to Dakar. Brazilian soldiers and the Brazilian Medical Mission continued their voyage to France. See also Cruz de Souza, chap. 7, in this volume.

4. Bertucci, *Influenza*, 96–99. In addition to the *Demerara*, other ships from European and African ports, where the epidemic was raging, docked in Brazil in the second fortnight of September.

5. "Bibliografia brasileira da grippe," supplement, *Archivos Brasileiros de Medicina* 9 (1919): 283–479.

6. Lucien Galliard, *La grippe* (Paris: Baillière, 1898); Grégoire André, *La grippe ou influenza* (Paris: Masson et Cie, 1908), 69–97.

7. Arthur Moses, "A bacteriologia da grippe," *Boletim da Academia Nacional de Medicina* 89 (1918): 681; Antonio Piga and Luis Lamas, *Infecciones de tipo gripal* (Madrid: Talleres tipográficos "Los Progresos de la Clínica" 1919), 1:63–65.

8. Moses, "Bacteriologia da grippe," 681; Fernand Bezançon and S. Israel de Jong, "Grippe, v.XVIII," in *Traité d'hygiène*, ed. Georges Brouardel and Louis Mosny (Paris: Baillière, 1912), 320–60.

9. Despite the fact that Spain was not the original source of the pandemic, as explained in the introduction, from the first outbreak, the flu was called "Spanish flu" in Brazil. In São Paulo, from as early as the beginning of July, the name "Spanish flu" was used. Bertucci, *Influenza*, 93.

10. Discussions about the causes of the flu, and its treatments, see also Sobral, Lima, and Silveira e Sousa's and Cruz de Souza's contributions to this volume in chapters 4 and 7, respectively, as well as María-Isabel Porras-Gallo, "Sueros y vacunas en la lucha contra la pandemia de gripe de 1918–1919 en España," *Asclepio* 60, no. 2 (2008): 261–88.

11. As Porras-Gallo and Davis have advanced in the introduction to this volume, the Oswaldo Cruz Institute and the Butantã Institute were the most important centers of research in Brazil during the pandemic, and they remain so today.

12. The question—"was it really the flu?"—is also dealt with by various other authors in this volume, including Sobral, Lima, and Silveira e Sousa (chapter 4), Porras-Gallo (chapter 5), Silveira (chapter 6), León-Sanz (chapter 8), and Feldman (chapter 10).

13. Carlos Luiz Meyer and Joaquim R. Teixeira, *A grippe epidêmica no Brazil e especialmente em São Paulo* (São Paulo: Casa Duprat, 1920), 58, 60.

14. The Oswaldo Cruz Institute and the Butantã Institute were set up to combat the bubonic plague that threatened Brazil in 1899, and both institutes expanded. The Manguinhos Sorotherapy Institute was established in 1900, between December 1907 and March 1908 it was renamed the Institute of Experimental Pathology, and later in 1908 the name was changed once again to the Oswaldo Cruz Institute. In the early decades of the twentieth century it was renowned for its work in protozoology. In 1900 the São Paulo State government set up an antiplague laboratory annexed to the São Paulo Bacteriological Institute, and in 1901 the laboratory paved the way for the Butantã Institute. In the first few years of the 1900s it was best known for its work in the field of ophidism. Among the most prominent researchers at the Oswaldo Cruz Institute and the Butantã Institute in the early twentieth century were, respectively, Dr. Carlos Chagas (who discovered Chagas disease and on June 24, 1912, was awarded the Schaudinn Prize for his discovery) and Dr. Vital Brazil (who, contrary to the theory of Albert Calmette, correctly defended the specificity of antiophidic serum according to the type of snake).

15. Jaime Larry Benchimol and Luiz Antonio Teixeira, *Cobras, lagartos e outros bichos* (Rio de Janeiro: Fundação Oswaldo Cruz, 1993). The following international institutions had a significant impact on the medical and scientific studies conducted in Brazil: the Pasteur Institute in Paris, the Hamburg School of Tropical Medicine, the Berlin Institute for Infectious Diseases, the Alfort Veterinary School, the Smithsonian Institute in Washington, and so on. In terms of international researchers, Brazilian scientists interacted with the likes of Stanislas von Prowazek and Max Hartmann. For further information, see Jaime Larry Benchimol, ed., *Manguinhos do sonho à vida* (Rio de Janeiro: Fundação Oswaldo Cruz, 1990); Benchimol and Teixeira, *Cobras*; Bertucci, *Influenza*, 68–90; and Luiz Antonio Teixeira, "Repensando a história do Instituto Butantan," in *Espaços da ciência no Brasil*, ed. Maria Amélia M. Dantes (Rio de Janeiro: Fundação Oswaldo Cruz, 2001), 159–82. It is also important to highlight the frequent exchanges that took place between Brazilian doctors and their Latin American colleagues. Marta de Almeida, "Das Cordilheiras dos Andes à Isla de Cuba, passando pelo Brasil: Os congressos médicos latino-americanos e brasileiros (1888–1929)" (PhD diss., University of São Paulo, 2003). In 1915 Dr. Arthur Neiva was invited by the Argentine government to organize and head the Zoology and Parasitology Section of the Buenos Aires Bacteriological Institute. Bertucci, *Influenza*, 75.

16. This debate also figures in the chapters of Silveira (6) and Cruz de Souza (7).

17. Ludgero da Cunha Motta, Eduardo Monteiro, Octavio de Carvalho, Caetano Petraglia, Porvença de Gouvea, Campos Seabra, Raul de Sá Pinto et al, "Sessão de 25 de setembro de 1918," *Annaes da Academia Paulista de Medicina* 1 (1919): 34.

18. Ibid., 34–36.

19. Ibid., 34–35.

20. Samuel Bradbury, "An Influenza Epidemic in Soldiers," *American Journal of the Medical* 46 (1918): 737–40; "Influenza and the Diferential Diagnosis of Sandfly

Fever," *Lancet* 195, no. I (1918): 645–46; "The Epidemic of Spanish Influenza," *Science* 48 (1918): 289. Some researchers have defended the hypothesis that the Spanish flu was a new disease. Other hypotheses claim German agents spread the Spanish flu to defeat their enemies or that "atmospheric fluid" modified by the war caused the epidemic. Bertucci, *Influenza*, 316, 370n70.

21. Carlos Seidl, "Conclusões relativas a grippe epidêmica ou influenza ora reinante no Brazil," *Boletim da Academia Nacional de Medicina* 89 (1918): 591–92. For more on individual prophylaxis, see Liane Maria Bertucci-Martins, "'Conselhos ao povo': Educação e higiene contra a influenza de 1918," *Cadernos CEDES* 23, no. 59 (2003): 103–17; María-Isabel Porras-Gallo, "Ateniéndose al consejo de los expertos: Los madrileños frente a la gripe durante las epidemias de 1889–90 y de 1918–19," in *De la responsabilidad individual a la culpabilización de la víctima: El papel del paciente en la prevención de la enfermedad*, ed. Luis Montiel and María-Isabel Porras-Gallo (Madrid: Doce Calles, 1997), 101–10.

22. Carlos Seidl, Garfield de Almeida, Adm. João F. Lopes Rodriguez, Daniel de Almeida, Theophilo Torres, Olympio da Fonseca, Henrique Autran, "Grippe epidêmica," *Boletim da Academia Nacional de Medicina* 89 (1918): 590–93.

23. Ibid., 593–99.

24. At the meeting of the National Congress on September 24, the admiral introduced the theory that the African epidemic was dengue fever, though he did not defend this hypothesis at the academy meeting on October 10. Meyer and Teixeira, *Grippe epidêmica*, 502.

25. According to some news sources, the first cases of Spanish flu in São Paulo were amateur football players from Rio de Janeiro who were visiting the city. The players took ill in São Paulo on October 9 and therefore would have been the carriers of the illness, which, a few days later, spread to other victims at the Hotel D'Oeste, where the team had been staying. But medical and governmental authorities did not confirm this information. Bertucci, *Influenza*, 100.

26. Meyer and Teixeira, *Grippe epidêmica*, 48, 529; Bertucci, *Influenza*, 100; Nara Azevedo de Brito, "La dansarina: A gripe espanhola e o cotidiano da cidade do Rio de Janeiro," *História, Ciências, Saúde: Manguinhos* 4, no. 1 (1997): 11–30, 20.

27. Other examples of social solidarity appeared during the pandemic as well; see chapter 6 by Silveira in this volume.

28. The Red Cross also played an important role during the pandemic in Portugal, other parts of Brazil, and Canada; see the chapters in this volume by Nunes (3), Silveira (6), Cruz de Souza (7), and Fahrni (12).

29. "A Espanhola," *A Gazeta*, October 19, 1918, 1.

30. "Gripe Espanhola," *O Estado de S. Paulo*, October 16 and 17, 1918, 4.

31. Spanish doctors reacted in a similar fashion, as Porras-Gallo shows in chapter 5 of this volume.

32. Aristides Marques da Cunha, Octávio de Magalhães, and Olympio da Fonseca, "Estudos experimentaes sobre a influenza pandêmica," *Memórias do Instituto Oswaldo Cruz* 10, no. 2 (1918): 175.

33. Olympio da Fonseca, "A pandemia de influenza de 1918 e as primeiras demonstrações da filtrabilidade do respectivo vírus," *Brasiliensia Documenta* 6, no. 2 (1973): 38.

34. "A Gripe," *O Estado de S. Paulo* December 2, 1918, 4.

35. "Duas entidades mórbidas,"*A Platéa*, November 5, 1918, 6.

36. Galeno de Revoredo, Rubião Meira, Eduardo Monteiro, Deolindo Galvão, Octavio de Carvalho, Raul de Sá Pinto et al., "Sessão extraordinária de 30 de novembro de 1918," *Annaes da Academia Paulista de Medicina* 1 (1919): 42.

37. Cunha, Magalhães, and Fonseca, "Estudos experimentaes," 174.

38. "Noticias diversas," *O Estado de S. Paulo* November 13, 1918, 7.

39. Oscar Rodrigues Alves, *Relatório do Secretário do Interior, anno 1918* (São Paulo, 1919), 149.

40. Moses, "Bacteriologia da grippe," 683–85. Dr. Carlos de Figueiredo, in Manguinhos, also conducted experiments with Pfeiffer's bacillus.

41. Ibid., 685.

42. Henrique Beaurepaire de Aragão, "A propósito da influenza," *Brazil-Medico* 45 (1918): 346–54.

43. Cunha, Magalhães, and Fonseca, "Estudos experimentaes sobre a influenza pandémica," *Brazil-Medico* 48 (1918): 1–2, The case of Minas Gerais is studied by Silveira in chapter 6.

44. Fonseca, "Pandemia de influenza," 38.

45. Cunha, Magalhães, and Fonseca, "Estudos experimentaes," 174, 189–91. In their report Cunha, Magalhães, and Fonseca also mention Aragãos's research and comment on the work of Keegan, who after a few experiments concluded there was no filterable flu virus (190–91).

46. Cunha, Magalhães, and Fonseca, "Estudos experimentaes," 175. The Noguchi medium is a medium of culture composed of fresh rabbit kidney tissue in sterile ascitic fluid under Petroleum Jelly in narrow tubes.

47. Three separate experiments used blood and mucus *in natura* and crushed and diluted bone marrow from a deceased patient affected by the disease. These experiments were conducted using human and animal serum.

48. Cunha, Magalhães, and Fonseca, "Estudos experimentaes," 178–79.

49. Ibid., 181–82.

50. Ibid., 179, 180–81.

51. Ibid., 185–87, 191.

52. Meyer and Teixeira, *Grippe epidêmica*, 48–49, 58–60, 496–98.

53. According to Johnson and Mueller, the recalculated rate of mortality was 6.8 per 1,000. Niall Johnson and Juergen Mueller, "Updating the Accounts: Global Mortality of the 1918–1920 'Spanish' Influenza Pandemic, *Bulletin of the History of Medicine* 76 (2002): 111.

54. Anny Jackeline Torres Silveira, *A influenza espanhola e a cidade planejada: Belo Horizonte, 1918* (Belo Horizonte: Argvmentvm, 2008), 277.

55. Ward J. MacNeal, "The Influenza Epidemic of 1918 in the American Expeditionary Forces in France and England," *Archives of Internal Medicine* 23 (1919): 687.

56. Serafino Belfanti, "A influenza e suas causas," *Archivos de Biologia* 37 (1919): 639.

57. Motta Rezende, "Considerações acerca da grippe," supplement, *Archivos Brasileiros de Medicina* 9 (1919): 380.

58. Ulysses Paranhos, "A influenza em S. Paulo," *Archivos de Biologia* 59–60 (1921): 933.

59. This situation was common throughout the world, as shown in chapters 4, 5, 6, and 7 of this volume.

60. S. Burt Wolbach and Channing Frothingham, "The Influenza Epidemic at Camp Devens in 1918," *Archives of Internal Medicine* 32 (1923): 600.

61. James McIntosh, "The Incidence of *Bacillus influenzae* (Pfeiffer) in the Present Influenza Epidemic," *Lancet* 195 (1918): 695–98.

62. "The cause of influenza," *British Medical Journal* II (1922): 138.

63. "The influenza pandemic, 1918," *British Medical Journal* I (1923): 560.

64. Miguel Couto, "Sessão de 22 de maio," *Boletim da Academia Nacional de Medicina* 95 (1924): 119.

65. William I. B. Beveridge, *Influenza: The Last Great Plague* (London: Heinemann, 1977), 7–10, 68–79; Michael B. A. Oldstone, *Viruses, Plagues, and History* (Oxford: Oxford University Press, 1998), 179–86. In the early 2000s studies proposed that the Spanish flu was the result of a disproportionate mutation of the flu virus. Mark J. Gibbs, John S. Amstrong, and Adrian J. Gibbs, "Recombination in the Hemagglutinin Gene of the 1918 'Spanish Flu,'" *Science* 293 (2001): 1842–45; Jeffery K. Taubenberger, Ann H. Reid, Raina M. Lourens, Ruixue Wang, Guozhong Jin, Thomas G. Fanning, "Characterization of the 1918 Influenza Virus Polymerase Genes," *Nature* 437 (2005): 889–93.

66. Pierre Lépine, quoted in Fonseca, "Pandemia de influenza," 39: "La grande pandémie de 1918–1919 permet de mettre en évidence dans les produits conta-gieux l'existence d'un virus filtrable (Selter 1918) transmissible au singe [Nicolle et Lebailly] . . . résultats retrouvés independamment à la même époque au Brésil (da Cunha, de Magalhães et da Fonseca)" (The great pandemic of 1918–19 allows us to highlight the existence of a filterable virus (Selter 1918) in contagious matter that is transmissible in monkeys [Nicolle et Lebailly] . . . results that were indepen-dently reproduced during the same period in Brazil (da Cunha, de Magalhães et da Fonseca). Fonseca also states that for years the reason the three Brazilians' experi-ments received such little recognition was that they had not carried out research with the ferret (*Mustella furos*), long considered by many as the appropriate animal for the type of experiments they conducted.

67. Some explanations about the main reasons can be found in the preceding chapter by Esteban Domingo.

Chapter Three

Ricardo Jorge and the Construction of a Medico-Sanitary Public Discourse

Portugal and International Scientific Networks

MARIA DE FÁTIMA NUNES

Despite the impact of the *peste pneumónica*—the Portuguese term for the Spanish flu—on Portuguese society, the memory of the pandemic in Portuguese historiography and in public opinion circles has been sparse, with the exception of family oral history and specific social contexts that have kept the tragedy alive (e.g., the death of the painter Amadeu de Sousa Cardoso or the death of the young Francisco Marto, one of the witnesses of the religious occurrence of 1917 known as the "Fátima miracle").[1] Only recently have scholars begun to offer a more systematic picture of the pandemic experience in Portugal. Paulo Girão and João José Cúcio Frada compare the extension and consequences of the pandemic in the Algarve region (in southern Portugal) and Leiria (in western Portugal), respectively, with the pandemic experience on the international scene.[2] Sobral and colleagues of the Institute of Social Sciences at Lisbon University (ICS) have recently published a collection of interdisciplinary essays on the history of the peste pneumónica that deal with such matters as development, demographic consequences, medical discourses, images, attitudes, and representations of the pandemic event.[3] In adducing a broad sample of primary materials—including national and local newspapers, municipal archives, the medical press, and creative literature—not only does this recent scholarship elucidate our understanding of the Spanish flu in Portugal, but much of it invariably points to the central role of Ricardo Jorge, the country's preeminent public health official at the time in his capacity as *director geral da saúde* (director general of health).[4]

Born in Oporto in 1858, Jorge studied medicine there, ultimately receiving his degree from the Escola Médico Cirúrgica (School of Medicine and Surgery), which, unlike the traditional Medical Faculty of Coimbra, was famous for its modern scientific training.[5] After presenting his graduate dissertation on neurology, Jorge became professor at the Escola Médico Cirúrgica of Oporto in 1880 and went to Strasburg and Paris—where he attended Jean-Martin Charcot's lectures—for further medical training. While abroad, his professional contact with Louis Pasteur proved a turning point in his scientific pursuits. In 1884 he began a lecture series titled Higiene Social Aplicada à Nação Portuguesa (Social Hygiene Applied to the Portuguese Nation), thus launching a professional phase in which his primary focus was hygiene.[6] In 1895 Jorge became professor of Higiene e Medicina Legal (Hygiene and Forensic Medicine) at the Escola Médico Cirúrgica of Oporto. Four years later, in 1899, he played an important role as hygienist during the bubonic plague that frightened the city and the entire Iberian Peninsula.[7]

At the turn of the century, Jorge helped found the Instituto Central de Higiene (Central Institute for Hygiene), a state department inspired by the German models with the aim of promoting the development of hygiene and public health in a scientific way. The institute would later be reorganized after the proclamation of the Portuguese Republic in 1910.[8] Jorge also belonged to Petrus Nonius—a Portuguese group for the history of science affiliated with Archeion, an international network for the history of science.[9] In 1934 he formed part of the organizing committee for the Third International Congress of the History of Science, which took place in the three largest cities of Portugal: Oporto, Coimbra, and Lisbon.[10] His many publications evince a wide-ranging interest in a number of fields, including public hygiene, history of medicine, and literary criticism.[11] Alongside his brilliant career in systematizing public health in Portugal, he maintained a program of intensive scientific activity that won him national and international recognition as an epidemiologist and a hygienist.[12] His national stature is reflected in his position as a member of the Faculty of Medicine at Lisbon University, a post from which he retired in 1929. Jorge also represented the Portuguese public health institutions at foreign missions during later decades of the monarchy (1899–1910), the First Republic (1912–26), and the dictatorship of the New State (Estado Novo) (1926–39).[13]

Before the influenza pandemic struck in 1918, Jorge had already acquired significant epidemiological experience in the 1894 cholera epidemic in Lisbon and the 1899 bubonic plague epidemic in Oporto.[14] In addition, he had edited (in French) a study of the impact of malaria in continental Portugal. By 1918 Jorge occupied the position of director of the Conselho Superior de Higiene (High Council for Hygiene), renamed the Direcção Geral de Saúde Pública (Directorate General of Public Health).

This position made him the foremost representative of the Portuguese state in matters of public health when the pandemic reached the country.[15] Given Jorge's stature, it comes as no surprise that he has been the subject of numerous biographical studies, all of which highlight his contributions to the history of medicine. Nevertheless, his biographers pay little attention to his role during the flu epidemic, a fact that may stem from Jorge's relatively modest contribution to Spanish flu scholarship. He wrote only three texts on the subject, between June 1918 and March 1919.[16] These essays, however, are important sources for understanding Portugal's experience with the Spanish flu pandemic. Moreover, it was his actions during the influenza pandemic that garnered him greater national and international prestige as a hygienist. The present chapter thus seeks to fill this critical void by elucidating the construction of a medicosanitary public discourse around the pandemic in Portugal. In doing so, I pay particular attention to the role Jorge played in establishing scientific connections between Portugal and other countries, especially in his capacity as the nation's representative to the Health Division of the League of Nations.[17]

The Beginning of the 1918–19 Influenza Pandemic and the Memory of Past Plagues

The Spanish flu showed the first signs of having struck the Portuguese population in early June 1918. After the second pandemic wave, between September and November of the same year, Jorge adopted the name of *influenza pneumónica* for the new variety of flu that was seriously affecting the lungs and respiratory tract.[18] Adding to the long list of historical epidemics, the pneumónica resuscitated the myth of the devastating public calamity associated with the plague in both the popular imagination and in scientific and political circles. In June 1918 the Portuguese government communicated to a number of its civil, military, religious, and municipal authorities throughout the country the preventive measures the population should take during the final months of summer and during the upcoming winter season. Jorge, in his position as *director geral da sáude*, stated that this was the moment to "demonstrate the scholarship of the history of medicine, of the history of the plagues and [their] respective impact in Europe—since the final stages of the Middle Ages" and that the outbreak of pandemic influenza, like these earlier plagues "must be faced down."[19] In other words, he encouraged people to bear up bravely against the casualties of the pandemic, adopting the motto of "daily hygiene," an important argument in the context of pandemic influenza. From Jorge's point of view, not only was pulmonary flu valuable for laboratory experiments, but it also provided an ideal opportunity to determine the role the state should play in the twentieth century in regard to legislation and public health institutions in helping the population to "face down" its own plagues.[20]

Furthermore, Portuguese collective memory immediately evoked images of the more recent medical and sanitary conditions of the late nineteenth-century plagues (e.g., the bubonic plague in Porto, 1899), which were viewed as uncontrollable scourges. The temporal proximity of these plagues may explain why the Portuguese called the Spanish flu *peste pneumónica*. These uncontrollable scourges raged over Portugal at a time when Jorge worked for the municipal sanitation department. Adding to the dark mood of the epidemic was the death of bacteriologist Câmara Pestana (1863–98), founder of the Real Instituto Bacteriológico (Royal Bacteriology Institute), following an autopsy carried out on a plague victim. Pestana, Jorge's friend and colleague, was asked to assist with bacteriological tests and the urgent implementation of sanitation measures.[21] His passing was a blow to the scientific cause of public health and undoubtedly had a profound impact on Jorge's professional and public work for the rest of his life.

As noted earlier, Jorge took a keen interest in public understanding of the history of plagues and epidemics. After first learning about the cholera epidemic of 1894 in Oporto (the Lisbon plague) and the bubonic plague of 1899 in the Douro riverside zone of Oporto, he took meticulous notes on the disease as part of a report submitted to the sanitation authorities of the municipality of Oporto. The report provided a new urban and hygienist vision of that part of Oporto, dismissed medieval-style fears, suggested policies for public and urban hygiene, and called for improved standards of living for the population—a basic condition for the prevention of epidemic outbreaks, which always propagate faster in areas of social poverty and hunger.[22] In general, Jorge sought to pinpoint in his medical reports the political, economic, military, and sometimes-ideological circumstances that contributed to the progress of a particular disease. A collection of scientific papers published together with the sanitation authorities shows that hygienists, scientists, and public health professionals all viewed the epidemic as a sobering phenomenon on a global scale.[23]

In addition to the Lisbon plague, it is worth noting Jorge's French-language report on the malaria outbreak of 1906 and his publications on the history of medicine and public health, particularly those in which he praises Francisco Ribeiro Sanches (1699–1703), a doctor from the European Enlightenment period, whose *Tratado da conservação dos povos* (Treaty on the conservation of peoples' health) was published in Paris in 1756.[24] In this treaty Sanches puts forward the new idea that the state should take preventive measures to improve "peoples' health" as a means of defending the well-being of society as a whole and of the states of enlightened philanthropic absolutism.[25] Jorge's ideas on the state's role in the organization and protection of public health reveal Sanches's influence on him and, more precisely, the prevalence of social hygiene at the time of the 1918 influenza pandemic.

Jorge's interventions in the public domain took many forms: official reports submitted to national and international organizations, books, public conferences, participation in medical and public health publications, newspaper articles, and manuscripts on the history of medicine (with particular emphasis on the history of epidemics).[26] Given his remarkable activity in the areas of medical science, culture, and social intervention, as a public health authority it is both natural that he would figure prominently in scholarly inquiry into the 1918–19 flu epidemic in Portugal and striking that more such scholarship has not been done. Any understanding of the system of intervention in citizens' public and private lives with regard to public health and the first attempts at coordinated actions during the epidemic in Portugal must take into consideration the paramount figure of Ricardo Jorge.[27] Indeed, it is within this context that the general framework of the social welfare state begins to take shape, even if health and welfare institutions at the time of the pandemic were still a long ways from providing the universal care that would later characterize the welfare state.[28]

Peste Pneumónica

Given his extensive work on epidemics at the national and international level and his position as *director geral da saúde*, Jorge was the authoritative source for information about the 1918–19 flu epidemic in Portugal.[29] From his perspective, the pneumónica became the test case for implementing sanitation policies and for improving international network strategies among the countries involved in World War I in the international health field, which was not yet established, in his opinion, on an institutional basis, notwithstanding the existence of the Office Internationale de Hygiène Publique in Paris since 1907 and the US-based International Sanitary Bureau since 1902.[30] The two major journalistic sources that communicated Jorge's knowledge about and understanding of the flu to the broader Portuguese society were *Diario de Noticias* and *O Seculo*.[31] On September 25, 1918, *Diário de Noticias* published on its front page an official note on public health written by Jorge: "Epidemic. Pulmonary influenza."[32] Jorge's name on the article gave the disease official weight, linking it to past plagues (e.g., the bubonic plague in Oporto) and more recent fevers (e.g., cholera and malaria) in which Jorge had played an important role in public intervention both through the implementation of legislative health measures and through public lectures, newspaper articles, and medical reviews.[33]

Through his column in *Diário de Notícias*, Jorge publicized the official scientific view of the strange epidemic that *Diário* had been covering since

August 1918. Moreover, he also advocated practical prophylactic measures that citizens should follow individually and collectively on a daily basis to avoid contamination, including refraining from kissing when showing affection! According to Jorge, the idea of impeding the circulation of people and goods was outdated and out of step with the contagious reality of the flu outbreak, though he did recommend isolating infected flu patients.[34] The news—subject to the rules of the Conselho de Saúde Pública (Department of Public Health)—pursued a two-fold objective: provide information on pneumónica occurrences in the country and, above all, avoid public panic.[35] The epidemic was a relatively silent affair compared to the commotion created by the high-impact news arriving from the frontlines of World War I and the plight of the Corpo Expedicionário Português (Portuguese Expeditionary Force) in the summer of 1918 in France and Belgium.

In June 1918 Jorge presented a report to the Conselho de Saúde Pública on the aspects of disease prevention and prophylactic measures to be put forward by the Portuguese state, the entity responsible for the scientific evaluation of all measures to be implemented.[36] In his report he avoided using language that, in discussing charitable, philanthropic, and humanitarian assistance, would have been seen as incompatible with the separation between church and state, one of the important objectives of the movement that led to the proclamation of the Portuguese Republic in 1910.[37] Instead, Jorge sought primarily to draw attention to the role the state should play in times of epidemic threats by strengthening the incipient public health structures still under development during President Sidónio Pais's military republic (1917–18).

In June 1918 Jorge, on behalf of the Conselho Superior de Higiene, released a note stating that, according to news coming from London, the fever had spread to the battlefields and that a ship that had docked in Lisbon on July 5 was carrying the flu.[38] The note offered some concise advice and practical rules to be followed as the end of summer approached, including avoiding visiting those sick with the flu; abolishing the traditional forms of greetings (i.e., hugs and kisses), which were considered repugnant actions from a hygienic point of view; and, in cities, maintaining good and salubrious habits.

As a general rule, the framework of control and prevention shaped the news information published in *Diário de Notícias* and *O Século*. *Diário de Notícias* portrayed the geographic spread of the disease by providing a variety of information at the regional level, giving information on the number of patients in the various districts of the country. In June *Diário* sought to relieve psychological tension by publishing interviews with doctors, who gave the impression that the epidemic was under control. The availability of a special unit in Lisbon's Hospital do Rego for those infected with the flu was announced. During the months of June and July, *Diário de Notícias*

continued to reflect the impact and the application of the measures, recommendations, and official positions issued by the Conselho Superior de
Higiene, which were recorded in Jorge's text of June 18, 1918. (As prophylactic measures, Jorge had recommended prohibiting fairs and processions and reducing attendance to mass and liturgy events.) It was not until
September that news of the first victims of the peste pneumónica began to
appear, as mentioned previously. With autumn temperatures dropping, the
newspaper reported the spread of the epidemic from south to north and
from Spain to the Atlantic coast, seeing as these were the two main entry
points of the epidemic into Portugal.[39]

The measures put forward by Jorge in his official note of September
25, 1918, were published repeatedly during the months of October and
November in official statements and informative articles. The goal was
to contain public opinion in order to avoid generalized social panic and
to educate the population—collectively and individually—in certain sanitary habits and routines, including isolating oneself and avoiding social
contact or public gatherings.[40] Although these measures were justifi-
able for medical and sanitary reasons, they also proved useful as tools
for political power. As noted in the introduction to this volume and in
chapter 4, the context of 1918 Portugal was one of great political, social,
and economic agitation, as witnessed not only by the presidential dictatorship of Sidónio Pais but also by Portugal's participation in World
War I, notably with the defeat in April 1918 of the Corpo Expedicionário
Português in the fields of La Lys. Portuguese authorities thus had little
interest in provoking popular unrest in these circumstances, and the
public health measures they advocated served these ends. Jorge's reputation as a man of science with the knowledge and tools to help authorities
in this regard may explain why he was able to survive under such different political regimes. But despite official efforts to calm the general
population, the distribution of ration coupons as well as the rise in the
price of food was followed by various cases of social unrest in Aveiro,
Coimbra, Évora, and Lisbon. The general sentiment was that Sidonismo,
the military phase of the First Republic, had run its course and it was
time for political change.[41]

As in other areas of the world, the month of October saw the most amount
of news coverage of the peste pneumónica. O Século, for example, published
numerous front-page stories, official statements by the Direcção Geral de
Saúde Pública (Directorate General of Public Health), and information
about prophylactic measures.[42] Certain businesses such as the Perfumaria
da Moda (a perfumery) and the Farmácia Estácio (a pharmacy) saw the flu
as a means to advertise their cosmetic and pharmaceutical products. In general, newspapers sought to avoid panic, reassuring their readers with phrases
such as "the epidemic is dying down" and "authorities are successfully

combating the epidemic and providing assistance to those affected by it"
and with news titles such as "Combating the Epidemic: Providing Assistance
to Those Affected by the Epidemic" or "Sanitary Measures Have Proven
Successful."[43] Similarly, some reports linked the official control of the situation to naming the flu *pneumónica* influenza.[44] A number of different stories about the geographic spread of the disease provide an update of the
situation in the various locations hit by the epidemic. On November 6 the
front page of *O Século* reads, "the aftermath; the epidemics; numbers keep
going down; assisting those affected by the epidemic; assistance and necessary actions; measures taken."[45]

By mid-November increased news coverage of the end of World War I and
the arrival of the Portuguese Expeditionary Corps at the Cais das Colunas in
Lisbon signaled a shift in public attention away from the epidemic. Although
newspapers continued to report on topics such as the assistance provided to
flu victims by the Red Cross, the White Cross, and the Portuguese State, the
epidemic had faded from the front page.[46] The attempted assassination of
the president of the republic, Sidónio Pais, on December 5, 1918, and his
death ten days later, marked the symbolic end of news coverage of the epidemic. Nevertheless, in the aftermath of the flu epidemic and World War I,
Jorge would continue to play an important role in Portuguese public health
affairs, representing the country's public health institutions at many international institutions as a spokesperson on matters concerning theoretical and
practical know-how on epidemics and plagues.[47] Despite the political import
of his work, especially given the positions he held, his status as *primarily* a scientist may have insulated him from the intense criticism faced by the political regimes under which he served.

Ricardo Jorge's Alter Ego

Under the pseudonym of Dr. Mirandela, Jorge published a series of articles
that addressed certain measures taken by Spain in response to the epidemic, including the closing of its border with Portugal.[48] These articles
provide important insights into his thinking on public health at the time
of the epidemic. Essentially, Jorge criticized Spain's public health policy for
its ignorance of "proper scientific sanitary prophylactic measures towards
the epidemic."[49] According to Dr. Mirandela, this constituted evidence that
Spain was considerably outdated in what regarded the international norms
in public health.[50] These were acute criticisms covering both public health
issues as well as the political context of the Iberian Peninsula, especially in
light of the war; issues Jorge would later make reference to in an international forum as part of the Sanitary Committee of the League of Nations
(Commission Sanitaire des Pays Alliés) in 1919.[51]

In an article titled "Diplomatic Problems: Spain Has Closed Its Borders after Creating the 'Sanitary Passport,'" Dr. Mirandela criticized "Spain's Wall of China," in other words, the establishment of a *cordon sanitaire* along the Spanish-Portuguese border to impede the circulation of people between the neighboring states. His rhetoric is sharp and blunt:

> The wall that Spain built around Portugal, thus imposing a sanitary blockade, not only prevents the Portuguese from crossing the immediate border into Spain but also from getting to the Pyrenees. . . . These are ridiculous and vexatious sanitation policies that treat the Portuguese like infected and leprous animals. . . . Even if we concede that our neighbors are entitled to defend themselves from us on a controversial whim, will their defense mean complete isolation, without a door or an escape hatch? Where has one seen such actions since the Middle Ages? What times are these in which we live? In 1844 when Portugal sought to protect itself from the eradication of cholera from Spain, it resorted to the system of the *cordon sanitaire*, anachronistic even then. . . . It seems Spain's only goal is to cut us off from France, where cholera is allegedly spreading. Who knows what concerns—other than those related to public health—are involved in this sanitary comedy, where hygiene is but a mask with holes and a game of dominos.[52]

By preventing the Portuguese from getting to the Pyrenees, Spain effectively and symbolically cut its neighbors off from the border to a cultivated, civilized Europe, mentor for the ideal of progress in public health institutions in general. One consequence of Spain's efforts was that it negatively impacted Portugal's participation in Spain's first National Medical Conference, making it difficult for Portuguese scientists and public health experts to attend and engage their counterparts in scientific dialogue.

Given that border closings were "ridiculous and vexatious health practices" from a scientific and epidemiological perspective, Jorge concluded that Spain's actions were motivated more by political and ideological reasons than by a concern for prophylaxis. In 1917 the First Constitutional Republic of Portugal was interrupted by the military dictatorship of Sidónio Pais (1872–1918), an avid Germanophile. His political leanings complicated the state of Portuguese international relations, since the country had begun World War I on the side of the Allies. Spain, perhaps in an effort to maintain its precarious neutrality during the war, and fearing a sort of political contagion from Portugal, opted to close its border with its neighbor. After the war Jorge was selected to represent Portugal on the Sanitary Committee of the League of Nations. It was in this capacity that in March 1919 he accused German scientists and hygienists of encouraging Spain to adopt its isolationist policy vis-à-vis Portugal and thereby using the peste pneumónica as a political weapon at the end of the war: "Exploiting the panic of the flu, the pro-Germanic Spanish press successfully took the most pompous measures against those arriving from Allied countries, this, of course, by doing violence to the opinions and advice of Spanish hygienists and, despite their [the hygienists'] protests, rendering them justice. One has reached the extreme point of maintaining the Portuguese border closed and of prohibiting all transit by way of a *cordon sanitaire*, which thus isolates us from overland contact with Europe."[53]

Ricardo Jorge and the Aftermath of the Peste Pneumónica

After the outbreak of the peste pneumónica, Jorge's diplomatic service at the League of Nations as a representative of the Portuguese state enhanced his professional and scientific career.[54] In this capacity, and at the request of the Allied Council, he prepared a report, *La Grippe*, for the council's international convention. In addition to reviewing information about past flu and other epidemics, the brief thirty-five-page report presented a new idea: "a specific vaccine is the only prophylactic hope to prevent a contagion of this type."[55] In this, Jorge was in agreement with his counterparts elsewhere, such as Manuel Martín Salazar, Spain's director general of health at the time.[56]

After World War I and the influenza pandemic, Western states began to invest more heavily in the domains of health and public hygiene, adopting measures to stimulate social well-being, which was increasingly considered the most effective measure against epidemics. Although Jorge's epidemiological experience began as early as the Oporto outbreak of plague, it was the peste pneumónica that gave him greater international visibility as well as a specific forum for expressing his views on matters of public health: the Division of Health of the League of Nations. After the New State period of 1926, Jorge worked to legitimate the new political power and promote the idea of security in national and international public circles. Moreover, his publications and articles, written over the decades of the twenties and thirties, right up to the moment of his passing away (July 29, 1939), together with the extremely rich documentation that can be found at the Espólio da Biblioteca Nacional de Portugal (Ricardo Jorge Archive, Archives of Portuguese Culture, National Library of Portugal), evidence the scope of both his geographic travels through Europe, the United States, and Latin America and, by extension, his professional stature.[57] Through his professional labors, he consistently connected Portuguese public health to the broader network of health and public hygiene as it was then developing in the West.

As the vast bibliography written about him attests, Ricardo Jorge led a life filled with public and scientific activities until the day he died. Although his biographers have largely overlooked his involvement in the peste pneumónica, the epidemic provided him with an opportunity not only to engage in scientific observation and experimentation but also to consider the role the state should play in the twentieth century in terms of legislation and public health institutions, an idea that was dominant at the time in Europe. The epidemic experience was also crucial to his growing international prestige as a hygienist. In addition to authoring a report on the epidemic to the Commission Sanitaire des Pays Alliés in March 1919, he also accepted a position in the Health Division of the League of Nations.[58] Although he lived through three radically different political regimes—the monarchy, the First Republic and the New State—he never ceased working to establish an international network of contacts.

Indeed, as a scientific authority who also occupied positions of political authority, Ricardo Jorge became a key figure in mediating between cutting-edge science and the political efforts to apply that science to the improvement of Portuguese society. In many ways he stands at a historical threshold. Prior to the epidemic, health care was hardly an integrated, statewide program (see chapter 9). In such a setting, individuals such as Louis Pasteur, Robert Koch, and, at least in Portugal, Ricardo Jorge, loomed large on the social landscape as somewhat heroic figures. Paul de Kruif immortalized the heroic persona of some of them in his international bestseller, *Microbe Hunters*, published only a few years after the influenza pandemic. After the pandemic, however, it was national and international institutions as much as individual scientists that would grow in prominence; for if the Spanish flu pandemic had revealed anything, it was the inadequacies of public health systems throughout the world. What the case of Ricardo Jorge allows us to see is the crucial role those towering figures of science—and the scientific networks they established—played in the slow but steady transition to what we call today the modern welfare state.

Notes

1. On the thirteenth day of the month for six consecutive months beginning in May 1917, the Virgin Mary allegedly appeared to Francisco Marto; his sister, Jacinta Marto; and their cousin, Lúcia dos Santos, in Fátima, Portugal. The apparitions garnered notoriety because of certain prophetic and eschatological elements, including intimations of a coming world war. More details on the "Fátima miracle" can be found in chapter 4 of this volume.

2. Paulo Girão, *A pneumónica no Algarve* (Lisbon: Caleidoscópio, 2003); João José Cúcio Frada, *A gripe pneumónica em Portugal continental 1918: Estudo socioeconómico e epidemiológico com particular análise do concelho de Leiria* (Lisbon: Sete Caminhos, 2005).

3. José Manuel Sobral, Maria Luísa Lima, Paula Castro, and Paulo Silveira e Sousa, *A Epidemia esquecida olhares comparados sobre a pneumónica 1918–1919* (Lisbon: ICS, 2009). Chapter 4 of this volume also expands our knowledge of the epidemic experience in Portugal.

4. In the absence of a health minister, the director general of health was the maximum authority on all public health matters. The situation was the same in Portugal's Iberian neighbor, Spain.

5. After the proclamation of the republic in 1910 it was renamed Faculdade de Medicina da Universidade de Lisboa (Faculty of Medicine of the University of Lisbon).

6. Augusto Silva Travassos, "A higiene, um grande epidemiologista: Ricardo Jorge," *Jornal da Sociedade das Ciências Médicas* 111, no. 4 (1947); Fernando da Silva Correia, *A vida, a obra, o estilo, as lições e o prestígio de Ricardo Jorge* (Lisbon: Instituto Superior de Higiene Dr. Ricardo Jorge, 1960), 3, 189.

7. In Spain the bubonic plague epidemic stimulated the creation of the Instituto de Sueroterapia, Vacunación y Bacteriología de Alfonso XIII, later renamed Instituto Nacional de Higiene (National Institute of Hygiene) that same year. María-Isabel Porras-Gallo, "Antecedentes y creación del Instituto de Sueroterapia, Vacunación y Bacteriología de Alfonso XIII," *Dynamis* 18 (1998): 81–105.

8. Sobral, Lima, Castro, and Sousa, *Epidemia esquecida olhares*, 70.

9. Augusto Fitas, Marcial Rodrigues, and Maria de Fátima Nunes, *Filosofia e história da ciência em Portugal no século XX* (Lisbon: Casal de Cambra, Caleidoscópio, 2008).

10. Ricardo Jorge, "La médicine et les médecins dans l'expansion mondial des portugais," in *Conférence faite le 2 octobre 1934 à l'Université de Coimbra, III Congrès International d'Histoire des Sciences* (Lisbon: Tipografia Seara Nova, 1935), 1–15.

11. Some of Jorge's literary articles deal with the work of Camilo Castelo Branco (1825–90), his close friend and the most famous literary writer of Romanticism in Portugal.

12. José Manuel Sobral, Maria Luísa Lima, Paula Castro and Paulo Silveira e Sousa, *Epidemia esquecida olhares*, 70.

13. On the chronology of Jorge's scientific endeavors in both national and international contexts, see Correia, *Vida*, 13–16. For more details, see chapter 4 of this volume.

14. Ricardo Jorge, *A peste bubónica no Porto, 1899: Seu descobrimento, primeiros trabalhos pelo medico municipal R. J.* (Porto: Repartição de Saúde e Hygiene da Câmara do Porto, 1899); F. Jorge Alves, "Ricardo Jorge e a saúde pública em Portugal: Um apóstolo sanitário," *Arquivos de Medicina* 22, no. 2–3 (2008): 85–90.

15. Correia, *Vida*.

16. Ricardo Jorge, *A influenza e a febre dos papatazes: Julho e Agosto de 1918* (Lisbon: Imprensa Nacional, 1918); Jorge, *A influenza, nova incursão peninsular: Relatório apresentado ao Conselho Superior de Higiene na sessão de 18 de Junho de 1918* (Lisbon: Imprensa Nacional, 1918); Jorge, *La grippe, préliminaire présenté à la Commission Sanitaire des Pays Alliés dans la session de Mars 1919* (Lisbon: Imprimerie Nationale, 1919).

17. An interesting book on this topic is Iris Borowy, *Coming to Terms with World Health: The League of Nations Organization, 1921–1946* (Frankfurt: Lang, 2009).

18. Jorge, *Grippe;* Frada, *Gripe pneumónica.* Jorge's initial characterization of the disease first appeared in a French-language publication in Lisbon: "Deux vagues épidémiques d'influenza ont passé sur le Portugal. La première s'est fait sentir des premiers jours de juin à la mi-juillet 1918. . . . Elle a été baptisée en raison de sa provenance immédiate, du nom de grippe espagnole. La seconde a sévi de la mi-août à la fin de novembre; épidémie secondaire, estivalo-automnale, de transmission plus lente,

hautement maligne et mortelle . . . elle a été nommée influenza pneumonique" (Two vague epidemics have entered Portugal. The effects of the first were felt from early June to mid-July. . . . This one has been dubbed the Spanish flu because of its immediate provenance. The second has raged from mid-August to the end of November; [this] second summer-autumnal epidemic, which spreads more slowly and is highly malignant and fatal, has been named pneumonic influenza.) Jorge, *Grippe*, 7.

19. Jorge, *Influenza, nova incursão peninsular*, 8.

20. Manuel Martín Salazar, director general of health in Spain at that time, shared Jorge's point of view. María-Isabel Porras-Gallo, "Una ciudad en crisis: La epidemia de gripe de 1918–19 en Madrid" (PhD diss., Faculty of Medicine, Complutense University of Madrid, 1994), 373–94. More details on Manuel Martín Salazar and on Spain's situation figures in chapters 5 and 9 of this volume.

21. Ricardo Jorge, *Saneamento do Porto relatorio apresentado à Comissão Municipal de Saneamento* (Porto: Tipographia de António José da Silva Teixeira, 1888); Jorge, *A epidemia de Lisboa de 1894: Impressões d'uma missão sanitária* (Porto: Typographia Occidental, 1895); Jorge, *Peste bubónica no Porto*; Jorge, *Demographia e hygiene na cidade do Porto*, vol. 1, *Clima, população, mortalidade, illustrado com quadros estatísticos, tabellares e graphicos, referentes ao Porto, Lisboa e Reino, e confrontos internacionais* (Porto: Repartição de Saúde e Hygiene da Câmara do Porto / Annuario do Serviço Municipal de Saúde e Hygiene da Cidade do Porto, 1899).

22. Alves, "Ricardo Jorge"; Ricardo Jorge, *Origens e desenvolvimento da população do Porto: Notas históricas e estatísticas* (Porto: Typographia Occidental, 1897); Jorge, *Peste bubónica no Porto*; Jorge, *Demographia e hygiene*; Jorge, *Sanidade em campanha conferências proferidas no acampamento de Tancos e na Faculdade de Medicina de Lisboa, Julho e Agosto de 1916* (Lisbon, 1917).

23. Jorge, *Saneamento do Porto*; Jorge, *Epidemia de Lisboa*; Jorge, *Peste bubónica no Porto*; Jorge, *Demographia e hygiene*.

24. Antonio Nunes Ribeiro Sanches, *Tratado da Conservação da Saude dos povos, com hum appendix: Considerações sobre os terremotos com a noticia dos mais consideraveis, de que fas menção a Historia, e dos ultimos que se sentiram na Europa desde o 1 de Novembro 1755* (Paris: [No/Ed], 1756). Jorge published numerous studies in French: *Le typhus exanthématique à Porto 1917–1919: Communication faite au Comité International d'Hygiène d'Octobre 1919* (Lisbonne: Imprimerie Nationale, 1920); Jorge, *Mission médica de la Société des Nations: Caderno dactilografado*, 1922, file 38, box 24, E-18 Legacy, Ricardo Jorge Archive, Archives of Portuguese Culture, National Library of Portugal, Lisbon; Jorge, *Les pestilences et la Convention Sanitaire Internationale* (Lisbonne: Institut Central d'Hygiène, 1926); Jorge, *Les anciennes épidémies de peste en Europe, comparées aux épidémies modernes Instituto Central de Higiene* (Lisbon: Imprensa Nacional, 1932); Jorge, "Médicine et les Médecins"; Jorge, *La peste africaine: Rapport présenté au Comité Permanant de l'Office International d'Hygiène Publique* (Paris: Office International d'Hygiène Publique, 1935); Jorge, *Summa epidemiologica de la peste épidémies anciennes et modernes* (Paris: Office International d'Hygiène Publique [Extraite du Bulletin Mensuel de l'Office International d'Hygiène Publique], 1935); Jorge, "Les 'Rodentia' domestiques et sauvages dans l'Evolution séculaire et mondiale de la Peste," *Extrait des Comptes Rendus du XII congrès International de Zoologie: Lisbonne 1935* (Lisbon: Tipografia Casa Portuguesa, 1937); Jorge, "Fièvre jaune," *Arquivos do Instituto de Higiene Ricardo Jorge* (Lisbon, 1938).

25. Sanches, quoted in Luís de Pina, *Ricardo Jorge e Ribeiro Sanches: Dois homens duas épocas* (Lisbon: Médica, 1941).

26. For reports submitted to organizations, see Jorge, *Typhus exanthématique*; Jorge, *Mission médica*; Jorge, *Pestilences*; Jorge, *Peste africaine*; Jorge, "Fièvre jaune." An example of his public conferences is Jorge, *Sanidade em campanha*. For his works on the history of medicine, see Jorge, *Anciennes épidémies*; Jorge, "Médicine et les médecins"; Jorge, *Summa epidemiologica*; and Jorge, "Rodentia."

27. Jorge was particularly active in international scientific meetings and in the actions of the Hygiene Institute in Lisbon, founded by him in 1899, which is now called the Ricardo Jorge National Institute of Health. Eduardo Coelho, *O Prof. Ricardo Jorge: Breve ensaio crítico seguido da resenha bibliográfica da sua obra* (Paris: Livrarias Aillaud e Bertrand, 1929); Travassos, "Higiene."

28. George Rosen, *Uma história da Saúde Pública*, 2nd ed. (São Paulo: Hucitec, 2006).

29. Chapter 4 of this volume deals extensively with the Portuguese's experience of the Spanish influenza.

30. Jorge, *Grippe*. The Versailles Peace Treaty of 1919 gave Allied countries the opportunity to begin organizing hygiene councils to have a common institutional basis to deal with epidemics, and Jorge was the Portuguese member of this committee.

31. Historians have widely used these periodical sources in their academic work, as they are valuable sources for issues related to the history of epidemics and their strategic role in the implementation of political concepts on public health. *Diario de Noticias* was founded in 1864 in Lisbon as a private enterprise based on the model of European professional newspapers. Many Portuguese intellectuals and scientific personalities regularly contributed to its pages. In Portugal it was the first newspaper to use news from agencies such as Havas and Reuters. *O Século*, founded in 1880 in Lisbon, presented itself as an alternative to the *Diario de Noticias*. The director had close ties to Masonic circles, and the newspaper followed the republican ideology linked to the Portuguese scientific circles.

32. As noted, Jorge uses the name "Pneumonica influenza" in the 1919 report.

33. Jorge, *Peste bubónica no Porto*; Jorge, *Demographia e hygiene*; Jorge, *La Malarie en Portugal: Premiers résulats d'une enquete* (Lisbonne: Imprimerie "Casa Portugueza," 1906).

34. Jorge, *Influenza, nova incursão peninsular*.

35. Newspapers regularly published official notes from departments such as Public Health. It was through this type of notes that newspapers communicated changes in the evolution of the epidemic. Authorities from many different countries expressed similar concerns about public panic. For example, see chapters 6 and 10 of this volume.

36. More details on the role of state are in chapters 4 and 9 of this volume.

37. In place of terms such as "charity assistance" and "philanthropic and humanitarian assistance," Jorge limited himself to hygienist and medical expressions. Thus he stated that people should have "fresh air, good hygiene, strict disinfection, [and] immunization practices." He also suggested that visiting flu patients "was not a good idea" and that "to avoid taking too many drugs is good for the flu patients and their budgets." Jorge, *Influenza, nova incursão peninsular*. See also Maria Fernanda Rollo

and Fernando Rosas, eds., *História da Primeira República Portuguesa* (Lisbon: Tinta-da-china, 2009). For the role of other paragovernmental health organizations in Spain during the 1918 flu epidemic, see chapter 8 of this volume.

38. Jorge, *Influenza, nova incursão peninsular.* The ship, named the *Demerara*, was linked to the introduction of the pandemic in Brazil, as noted in chapters 2, 6, and 7 of this volume.

39. Girão, *Pneumónica no Algarve*; Frada, *Gripe pneumónica.*

40. On the effect of social panic in Brazil and Argentina, see chapters 6 and 10, respectively.

41. Rollo and Rosas, *Primeira República Portuguesa*; Armando Malheiro da Silva, *Sidónio e Sidonismo*, 2 vols. (Coimbra: Imprensa da Universidade, 2006); Tom Gallagher, *A Twentieth-Century Interpretation of Portugal* (Manchester: Manchester University Press, 1983).

42. The Direcção Geral de Saúde Pública (Directorate General of Public Health), of which Jorge was a member, presided over public health in Portugal and was closely linked to the Conselho Superior de Higiene (High Council for Hygiene).

43. "In Lisbon," *O Século*, October 13, 1918; "Combating the Epidemic: Providing Assistance to Those Affected by the Epidemic" and "Sanitary Measures Have Proven Successful," both in *O Século*, October 20, 1918.

44. "Public Health. The Flu," *O Século*, October 28, 1918. Concerning the important relationship between naming and controlling a disease, see Charles E. Rosenberg, *Explaining Epidemics and Other Studies in the History of Medicine* (Cambridge: Cambridge University Press, 1992), 258–318.

45. "The aftermath," *O Século*, November 6, 1918.

46. The Red Cross also played a key role during the pandemic in Brazil and Canada, as noted in chapters 2, 7, and 12 of this volume.

47. Jorge, *Grippe*; Jorge, *Typhus exanthématique*; Jorge, *Mission médica*; Jorge, *Pestilences*; Jorge, *Peste africaine*; Jorge, "Fièvre jaune."

48. For Spain's perspective on closing the border, see Ryan A. Davis, *The 1918 Spanish Flu: Narrative and Cultural Identity in Spain* (New York: Palgrave MacMillan, 2013).

49. Signed by Dr. Mirandela, three of these articles are collected in file 1, box 5, E-18 Legacy, Ricardo Jorge Archive, Archives of Portuguese Culture, National Library of Portugal, Lisbon. The titles of the articles are "Isolated by Spain: I (The Current Epidemic)," October 19, 1918; "Isolated by Spain: II," October 21, 1918; and "Epidemic War in Spain," October 25, 1918.

50. As noted in the introduction to this volume and in chapters 5, 9, and 11, Jorge's claims of Spanish backwardness were not unfounded, though other countries also evinced similar backwardness in matters of science. For the case of Portugal, see Sobral, Lima, and Silveira e Sousa, chap. 4, in this volume.

51. Jorge, *Grippe.*

52. Dr. Mirandela [Ricardo Jorge], "Diplomatic Problems: Spain Has Closed Its Borders after Creating the 'Sanitary Passport,'" *Diário Notícias*, October 21, 1918, 1–2, file 1, box 5, E-18 Legacy, Ricardo Jorge Archive, Archives of Portuguese Culture, National Library of Portugal, Lisbon.

53. Jorge, *Grippe*, 33. The original in French reads, "Exploitant la panique de la grippe, la presse pro-germanique espagnole réussit à faire prendre les mesures les

plus pompeuses contre les provenances des Pays alliés, cela, bien entendu, en fai-sant violence à l'opinion et aux conseils des hygiénistes d'Espagne, et malgré leurs protestations, rendons-leur justice. On en est arrivé à cette extrémité de maintenir les frontières portugaises fermées et d'interdire tout transit par un cordon sanitaire, nous isolant ainsi de l'Europe para la voie de terre."

54. Jorge, *Grippe*; Jorge, *Pestilences*.

55. Jorge, *Grippe*, 35.

56. See María-Isabel Porras-Gallo, "Sueros y vacunas en la lucha contra la pan-demia de gripe de 1918–1919 en España," *Asclepio* 60, no. 2 (2008): 261–88; and chapter 5 of this volume.

57. For the Espólio sources, see E-18 Legacy, Ricardo Jorge Archive, Archives of Portuguese Culture, National Library of Portugal, Lisbon; Correia, *Vida*; Travassos, "Higiene"; Coelho, *Prof. Ricardo Jorge*.

58. Jorge, *Grippe*.

Part Two

Social Responses

Human and Institutional Actors

Chapter Four

And to Make Things Worse, the Flu

The Spanish Influenza in a Revolutionary Portugal

José Manuel Sobral, Maria Luísa Lima,
and Paulo Silveira e Sousa

In the first decades of the twentieth century, although Portuguese society was undergoing a transformation process marked by a growing population, industrialization, and urban development, the country remained predominantly rural. At the start of the decade in which the epidemic outbreak known internationally as the Spanish influenza occurred, nearly 80 percent of the population was tied to agriculture, the vast majority being small agricultural landowners and poor rural workers.[1] In 1920, the census year closest to the pandemic, Portugal's population was 6,032,991; of this number, only 676,107 lived in the country's largest cities of Lisbon and Porto, while 4,929,365 lived in the so-called rural zones, which included smaller cities.[2]

To reconstruct the context in which the epidemic occurred, we must include a number of facts involving the economic and social structure of Portugal, together with its political, ideological, and health and welfare domains. The establishment of a republican regime in 1910 through a revolution had alienated a segment of the population sympathetic to the monarchy. Moreover, the radical separation achieved between the church and state, following the model of the Third French Republic, was an affront to the Catholic Church.[3] In fact, the new regime directly offended the church by attempting to impose an official lay culture of positivist inspiration by separating it from the state, by depriving the church of means and influence, by making spiritual and religious group activities subject to strict control, and by expropriating its property. Meanwhile, the republican regime, which had been fully embraced by the predominantly urban workforce, often reacted ruthlessly against social movements involving strikes. This intensified discontent with the republic's most influential parties, particularly the most important, the Democratic Party. Portugal's involvement in World War I on the side of the Allies—in which this party played a key supporting role—further divided the Portuguese, who had not faced a mass military mobilization in nearly a century. Among various social groups, particularly the monarchists, sympathy for the cause of the empires against which Portugal fought was notorious.

As noted in the introduction to this volume, the wartime circumstances also aggravated situations of hunger, food shortages, and the cost of living, with mounting social and political conflicts, including assaults on warehouses and establishments for essential needs in May 1917. The military coup of December 5, 1917, led by the conservative republican army officer Sidónio Pais, marked the initial attempt at a regime change, though it was cut short by Pais's assassination the following year. The coup temporarily halted the supremacy of the Democratic Party, which had promoted involvement in the war. In its place, an increasingly authoritarian presidential regime was installed, supported by conservative republicans, Catholics, the aristocracy, the upper bourgeoisie, and by wealthy factions of the urban and rural middle classes and agricultural landowners. The formation of this coalition was facilitated by the messianic expectations surrounding Pais's authoritarian approach, which he and his followers cultivated. It was only after some years of conflict that this regime reestablished ties with the Catholic Church.[4]

In terms of public health, Ricardo Jorge, the *director geral de saúde* (director general of health), was nominated the *comissário geral do governo* (state commissioner general) to lead the fight against the pandemic.[5] In a report about it he described how the flu had arrived at a time of widespread shortages in food, medicine, transportation, and doctors.[6] In fact, Portugal's collection of health and welfare institutions at the start of the twentieth century still fell far short of the universal care that would later come to characterize the modern social and health services of the welfare state.[7] Following the more global progress of the state apparatus since the second half of the nineteenth century, state-run services began to supplement former assistance networks traditionally based on religious establishments with specialized civil hospitals, vagrant and infant assistance, and the first health-control networks.[8]

At another level, since the end of the nineteenth century, efforts were pursued to professionalize health services with the creation of nursing and medical schools. In 1920 there were 2,580 active doctors throughout the country, or one doctor per 2,338 residents. There were also 1,577 pharmacies, or one pharmacy per 3,825 residents. But these averages are deceiving, since doctors and pharmacies were concentrated in cities, mainly the largest ones.[9] In rural areas, shortcomings were severe. In 2,848 provincial parishes, comprising a population of 2,613,332 people, there existed no medical assistance or pharmacies.[10]

In the decade of the flu outbreak, and specifically with the impact of bacteriological discoveries, there was a sound awareness in Portugal (as elsewhere in the world) of the importance of basic hygienic, health, and preventive measures to avoid the emergence and propagation of epidemics.[11] But the implementation of concrete measures would, for the time being, be highly limited. Little progress had been made in terms of infrastructure— the construction of water and wastewater distribution equipment, improved living conditions, urban sanitation or new prevention and monitoring services—and what progress was made was limited to Lisbon, Porto, and a handful of district capitals. The situation was no better in the area of public health and preventive medicine. The public dissemination of principles involving personal hygiene, or the organization of medical and nursing services into accessible, coordinated networks with early diagnosis and treatment capabilities, were realities confined to the dialogues of doctors and some civil servants. In this scenario, diseases such as malaria, typhoid fever, typhus fever, anthrax, smallpox, tuberculosis, and diphtheria were common. The flu epidemic of 1918–19 occurred in a context of multiple, recurring epidemics. Some twenty years later—an important indicator in comparative terms—Portugal still had the highest mortality rates in Europe due to smallpox, diphtheria, and typhus fever.[12]

The flu pandemic, or simply *pneumónica* (the most common name of the Spanish influenza in Portugal), thus occurred in this challenging socioeconomic and political context. In this chapter we present an overview of the way this pandemic was experienced in Portugal, focusing particularly on the response of state agencies and civil organizations and on the role of the Catholic Church and Christian beliefs. We also comment on the politicization of the pandemic, which occurred at a time of acute political conflict.

The Flu Outbreak of 1918–19

The characteristics and time frame of the Spanish flu in Portugal were similar to those seen on a worldwide scale, including the progression of the epidemic in three successive waves.[13] The first wave penetrated Portugal at the end of May with agricultural workers returning from Spain, where it had already been confirmed.[14] The contagion likely originated from hubs in Badajoz and Olivenza, with the first cases diagnosed in Vila Viçosa (in the southeastern region of Alentejo, close to the Spanish border). From there, it spread to other settlements in the region and to the rest of the country.[15] It peaked at the end of June 1918, affecting the cities of Lisbon and Porto, and then suddenly declined. Although short-lived and relatively benign, the first wave still resulted in an overall increase in urban mortality. The second wave began to appear in the zone of Porto (Gaia) in northern Portugal in

August and immediately progressed to the northwest and along both sides of the Douro River valley up to the Spanish border, with other hubs in the center of the country. The coast, center, and south remained unaffected in mid-September, although it reached the Algarve, the country's southern-most province, in early October. This outbreak had a much greater impact on the population, with a higher mortality rate and greater virulence than any other major epidemic previously experienced.[16] A third wave occurred in April and May 1919, though without the particularly lethal effects of the prior wave.[17]

Five population flows—which are key factors in propagating the epidemic on a worldwide scale—have been identified as the cause of contagion among the various regions of the country: military migration, tied to the deployment of troops in a country at war; agricultural migration, due to the large-scale relocation of workers for the grape harvest in the Douro valley and southern Portugal in September; popular migration, tied to fairs and pilgrimages that peak in July, August, and September; spa and beach migration, with people traveling and gathering at the seaside and in the countryside; and maritime migration, due to transport by sea.[18] Each of these modes of migration contributed to the spread of the epidemic in Portugal.

As noted in the introduction to this volume, the actual mortality of the pandemic on a global scale remains uncertain, although estimates range from 30 million to upward of 100 million people.[19] As regards Portugal, a total mortality figure of 59,000 people has been cited, with a mortality rate of 9.8 per 1,000, which was only surpassed in Europe by Spain and Italy (traditional partners of Portugal in other epidemics) and Hungary. This was in marked contrast to northern Europe, where the rate was little more than 5 per 1,000 in Norway and Sweden.[20] These figures, however, were based on the published death toll (55,780 people died from the flu in 1918 and 3,097 in 1919), which grossly underestimated mortality. In fact, when the number of cases of excess mortality due to respiratory tract infections and to illnesses of unknown cause is taken into account, the estimates are completely different. Using this approach, Fernando da Silva Correia claims that the number of flu deaths in Portugal may have reached a figure slightly higher than 100,000.[21] In the same vein, the demographer Mário Leston Bandeira estimates that in 1918 and 1919 the flu hypothetically caused an excess mortality of 135,257 deaths (in mainland Portugal and the district of Ponta Delgada, in the Azores islands).[22] For Spain, a much more populous country, a total of 257,082 deaths was recently suggested.[23] These figures seem to justify the claim by Machado that the mortality rate in Portugal was higher than that of countries such as Spain and Italy. But regardless of the exact number of deaths, the pandemic's brutality remains constant. It was a veritable massacre, causing a sharp rise in mortality in Portugal in the five-year period from 1916 to 1920.[24]

The majority of deaths from the Spanish flu occurred in October and November, and the age groups most affected in terms of mortality were young adults; both of these features are in line with what generally occurred on an international scale.[25] Specifically, it affected those believed to be most capable of resisting, and its impact was fulminating.[26] As regards gender, contrary to what was found for the pandemic in global syntheses—that is, higher male mortality—recent calculations suggest an excess female mortality due to the flu in Portugal.[27]

No clear picture of the different frequencies of morbidity and mortality among different social classes, all of which were affected by the epidemic, has emerged. There seems to be no international consensus in this regard either. Howard Phillips and David Killingray confirmed that the poor, living in crowded, unsanitary housing, generally had poor nutrition and health and were the most vulnerable to disease.[28] Killingray reached the same conclusion for the Caribbean and a number of authors share this opinion.[29] Others, however, argue against this correlation between the epidemic's effects and social status, asserting the flu disregarded differences of class and admitting the wealthy had a slight advantage at best.[30] The epidemic's allegedly indiscriminate nature is seen in the fact that it affected the prime ministers of Germany, France, and England, the president of the United States, the president elect of Brazil, the prime minister of South Africa, and the maharaja of Jaipur.[31] As Mark Honigsbaum has recently written, "although the tension and constraints of the war may have contributed to the flu's high morbidity, particularly among the poor, the illness did not respect social classes and was democratic in its choice of victims."[32] For example, in a study on the city of Madrid, María-Isabel Porras-Gallo asserts that it is difficult to speak of differentiated mortality for the flu between districts of different socioeconomic levels, although this did occur in the case of tuberculosis.[33]

In Portugal, there is no exact consensus regarding differential mortality and morbidity rates. Victims came from the upper classes, the highest segments of the middle class, and, notoriously, from among members of the artistic community, who were mostly of middle-class origin. But along these lines, the director general of health, Ricardo Jorge, wrote, "If all the classes paid their dues, it weighed most heavily on the most underprivileged; the horrors of the epidemic once again joined those of poverty." He relates that mortality was stratified by class in the voyage of the steamship *Moçambique*, which traveled between the Portuguese colony of Mozambique and Lisbon in September 1918. It carried 952 passengers, and the overall mortality was 22 percent. But mortality among the 558 soldiers in fourth class was 180 individuals, more than 30 percent. In first, second, and third classes, where 261 officials, sergeants, and civilians traveled, only 7.2 percent died. Not one official died.[34] Similarly, a doctor (and a reader of the *Lancet*) who fought the outbreak during his summer vacations in the Ave River valley, a rural industrial zone in northern Portugal, wrote what one might call a short eth-nography of the epidemic. He treated more than 500 patients, finding that the epidemic's most serious manifestations were found among those with the worst living conditions in terms of housing.[35]

Almeida Garrett, a subordinate of Jorge who was in charge of direct-ing the fight against the epidemic in late September (the second wave) in northern Portugal, held a different position from Jorge's. In reference to the second wave in Porto, he gave his impression that the poorer classes were not punished more than the rich, but he provides no evidence for his view.[36] The demographic analysis by Mário Leston Bandeira (2009) concluded that the flu's lethal effects were lower in the cities of Porto and Lisbon compared to all other mainland districts, suggesting that the fight against the epidemic may have been more effective in locations with a greater presence of health services and more efficient administrative control, as occurred in Spain.[37] Comparatively speaking, the rural, poorer part of the country suffered the most.

The Response of Public Health Authorities

According to a note published in the newspapers of May 28, 1918, Ricardo Jorge informed the Conselho Superior de Higiene (High Council for Hygiene) that the disease had spread quickly throughout all of Spain. He reiterated the diagnosis of influenza or flu, caused by a "filter-passing virus," in a report submitted to the same council on June 18.[38] This report men-tioned the extreme contagiousness of the disease, together with the fact that its benign nature was merely superficial, as it was a lethal epidemic.[39] On August 31 he identified the epidemic as *Influenza pneumónica*, the so-called Spanish influenza, a name whose origin may stem, as Nunes suggested in the previous chapter, from the presence of various plagues that gripped Portuguese society in the years just prior to the influenza epidemic.[40] Health authorities took little action during the summer; however, the sit-uation would change with the characteristics of the flu's second wave. On September 29 the director general of health issued the first official instruc-tions specifically aimed at coordinating the fight against the epidemic. On October 2 these were converted into an order of the *secretaria de estado do trabalho* (order of the secretary of state for labor) published on October 4 in the *Diário do Governo*.[41] A new decree was enacted on October 4, with the endorsement of the Directorate General of Health. In view of the country's "health status," "the exit of all medicinal drugs from the country, whether by [land] . . . or by sea," was prohibited.[42] On October 6, 1918, decree 4,872 of the Directorate General of Health clearly alluded to the "current flu epidemic that has disseminated throughout the country," with attempts to establish a clear intervention program based on the traditional epidemiological response.[43] Through this decree a state commissioner general, Ricardo Jorge, was appointed with exceptional powers, including the ability to requisition public services and solicit aid and assistance from public and private collectives, which could not be refused.

Responding to the epidemics of 1918 required an enormous financial effort, although such resources would always be scarce.[44] In a short period the Directorate General of Health attempted to take up various measures to confront the catastrophe, including the reallocation of doctors from military service to civilian clinics, the reinstatement of retired doctors, the mobilization of senior students from faculties of medicine, and the requisition of private automobiles for medical health service. Foodstuffs (such as bread and sugar) and recommended remedies (such as quinine and other drugs) were distributed. Monetary subsidies were given to the poor, and "emergency commissions" were established to collect donations and provide charity.[45] Efforts were made to furnish pharmacies with common medications, control their prices, and distribute subsidies among the districts affected by the epidemic.[46]

Despite this mobilization, the authorities, tremendously lacking in resources of all kinds, were overwhelmed by the epidemic's speed and intensity. A study of the Algarve, the southernmost region of Portugal, concluded that the measures taken by the central government had little effect. In a setting of widespread shortages, there was a breakdown in administrative and health services, which were powerless against the epidemic, while the public remained gripped with panic.[47] Another study on the municipality of Leiria, which witnessed a high level of mortality, found every type of shortcoming, from public food shortages to deplorable sanitary conditions to a lack of doctors and medications.[48] The director of Lisbon's civilian hospitals—the country's most modern hospital network—stated that decommissioned hospitals had to be reinstated and that public establishments (schools and convents) had to be converted into hospitals.[49] The scenario described is one of a lack of means, of disorientation among many of the agents involved in fighting the disease, and of alarm among the authorities and the public.[50] Indeed, the inability of the public health infrastructure to deal with the catastrophe was a common problem in many countries, including Spain, the United States, Brazil, and Great Britain.[51]

If sporadic references exist in the official guidelines to the closing of schools, places of worship, factories, large warehouses, public transport, theaters, and cinemas, it is also true that some public transportation continued to operate. The closing of railway stations can be attributed to the sick status of workers more than to any other quarantine or *cordon sanitaire* guidelines.[52] The director general of health defended the adoption of some measures to curb the contagion (closing major fairs and pilgrimages or schools) but opposed a broadening of prohibitions, including closing theaters and cinemas or, subsequent to these, presumably cafés, churches, public transport, markets, public offices, warehouses, and factories.[53] In addition, the complete prohibition of all major gatherings would contradict the regime's political practice, which used mass public mobilization around its leader as a means of propaganda. But the failure to observe measures such as closing public places or prohibiting gatherings, or contradictory provisions authorizing a specific type of gathering while prohibiting others, were in no way limited to Portugal; this strategy also occurred in Spain, the United States, the United Kingdom, and Brazil.[54] In general, quarantine measures were imposed, "but only in some places, and in some countries, half-heartedly and with little success."[55]

The speed and intensity of the second flu outbreak were not the only factors that hampered the formation of a structure capable of providing a concerted institutional response. Many doctors were absent, assigned to military service outside the country. Medical knowledge and capacities were being questioned, despite the successes of bacteriology, which had detected the origin of specific diseases in the activity of microorganisms at the end of the nineteenth century.[56] In Portugal, as everywhere, the origin of the infectious agent was debated, but Portugal's highest health authority was among those that correctly believed that the cause of the flu was an unidentified "filter-passer" virus (*virus filtrante*) and that the only remedy would be the discovery of a specific vaccine, as had occurred in the case of smallpox.[57] The majority of Spanish doctors, among others, thought the same.[58] Classic disinfection procedures, however, were not completely overlooked (in terms of public transportation and establishments), and cleaning homes and settlements and isolating the sick (whether at home or in hospitals, shelters, schools, prisons, or hospices) were recommended.[59]

The Response of Political Agents: Church, State, and the Political Opposition

The fight against the epidemic was conducted in a top-down, hierarchical manner through a circuit combining bureaucratic channels and health services. The base health structures would report the existence of epidemics to the Directorate General of Health. The public opinion was informed through notes published by the directorate or through news from local correspondents.[60] Local initiatives complied with appeals originating from the political center. This system was put in place only at the beginning of October, when the effects of the second wave were felt.[61] The state's response, however, was insufficient.

An analysis of the response of political and administrative agents of the state requires a consideration not only of structural circumstances, such as the status of health and welfare in Portugal, but also of its specific context. This includes the highly personalized and authoritarian type of regime of the time and its alliances, political and social conflicts, scarce financial resources, and the available means to fight the illness. Despite the political changes caused by the coup that brought Sidónio Pais to power, public health and welfare policies remained within the traditional republican model (i.e., a lay system as opposed to one grounded in religion).[62] These policies were not supplemented until the reinstatement of several religious orders and the development of charitable works of a more traditional propensity.[63] Led by key figures from the bourgeoisie and the Catholic community, these works were directly supported by Sidónio Pais, allowing a centralized, personalized network of clientele to be assembled. In the context of the epidemic, Pais presided over a central emergency commission led by some of the country's most affluent individuals, who were assisted by their wives. Many of them were known for showing hostility toward the republic or for defending conservative positions within it. During this organization's first meeting at the presidential palace, donations were taken from those present, resulting in a substantial monetary amount, a testament to how power entailed not only formal structures but also the network of informal relationships surrounding the president.[64] For his part, the president of the republic traveled throughout the country distributing provisions, either leaving them for others to distribute or handing them out himself.[65] In this way, he sought to enhance his charisma by using the speed of his efforts as a political tool. Nonetheless, Pais's power faced structural constraints that could not be overcome by personal will, hence the state's limited response to the catastrophe.

Meanwhile, the measures taken against the pandemic inevitably became a topic of political struggle amid the setting of intense political conflict. *O Mundo*, a newspaper of the opposing Democratic Party (subject to censorship, like all others), criticized the government as one "of the wealthy exploiting the poor," calling attention, along with others, to the need to isolate the sick and take preventive measures. The newspaper criticized the authorities for not taking the necessary measures and insisted on the insufficiency of resources in terms of medical personnel, medications, and food. It accused Pais's government of canceling the official celebrations of October 5—the date of the proclamation of the republic—to win the support of monarchists, not to avoid contagion from the epidemic, as it had stated, since it had allowed popular celebratory sessions to take place and had left theaters and cinemas open.[66]

The church—a political agent in itself—joined forces with the monarchists, which opposed the well-known anticlericalism that had characterized republican governments since 1910.[67] On November 5, 1918, the leading figure of the Portuguese Catholic Church published a note on the epidemic. In it, the cardinal delights in the action of the head of state, "who, with such commitment and untiring work, has pursued the praiseworthy purpose, through effective and prompt measures, of coming to the aid of our country, currently wounded by the cruelest of calamities."[68] Using the leading Catholic publication of the time, *Vida Católica*, Sobral and collaborators have shown that the church claimed a key role in fighting the pandemic for itself and the network of lay organizations under its control.[69] In terms of direct assistance to the sick, this involved intervening in treatment and assisting them with basic expenses. In addition, the church would provide the religious means to cope with the catastrophe, such as prayer and other suitable worship activities. The circumstances also served to celebrate values tied to Christianity—for example, charity—and for the church to organize public demonstrations of power, both as an auxiliary to the state in fighting the illness and an interpreter of its meaning.[70]

The types of explanations for the flu put forward by the church combine natural and supernatural reasons.[71] Naturalist explanations were based on medical and health knowledge, with the church assuming the role of intermediary, as a collaborator of political and health agents, disseminating procedures outside of its jurisdiction and acknowledging the importance of scientific knowledge. A collection of specific instructions was thus publicized for the churches and their facilities to keep them from becoming places of transmission of the disease (for instance, washing floors with soap and water, disinfecting them daily or before major gatherings, cleaning confessional boxes, and drying holy water fonts).[72]

The supernatural interpretation gave the church primacy as a representative of divinity in the world. Capable of interpreting divine will, the church was the only one with the ability and legitimacy to appease God's anger through the appropriate ritual practices. Allusions to the epidemic evil as a "punishment of God" were updated for the Portuguese historical context. As written in the publication *Vida Católica*: "the blood that has flowed in our country from revolutions and offences, the crimes against religions and its ministers . . . through which we have deserved the great punishment of plague, hunger and war."[73] The medical historian Charles Rosenberg recalls that "accepting the existence of an epidemic implies—and in some sense demands—the creation of a framework within which its dismaying arbitrariness can be managed."[74] The Catholic Church in Portugal did just this. The explanations of the pandemic it produced have a lineage that predates the 1918–19 influenza pandemic.

The use of the "punishment from God" explanation in Portugal echoes identical stances of the Catholic Church in other countries where Catholicism was the primary religion, such as in Spain and Brazil.[75] Without discounting the specific weight of the circumstances that allowed the Portuguese church to find culprits for the unleashing of divine anger in the Portuguese context, this explanation should be understood as part of a broader phenomenon. In Brazil Protestants offered similar explanations to those of their Catholic counterparts.[76] According to Tom Quinn, in the United States people belonging to what is now called the "religious right" believed that the pandemic was a biblical calamity sent by God to annihilate humanity before the Second Coming and Final Judgment. In the southern and southeastern region called the "Bible Belt," socially conservative evangelical Protestants considered the pandemic a punishment for the immorality of men.[77]

The religious explanation of the pandemic was nothing new, nor was the repertoire with which to cope with the catastrophe. If disease is a punishment, it is redeemable through atonement and the righting of wrongs by sinners.[78] This entails showing signs of repentance in an attempt to appease divine anger manifested by the epidemic and restore good relationships with the supernatural. In response to the pandemic, rituals of repentance, specifically public processions, increased in number in Portugal, and many of them had broad participation throughout the country. For example, the patriarch cardinal decided to hold prayers for three days in the Lisbon cathedral, with the Exposition of the Blessed Sacrament.[79] In Lisbon participants in the Senhor dos Passos da Graça procession included members of groups most closely tied to the church but also to Sidónio Pais.[80] Prayers from the times of the cholera epidemics of the nineteenth century were brought back, such as the following: "By your wounds / By your cross / Free us from plague / Oh holy Jesus."[81] In Portugal a vast number of intercessors with the divine were used to help humans reconcile with divinity. Saints specializing in antipestilence, such as Saint Sebastian, were invoked, together with local patron saints, Christ, and the Virgin.[82]

This overall context of affliction among devout Catholics should be borne in mind to explain the initial success of the Marian apparitions of the Virgin of Fátima, which took place in 1917. Three children from a poor and mountainous region said the Virgin Mary had appeared to them while they were herding their flock. The children were submitted to harassment by local authorities and initially were not taken seriously by the church. But they attracted an increasing number of followers, mainly from the peasantry, but also some individuals from the upper classes. Although occurring before the flu, the apparitions contain abundant references to curing a number of diseases that afflicted the population. Two of the three children died shortly after the apparitions: Francisco on April 4, 1919, and Jacinta on February 20, 1919. They were diagnosed with the "flu."[83] The Virgin of Fátima is specifically named as the agent of cure for those believing to have been irreversibly affected by the epidemic.[84] It was the beginning of an enormous success that would eclipse other Marian invocations in Portugal and the cult of saints in general. The Catholic Church, which built a great sanctuary and organized an increasingly international cult, officially recognized the apparitions as legitimate, and the Virgin of Fátima became one of the most important Marian cults in the contemporary Catholic world. The children who died from the flu were beatified in 2000.

The Challenges of Flu Epidemics in Portugal

The flu epidemic occurred in a Portugal that faced tremendous economic, political, and public health challenges. The country's economic fragility was aggravated by wartime circumstances and the lack of all kinds of resources: financial, food, medicinal, and human (i.e., medical personnel). In October adversaries of the regime of Sidónio Pais—which was politically in its death throes—attempted military insurrection, followed by a general strike in November. With the armistice taking place on November 11, 1918, the end of the war foretold the coming of change. Pais was shot on December 14, 1918. And to make things worse, the flu had reached its peak.

In addition to contextual factors, the crisis brought about by the pandemic revealed the long-term structural deficiencies of a poor country. The existence of relevant figures and institutions in the health and medical domain, rising to the forefront in the fight against the pandemic, starkly underscored the shortcomings that continued to be felt. In this way, the responses of the government and other agents responsible for public health were strictly determined by the unforeseen, extremely rapid nature in which the pandemic was propagated. The highly limited effects of the actions of doctors and public health authorities revealed the impotence of scientific knowledge in overcoming the catastrophe, in Portugal and everywhere else.[85] The pandemic uncovered the insufficiency of the weak Portuguese public health system, which was making its first attempts at universal care. It demonstrated the ineffectiveness of political efforts, despite the commitment of the president himself, who ventured his own charisma in personally mobilizing resources. Finally, it revealed deep political and ideological gaps, where the regime's adversaries and supporters capitalized on the epidemic to combat those in power.

Notes

This chapter was the result of a research project titled "The Spanish Flu in Portugal: Risk Management and Public Health," an FCT-funded project, 2005–7, POCTI/HCT/60718/2004.

1. António Henrique de Oliveira Marques, *História da 1a República Portuguesa: As estruturas de base* (Lisbon: Iniciativas Editoriais, 1978).

2. Arnaldo Sampaio, *Subsídios para o estudo da epidemiologia da gripe* (Lisbon: Edição de Autor, 1958), 127.

3. In chapter 3 Nunes shows the effects of this separation on the measures Ricardo Jorge proposed to combat the Spanish flu.

4. David Ferreira, "Sidónio pais," in *Dicionário de história de Portugal*, ed. Joel Serrão (Porto: Livraria Figueirinhas, n.d.), 4:517–24.

5. Chapter 3 of this volume deals extensively with Jorge's role during the pandemic.

6. Ricardo Jorge, *La Grippe* (Lisbonne: Imprimerie Nationale, 1919), 35.

7. The concern for public health emerged internationally over the course of the nineteenth century, with the perceived connection between the influence of the environment—poverty, lack of hygiene, and so on—on illness and epidemics in particular. Dorothy Porter, "Public Health," in *Companion Encyclopedia of the History of Medicine*, ed. William F. Bynum and Roy Porter (London & New York: Routledge, 1993) vol. 2, 1231–61. Note that, in comparative terms, a Ministry of Health was not created in the United Kingdom until 1919 in a specific postwar context marked by poverty, disease, and unemployment. Roy Porter, *The Greatest Benefit of Mankind* (London: Fontana, 1999), 642. In Portugal an equivalent institution was not created until 1958, nearly forty years later. António Correia de Campos, "Saúde Pública," in *Dicionário de História de Portugal Dictionary of the History of Portugal*, ed. António Barreto and Maria Filomena Mónica, vol. 9 (Porto: Livraria Figueirinhas, 2000), 405–6. But, as pointed out by Nunes in chapter 3 in this volume, we can consider the experience of the Spanish flu and Ricardo Jorge's thoughts on the role the state should play in times of epidemic and in the twentieth century in general as the starting point to the changes that would ultimately lead to the welfare state.

8. Maria de Lurdes Akola Neto, "Assistência pública," in Serrão, *Dicionário*, 1:234–36. Pilar León-Sanz deals with this topic as it relates to Spain in chapter 8 of this volume.

9. Fernando da Silva Correia, *Problemas de higiene e puericultura* (Coimbra: Imprensa da Universidade, 1934); Paulo Jorge Marques Girão, *A pneumónica no Algarve* (Casal de Cambra: Caleidoscópio, 2003), 30–31, 102–3.

10. Correia, *Problemas de higiene*, 219–74.

11. George Vigarello, *Histoire des pratiques de santé: Le sain et le malsain depuis le Moyen Âge* (Paris: Éditions du Seuil, 1999), 240–43, 260–65; Gina Kolata, *Flu: The Story of the Great Influenza Pandemic of 1918 and the Search for the Virus That Caused It* (1999; repr., New York: Touchstone, 2005), 47. See also the introduction and chapters 2 (for Brazil) and 5 (for Spain) of this volume.

12. Fernando da Silva Correia, *Portugal sanitário (subsídios para o seu estudo)* (Lisbon: Ministério do Interior e da Saúde Pública, 1938), 499–507, 192.

13. Howard Phillips and David Killingray, eds., *The Spanish Influenza Pandemic of 1918–19: New Perspectives* (London: Routledge, 2003), 5–7.

14. Indeed, the flu became epidemic in mid-May 1918. María-Isabel Porras-Gallo, *Un reto para la sociedad madrileña: La epidemia de gripe de 1918–19* (Madrid: Complutense / Comunidad Autónoma de Madrid, 1997), 41.

15. Sampaio, *Subsídios*, 121. In fact, the Spanish region of Extremadura, which borders the Beira Baixa and Alto Alentejo regions, was among the zones with the highest mortality rates during this first wave. Beatriz Echeverri Dávila, "Spanish

Influenza Seen from Spain," in *The Spanish Influenza Pandemic of 1918–19: New Perspectives*, ed. Howard Phillips and David Killingray (London: Routledge, 2003), 173–90, p. 178.

16. Jorge, *Grippe*, 14–15. According to one of its first researchers, the pandemic had two waves with high points in July and October. The difference between the mortality rate of the first wave—6.6 per 100,000—and that of the second wave—561.4 per 100,000—highlights the dramatic gap between the two. Sampaio, *Subsídios*, 121.

17. Jorge, *Grippe*, 18.

18. On the factors involved in propagating epidemics on a worldwide scale, see Roy Porter, *The Greatest Benefit of Mankind* (London: Fontana, 1999), 483. On maritime migration specifically, see Jorge, *Grippe*, 21–23.

19. Phillips and Killingray, although admitting the lack of data and exact sources made their figure merely an informed estimate, point to a total of thirty million deaths, many more than those caused by World War I. *Spanish Influenza Pandemic*, 4.

20. Niall Johnson and Juergen Mueller, "Updating the Accounts: Global Mortality of the 1918–1920 'Spanish' Influenza Pandemic," *Bulletin of the History of Medicine* 76, no. 1 (2002): 113.

21. Correia, *Portugal sanitário*, 233, 479–80.

22. Mário Leston Bandeira, "A sobremortalidade de 1918 em Portugal: Análise demográfica," in *A pandemia esquecida: Olhares comparados sobre a pneumónica (1918/19)*, ed. José Manuel Sobral, Maria Luisa Lima, Paulo Silveira e Sousa, and Paula Castro (Lisbon: Imprensa de Ciências Sociais, 2009): 131–54.

23. Beatriz Echeverri Dávila, "Spanish Influenza Seen from Spain," in Phillips and Killingray, *Spanish Influenza Pandemic*, 183.

24. José Timóteo Montalvão Machado, *Como nascem e morrem os Portugueses: Estudo demográfico* (Lisbon: Depositários Gomes e Rodrigues, 1959), 185.

25. Mark Honigsbaum, *Living with Enza: The Forgotten Story of Britain and the Great Flu Pandemic of 1918* (London: Macmillan, 2009), 5.

26. Jorge, *Grippe*, 25; Augusto Lobo Alves, "Relatório do director geral dos Hospitais Civis: A. Lobo Alves," in *Relatórios e notícias sobre a epidemia de gripe pneumónica*, ed. Hospitais Civis de Lisboa, Repartição do Boletim e Serviços de Estatística Clínica, 3–22 (Lisbon: Imprensa Nacional, 1920); Alfred Crosby, *America's Forgotten Pandemic: The Influenza of 1918* (1989; repr., Cambridge: Cambridge University Press, 2003), 322; Beatriz Echeverri Dávila, *La gripe española: La pandemia de 1918–19* (Madrid: Centro de Investigaciones Sociológicas / Siglo XXI, 1993), 122–23; Porras-Gallo, *Reto*, 65–67; Honigsbaum, *Living with Enza*, 19; Leston Bandeira, "Sobremortalidade"; Phillips and Killingray, *Spanish Influenza Pandemic*, 8–9; Anny Jackeline Torres Silveira, *A influenza espanhola e a cidade planejada: Belo Horizonte, 1918* (Belo Horizonte: Argumentum, 2008), 24; Jeffery K. Taubenberger and David M. Morens, "1918 Influenza: The Mother of All Pandemics," *Emerging Infectious Diseases* 12, no. 1 (2006): 19.

27. On male mortality, see Phillips and Killingray, *Spanish Influenza Pandemic*, 8–9. On excess female mortality in Portugal, see Leston Bandeira, "Sobremortalidade."

28. Phillips and Killingray, *Spanish Influenza Pandemic*, 9.

29. David Killingray, "The Influenza Pandemic of 1918–19 in the British Caribbean," *Social History of Medicine* 7, no. 1 (1994); John M. Barry, *The Great Influenza: The Epic Story of the Deadliest Plague in History* (London: Penguin Books,

2005), 408; Liane Maria Bertucci, *Influenza: A medicina enferma* (Campinas: Universidade Estadual de Campinas, 2004), 118–19; Echeverri Dávila, *Gripe española*, 103–7; Echeverri Dávila, "Spanish Influenza"; Niall Johnson, *Britain and the 1918–19 Influenza Pandemic: A Dark Epilogue* (London: Routledge, 2006), 105; Svenn-Erick Mamelund, "A Socially Neutral Disease? Individual Social Class, Household Wealth and Mortality from Spanish Influenza in Two Socially Contrasting Parishes in Kristiania, 1918–19," *Social Science and Medicine* 62 (2006): 923–46; Kevin McCracken and Peter Curson, "Flu Downunder: A Demographic and Geographic Analysis of the 1919 Epidemic in Sydney, Australia," in Phillips and Killingray, *Spanish Influenza Pandemic*, 110–31; Christiane Maria Cruz de Souza, "A gripe espanola em Salvador, 1918: Cidade de becos e cortiços," *História, Ciências, Saúde: Manguinhos* 12, no. 1 (2005): 71–99.

30. Crosby, *America's Forgotten Pandemic*, 323.

31. Michael B. A. Oldstone, *Viruses, Plagues, and History* (Oxford: Oxford University Press, 2000), 174–75; Bertucci, *Influenza*, 352; Tom Quinn, *Flu: A Social History of Influenza* (London: New Holland), 145.

32. Honigsbaum, *Living with Enza*, 63.

33. Porras-Gallo, *Reto*, 57–60.

34. Jorge, *Grippe*, 25, 23–24.

35. Joaquim A. Pires de Lima, "Notas sobre a epidemia gripal," *Separata do Portugal Médico*, 3rd ser., 4, no. 11 (1918): 12. On the relationship between flu mortality and poor living conditions in Alicante, Spain, see chapter 11 of this volume, which includes various figures.

36. Almeida Garrett, "Contra a epidemia de gripe pneumónica, em 1918, no norte do país (Relatório)," *Portugal Médico* 11 (1919): 653–73.

37. Mario Leston Bandeira, "Sobremortalidade"; Echeverri Dávila, *Gripe española*, 170.

38. Viruses were first discovered at the end of the nineteenth century. Oldstone, *Viruses, Plagues, and History*, 12–14. At the time, the uses of the term "virus" were different from today. According to Honigsbaum, "bacteriologists had no concept of viruses invad[ing]e and tak[ing]e over the machinery of animal cells in order to replicate and make multiple copies of themselves. Instead, they tended to conceive of such filter-passers as specialized forms of bacterial 'poison'—ultramicrobes that had evolved from bacteria by increasing parasitism and that, like larger bacteria, multiplied by means of binary fission." *Living with Enza*, 109. In line with what occurred on an international scale, Bertucci deals extensively with the problem of identifying the specific agent of the flu pandemic in Brazil in chapter 2 of this volume, and some mention on the Spanish case figures in chapter 5.

39. Ricardo Jorge, "A nova incursão peninsular da influenza," *Portugal Médico*, 3rd ser., 4, no. 6 (1918): 436–43.

40. "Tifo exantemático," *Portugal Médico*, no. 8, August 4, 1918, 528.

41. This is the oficial journal where Laws and Decrees are published. There is no name of the author nor a title. *Diário do Governo*, ser. 2, no. 233, October 4, 1918, 3255–56.

42. Decree no. 4,871, *Diário do Governo*, ser. 1, no. 217, October 4, 1918, 1754.

43. Decree no. 4,872, *Diário do Governo*, ser. 1, no. 218, October 7, 1918, 1755.

44. Chapter 8 deals with the financial challenges of providing health care during the epidemic in Pamplona, Spain.

45. Jorge, *Grippe.*

46. See "Instructions from the director general of health,"*O Comércio do Porto,* October 1, 1918, 1. It is not signed. The director was Ricardo Jorge at the time.

47. Girão, *Pneumónica no Algarve,* 140–41.

48. João José Cúcio Frada, *A pneumónica em Portugal Continental: Estudo socioeconómico e epidemiológico com particular análise do concelho de Leiria* (Lisbon: Sete Caminhos, 2005). These circumstances are similar to those described in chapters 8 and 11 of this volume.

49. Alves, "Relatório do director," 6–7.

50. Arruda Furtado, "Relatório do inspector de higiene dos Hospitais Civis de Lisboa," in Hospitais Civis de Lisboa, *Relatórios e Notícias,* 23–30, 24–27.

51. On Spain, see Echeverri Dávila, *Gripe española,* 140; Porras-Gallo, *Reto,* 90–96. On the United States, see Crosby, *America's Forgotten Pandemic,* 49; Quinn, *Flu,* 143; and Davis, chap. 9, in this volume. On Brazil, see Adriana da Costa Goulart, "Revisitando a espanhola: A gripe pandêmica de 1918 no Rio de Janeiro," *História Ciências Saúde: Manguinhos* 12, no. 1 (2005): 101–42; Silveira, *Influenza espanhola,* 65; and Bertucci, chap. 2; Silveira, chap. 6; and Cruz de Souza, chap. 7, all in this volume. On Great Britain, see Honigsbaum, *Living with Enza,* 119; and Sandra M. Thomkins, "The Failure of Expertise: Public Health Policy in Britain during the 1918–1919 Influenza Epidemic," *Social History of Medicine* 5 no. 3 (1992): 435–54.

52. Nunes points out in chapter 3 of this volume that Ricardo Jorge, the director general of health, considered the establishment of a *cordon sanitaire* outdated and inadequate to the reality of the flu outbreak.

53. Jorge, *Grippe,* 32.

54. On Spain, see Echeverri Dávila, *Gripe española,* 143–45; Porras-Gallo, *Reto,* 80; and Porras-Gallo, chap. 5, in this volume. On the United States, see Quinn, *Flu,* 136–37. On the United Kingdom, see Johnson, *Britain,* 122–30. On Brazil, see Bertucci, *Influenza,* 106–13; Silveira, *Influenza espanhola,* 146–48; and chapters 2, 6, and 7 of this volume.

55. Quinn, *Flu,* 137.

56. María-Isabel Porras-Gallo, "Sueros y vacunas en la lucha contra la pandemia de gripe de 1918–1919 en España," *Asclepio* 60, no. 2 (2008): 261–88; R. Porter, *Greatest Benefit,* 428–61.

57. On the scientific debates about the agent, see Jorge, "Nova incursão," 437–38; Jorge, *Grippe,* 8–10; and Bertucci, chap. 2, in this volume. On the relation to smallpox, see Jorge, *Grippe,* 34.

58. Porras-Gallo, *Reto,* 106; Porras-Gallo, "Sueros y vacunas"; Porras-Gallo, chap. 5, in this volume.

59. Jorge, *Grippe,* 33–34.

60. In chapter 3 of this volume, Nunes deals extensively with Ricardo Jorge's role in this regard.

61. This is the oficial journal where Laws and Decrees are published. There is no name of the author nor a title. *Diário do Governo,* 2nd ser., 233 (April 10, 1918): 3255–56.

62. Nunes shows in chapter 3 how the director general of health, Ricardo Jorge, tried to adapt disease prevention and prophylactic measures against the flu outbreak to this new idea.

63. These religious orders had been expelled following the republican revolution of 1910.

64. "Contra a epidemia. A influenza Pneumonica," *O Século*, no. 13243, October 22–31, 1918, 1–2 and November 6, 1918.

65. Cf. "A influenza pneumonica," *O Comércio do Porto*, October 1, 1918, 1.

66. "Por causa da epidemia o governo não festeja a republica," *O Mundo*, no. 6438, October 8, 1918, 2.

67. For the Catholic Church's role, see also chapters 7 and 12 of this volume.

68. António Cardeal Patriarca, "Provisão," *Vida Católica* 4, no. 77 (1918): 129.

69. José Manuel Sobral, Maria Luísa Lima, Paulo Silveira e Sousa, and Paula Castro, eds., *A Pandemia esquecida: Olhares comparados sobre a pneumónica, 1918–1919* (Lisbon: Imprensa de Ciências Sociais, 2009).

70. On the role of mutual benefit societies as auxiliaries to the state during the flu pandemic, see chapter 8 of this volume.

71. Paul Slack, *The Impact of Plague in Tudor and Stuart England* (1983; repr., Oxford: Oxford University Press, 2005), 22–36.

72. "Instrucções para o Povo," *Boletim da Dioces e do Porto* 4, no. 13, February 15, 1918, 260.

73. "A epidemia," *Vida Católica* 4, no. 77, November 5, 1918, 138. The same sentiment was reiterated several days later in *O Mensageiro: Órgão dos Católicos do Distrito de Leiria* (November 11, 1918): "May God help us and open our eyes to His divine law which, because of our disdain, has brought us such punishments of hunger, war and plague." Hunger, plague, and war tend to be symbolically associated with the horsemen of the apocalypse, a sacred text announcing the final judgement. Cf. Apocalypse of Saint John, in Biblia Sagrada (Sao Paulo: Edição Paulinas, 1959), 1479–98. Hunger, plague, and war are repeatedly referred to as punishments of God, as demonstrated by the words of an archbishop of Évora at the end of the sixteenth century with regard to the city's plague at the time. Laurinda Abreu, "A Cidade em Tempos de Peste: Medidas de Protecção e Combate às Epidemias em Évora, entre 1579 e 1637 (The city in times of pestilence: the fight against epidemcs in Évora, 1579–1637)." In http://www.ugr.es/~adeh/comunicaciones/Abreu_L.pdf, retrieved 07-07-2009.

74. Charles E. Rosenberg, *Explaining Epidemics and Other Studies in the History of Medicine* (Cambridge: Cambridge University Press, 1992), 282.

75. On Spain, see Echeverri Dávila, *Gripe española*, 11, 12, 146. On Brazil, see Silveira, *Influenza espanhola*, 57–59; and chapter 7 of this volume.

76. Bertucci, *Influenza*, 243–44.

77. Quinn, *Flu*, 142–43.

78. Bertucci, *Influenza*, 243; Silveira, *Influenza espanhola*, 197.

79. "Influenza Pneumonica. O decrescer da epidemia," *O Século*, no 13237, October 16, 1918, 3.

80. "Procissão de penitencia," *O Século*, no 13249, October 28, 1918, 1.

81. "Epidemia," *O Mensageiro: Órgão dos Católicos do Distrito de Leiria*, November 1, 1918, 2.

82. "Procissão do Terço," *O Mensageiro: Órgão dos Católicos do Distrito de Leiria*, October 25, 1918, 2; November 6, 1918; November 8, 1918; December 6, 1918. On saints associated with antipestilence in Brazil, see chapter 7 of this volume.

83. See José Geraldes Freire, ed., *Documentação crítica de Fátima*, vol. 1, *Interrogatórios aos Videntes, 1917* (Fátima: Santuário de Fátima, 1992); Freire, ed., *Documentação crítica de Fátima*, vol. 2, *Interrogatórios aos Videntes, 1917* (Fátima: Santuário de Fátima, 1999). Information provided by Pedro Pereira.

84. "Correspondências," *O Mensageiro: Órgão dos Católicos do Distrito de Leiria*, November 16, 1918.

85. See also chapters 2 and 5 of this volume.

Chapter Five

Between the Pandemic and World War I: The 1918–19 Influenza Pandemic in the Spanish Army, through the Eyes of the Press

María-Isabel Porras-Gallo

As noted in the introduction to this volume, the 1918–19 influenza pandemic started when Spain was very backward in public health matters and when the political crisis and adverse socioeconomic conditions made it difficult to answer the call for modernization from different medical sectors and health authorities.[1] The Military Medical Service, having undergone a radical transformation during the reign of Isabel II (1833–68), was fighting to achieve scientific supremacy vis-à-vis an impoverished Civilian Public Health Service.[2] But the Spanish army needed to reorganize and improve some of its infrastructure for this to occur. For instance, the hygienic conditions of the barracks and the food the soldiers were receiving were rather poor. As we shall see, these conditions would become prominent during the pandemic and, for some people, responsible for its existence and gravity.

As Charles Rosenberg has noted, an epidemic offers a cross-section of society, helping to highlight the existing and latent problems a given community has at the time of the outbreak. Moreover, an epidemic as a social phenomenon takes the form of a theatrical drama.[3] In a limited time and space, different social groups are forced to modify their usual dynamic and to perform various activities to address the critical situation. This results in the mobilization of their members to perform propitiatory rituals, incorporating and reaffirming their fundamental social and cultural values.

Taking Rosenberg's approach as a starting point and using as my main sources military scientific journals and newspapers, as well as the general and popular press, this chapter explores the reactions of Spain's Military Medical Service to the 1918–19 influenza pandemic.[4] In what follows I focus on the social impact of debates as well as on tensions and conflicts between different sectors of society. For this reason I assess whether the Military Medical Service defended scientific opinions that were more modern than those of the Sanidad Civil (Civilian Health Service) and whether there were any conflicts of interest between the measures they both took in response to the epidemic, especially as related to soldiers. My previous research on the Spanish influenza has focused on the social, economic, demographic, and sanitary impact of the pandemic in Madrid as well as on the more general social reactions from laypeople, politicians, and members of the Civilian Health Service, not on Spain's Military Medical Service.[5] Given Spain's neutrality, it seemed logical to focus on the Civilian Health Service; however, since Spain's neutrality did not mean the two services operated in isolation of each other, a comparative view is in order.

The relation between the pandemic and the military has not to date been analyzed within the Spanish context, with the exception of Beatriz Echeverri, who limits herself to providing an evaluation of the demographic impact the pandemic had on the Spanish army and navy.[6] More attention has been paid to the US case by Alfred Crosby, though his primary focus also lays elsewhere, and, especially, by Carol R. Byerly, whose interesting and broad-ranging monograph explores the impact of the 1918–19 influenza on the United States army.[7] Byerly's work begins to address the glaring gap in scholarship, already noted by Howard Phillips and David Killingray in 2003, that deals specifically with the relationship between World War I and the influenza pandemic.[8] Byerly argues that "the war *created* the influenza epidemic by producing an ecological environment in the trenches in which the flu virus could thrive and mutate to unprecedented virulence."[9] She also examines how army medical officers responded to the sanitary crisis in an ambiance of unprecedented confidence in medicine's ability to keep soldiers healthy after medical advances in the prewar years and how the pandemic experience was a professional disaster for physicians and especially army medical officers.[10] She studies the nature of military medicine and the special role of medical officers who served both government aims and the soldiers under their care, and she shows how army medical officers experienced tensions stemming from their condition as both physicians and soldiers.[11]

Scholarship like Byerly's, and similar research that will surely follow, directly (if perhaps implicitly) engages the ideas of Thomas Robert Malthus,[12] who held that war and epidemics went hand in hand. From a suggestive and constructivist perspective, Roger Cooter has argued that wars and epidemics are "unnatural couplings" and sees in these couplings "problematic conceptions."[13] The present chapter addresses this issue by exploring the case of Spain, which remained neutral throughout World

War I but acted as the point of connection, both epidemiologically and discursively, between Europe and the Americas.[14] Epidemiologically, Portuguese soldiers and Spanish workers returning from central Europe and France served as vectors for introducing the pandemic into these countries.[15] The discursive import of Spain is reflected in the nickname of the disease, as we have explained in the introduction. Specifically, I argue that we can apply Cooter's argument—given the special situation of Spain—but also some of the key points pointed out by Byerly's work. Like their American counterparts, Spanish military doctors shared an unprecedented confidence in medicine's ability to combat an infectious disease epidemic, even though the experience of the 1918–19 pandemic would undermine this confidence, and though not directly involved in the war, they also experienced tension because they were both physicians and army officers. Their decision to discharge soldiers—in theory, a preventive measure—became a major source of spreading the epidemic into the civilian population and highlighted inequalities in the medical attention Spanish army soldiers received. For all these reasons, studying the case of Spain allows us to understand more precisely the relationships between the 1918–19 influenza pandemic and World War I, thus expanding scholarship like Byerly's and that which will surely follow.

The Development of the Influenza Pandemic of 1918–19 within the Army

As in most countries throughout the world, the 1918–19 influenza pandemic occurred in three waves in Spain: the late spring of 1918, autumn of 1918, and the spring of 1919. The second wave was the most serious in the majority of the country, except for Madrid and other central regions of Spain, where the first wave was the worst.[16] Its appearance in the army was noted by the political-military newspapers of the time, such as *El Heraldo Militar* and *La Correspondencia Militar* but also in the *Revista de Sanidad Militar* (the main professional scientific journal of the Military Health Service) and the popular press. Their pages indicated the mildness of the first outbreak and gave greater importance to the second, pointing out "its wide spread" and "the serious set of symptoms which accompanied it."[17]

In the army the first outbreak of the pandemic was recorded during May and June and the second in September and October (both of which were later than on the war front in France). As indicated by Echeverri, the pandemic spread faster in the army than among the civilian population, a feature of closed communities, where individuals live in overcrowded conditions, thereby providing a rapid spread of the epidemic until it exhausts the available hosts and dies out.[18] Levels of hospitalization were the same in both outbreaks, and the morbidity rates due to influenza among rank-and-file troops who were hospitalized were between eight and twenty times the rates of the corresponding months of 1917 and between four and eight times those of the preceding months of 1918 (see table 5.1).[19]

Echeverri has attributed the high hospitalization rate during the first outbreak, similar to that of the second, to the principle of isolation of the sick rather than the severity of cases, given the benign nature of this outbreak.[20] Her interpretation is supported by the declarations of the military doctor G. Sierra, who stated that during the first outbreak more rigorous isolation was carried out in the Medical Corps than in the Civilian Health Service.[21] At the same time, Echeverri has criticized the army's data regarding morbidity and mortality among its troops during the 1918–19 influenza pandemic. According to their sources, 106 of every 1,000 soldiers caught influenza in 1918 and, of these, 3 died. In this view, a case fatality rate of 3 per 1,000 is within the limits of what Wade Hampton Frost observed for American communities; however, given that this rate approximates the national average, it seems low. Unlike the general population, the army provided the ideal conditions for the development of a catastrophic epidemic in its midst. Indeed, as Echeverri has also noted, between 1909 and the emergence of the epidemic, an average of almost 50 percent of the troops was hospitalized at one time or another, which points to the generally insalubrious conditions of the barracks.[22]

In fact, the poor sanitary conditions of the barracks were denounced during the epidemic and linked to its outbreak. Moreover, the need for major improvements was stressed to avoid a future recurrence of situations similar to those that had occurred during the pandemic.[23] Echeverri has given two reasons to justify this lower-than-expected mortality. First, part of the army population may have acquired immunity during the first outbreak, a view espoused by the military doctors José Alberto Palanca and Santos Rubiano.[24] Second, military statistics may have underreported the number of deaths of soldiers who had been discharged while still sick.[25] The general press registered numerous complaints about the underreporting, most notably by Dr. Gonzalo R. Lafora.[26] The discharge of (healthy) soldiers, however, was considered by some military doctors as one of the best prophylactic measures to combat the epidemic in the army.

A Theoretical Framework for Action

When the pandemic hit, military doctors debated various aspects of the disease (etiology, clinical characteristics, transmission, etc.) to determine which measures to adopt to combat it. Their discussion echoed the methodology and major scientific ideas of the time but also highlighted some

Table 5.1. Influenza morbidity rates for hospitalized soldiers (per 1000)

Month	1917	1918
January		4.0 (including recruits)
February		4.4
March		4.2
April		3.4
May	1.7	12.7
June	0.9	23.7
July		4.7
August		1.8
September	0.7	22.3 (including recruits)
October	1.7	16.9
November		3.9
December		3.2

Note: Hospitalization occurred in different Spanish military hospitals during the month indicated in the table.

Source: Adapted from table 22 of Beatriz Echeverri Dávila, *La gripe española: La pandemia de 1918–19* (Madrid: Centro de Investigaciones Sociológicas / Siglo XXI, 1993), 111. Reproduced with permission from the author.

inconsistencies and lack of agreement among military medical profession-als on certain aspects of the disease. One of these inconsistencies con-cerned the etiological agent of influenza. From the very beginning of the pandemic, both military and civilian doctors participated in the intense debate that arose on the subject in Spain, a debate that was held in numer-ous countries.[27] Military doctors formed their own Scientific Committee with members from the Instituto de Higiene Militar (Military Institute of Hygiene).[28] Some remained faithful to the Pfeiffer's bacillus hypothesis, although the laboratory was unable to confirm its role as the specific agent of influenza.[29] This opinion was shared not only by other Spanish civilian doctors but also by those of other countries, as well as by the Committee of the British Military Health Service in France.[30] Spain's *director general de sani-dad* (director general of health), the military doctor Manuel Martín Salazar (1854–1936), defended this hypothesis at the beginning of the epidemic, although over the course of its development he abandoned it in the face of his inconclusive laboratory results.[31]

In accordance with these laboratory results, four other etiological hypotheses, similar to those that emerged in other countries, arose.[32] The first proposed that a different bacterium from the Pfeiffer bacillus, unique for all cases of influenza (a view supported by the military doctor Rafael Criado Cardona), was responsible.[33] The second promoted a bacterial association (initially defended by Martín Salazar).[34] The third introduced a "filterable virus." Martín Salazar abandoned his support of bacterial association in favor of this hypothesis after learning of Charles Nicolle's research at the Institut Pasteur in Tunis.[35] This was also the opinion of some military and civilian commissions outside Spain.[36] The fourth assumed an unknown agent, which both Martín Salazar and Palanca defended.[37] This theory had more followers outside Spain than inside.[38]

The inability of laboratories to solve the problem of the etiology of influenza during the course of the pandemic had a negative impact not only on how to tackle treatment and prophylaxis but also on diagnosis. In fact, some doctors—both military and civilian—suggested such divergent diagnoses as cholera, dengue, epidemic typhus, and typhoid fever.[39] There was even talk of the plague.[40] The friction between clinicians and bacteriologists exacerbated the situation.[41] Disagreements were evident not only in the sessions of the Real Academia de Medicina (Royal Academy of Medicine) but also in the pages of the *Revista de Sanidad Militar* and of the military newspapers, especially *La Correspondencia Militar*.[42] While clinicians clearly identified the disease as influenza, bacteriologists and clinicians who wanted to make use of bacteriology for diagnosis found problems in doing so. This situation prompted the military doctor Palanca to state, "[if] it had been possible to suppress bacteriological knowledge, no one would have doubted that it was flu." In his opinion, what was happening was an example of "the possibility of the paradox that an excess of bacteriology might be damaging." In support of his opinion, he cited the examples of other viral diseases: "nobody worries about the laboratory diagnosis of smallpox, measles, scarlet fever, etc.; and yet all of these conditions are easily diagnosed. They may have their specific agents, but it is unnecessary to see them to prove they are there."[43]

For Palanca, the experience of the influenza pandemic of 1918–19 confirmed that "the laboratory was a most important ancillary to the clinic; but if maximum utility was required from the laboratory, it was essential to guide it and back it up with clinical data."[44] Similarly, the health crisis of 1918–19 highlighted the difficulties in achieving consensus among Spanish doctors, both civilian and military, on the etiological agent of influenza. It could be argued that the lack of appropriate technical resources—such as the fact that electron microscopy was not yet available—and the consequent inability to see the influenza virus led to this lack of consensus. But, as Palanca suggested, in diseases such as smallpox or measles, what was important was not seeing their specific agents but rather achieving professional consensus about them.[45]

The need to address the existing serious health problem called for the formulation and adoption of various prophylactic and therapeutic measures to limit the spread of the epidemic and minimize its effects.[46] Although some of these were common to the Civilian and Medical Health Services, the peculiarities of the latter, and its preoccupation with acting quickly to combat the rapid spread within the army, gave rise to certain differences. Military doctors were clear proponents of the resources of public health, such as isolating the sick, which they regarded as one of the major public preventive measures against the influenza of 1918–19. In fact, the Comisión de Higiene Militar (Military Health Commission) was in favor of isolating the sick "until at least a month after the beginning of convalescence," although the circumstances of the time made it impossible to put this into practice.[47] In turn, for the deputy medical inspector, José Valderrama, "the only prophylactic measure for this infection within the Army" was "to discharge [rapidly] the largest possible number of individuals."[48] The Health Commission shared this opinion, although it recognized the difficulties of carrying it out in the case of the influenza.[49] It was likewise difficult to improve the sanitary conditions of the barracks, another of the preventive measures proposed, which some military doctors were confident could be achieved after the approval of the Law of Military Reorganization and Reform, then under discussion in Parliament.[50] But the only measure that seemed viable, in the opinion of Deputy Medical Inspector Valderrama, was "to disinfect and whitewash all the barracks."[51]

These four measures—isolating the sick, discharging the greatest number of soldiers, improving the sanitary conditions of the barracks, and disinfecting and whitewashing all the barracks—all of which were difficult to put into practice, were the main preventative measures proposed by military doctors to mitigate the effects of the 1918–19 pandemic in the Spanish army. Although the sources I consulted contain no references to doctors feeling "defenseless" against influenza—a suggestion Martín Salazar (*director general de sanidad*) had made to the Real Academia de Medicina (Royal Academy of Medicine)—it is nevertheless conceivable that many doctors did, in fact, feel this way. First, the resources that the Public Health Service routinely used to combat epidemics did not seem to be very effective against the pandemic. Second, as emphasized by the inspector general, there was "no specific vaccine or preventive measure against the flu," since the issue of the etiological agent of this disease had not been resolved.[52] In spite of this, the Military Medical Service—especially the hospital in Carabanchel, Madrid—collaborated in the preparation of a vaccine that would fight the influenza or, more precisely, avoid its complications.[53] In fact, patients from the Carabanchel hospital, Madrid's provincial hospital run by Drs. Francisco Huertas,[54] José Codina,[55] and the renowned Gregorio Marañón,[56] contributed to the development of the vaccine developed by the Laboratorio Municipal de Madrid (Madrid Municipal Laboratory),[57] then headed by the pharmacist César Chicote.[58] But according to the sources consulted, there is no evidence that military doctors recommended vaccines as a prophylactic resource or that they ever used them. Perhaps the latter was because, by the time the vaccines were ready, the second outbreak in the army was already over.[59]

As was the case in the Civilian Health Service, disinfection was considered to be the key to public and individual prevention of influenza. The Instituto de Higiene Militar (Military Hygiene Institute) recommended disinfecting not only the clothes and personal items of the sick soldiers but also their respiratory excretions. It also recommended disinfecting the mouth with appropriate antiseptic solutions and the nostrils with germicide creams based on boric acid, menthol, salol, gomenol, and the like.[60] Deputy Inspector José Valderrama advocated "the proper cleaning of the skin," avoiding colds and physical fatigue, and "the improvement of soldiers' diet."[61] Civilian health authorities proposed similar measures, and in both cases they were difficult to enforce in the Spain of the time. Not only did the chronic shortage of basic goods worsen during the pandemic, but the poor conditions of most of the barracks did not allow the soldiers to keep themselves properly clean, since they had no baths or showers.[62]

The lack of any specific treatment against influenza led military doctors, like those of the Civilian Health Service, to recommend a wide range of remedies, which included commonly used resources of a symptomatic nature, such as expectorants, analgesics, and tonics, as well as autoserotherapy and serums like equine, antidiphtheria, and antipneumococcal.[63] Although serums were recommended mainly for the treatment of the pulmonary complications of influenza, diphtheria serum was considered by some military physicians as "the indicated pharmacological treatment" for the disease.[64] Tomás Maestre Pérez (1857–1936), a physician and professor of forensic medicine, energetically defended this view.[65] But it is remarkable that, among military health professionals, there was no great debate about the usefulness of serum and, especially, about the controversial use of antidiphtheria serum, like that which took place between doctors of the Sanidad Civil (Civilian Health Service). Not only was it discussed at meetings of the Real Academia de Medicina (Royal Academy of Medicine) and in major medical journals but also in the Congreso (Chamber of Deputies or Congress) and the Senado (Senate).[66] The debate even moved to the pages of the general press. At that time Spanish doctors held two basic positions on serums: while some still considered them simply as resources to activate the body's general defenses, others pointed to immunological specificity.[67]

Contradictions and Inequalities in Soldiers' Medical Attention

Despite various challenges, an attempt was made to apply the proposed preventative and therapeutic measures to lessen the impact of influenza in the barracks. In fact, in the words of one of Barcelona's major newspapers, the regional *inspector de sanidad militar* (military health inspector) gave orders for "the isolation of suspected cases as much as possible" and for "the maximization of the hygienic practices of ventilation, exposure to sunlight and hosing down of all premises and effects," as well as "periodical thorough disinfection, taking care to carry out all personal hygiene procedures, especially of the mouth."[68] Similar action was taken in the other military regions of Spain as they were hit by the flu. Moreover, in the second outbreak of the epidemic, when it reached its peak, military authorities proceeded to discharge surplus reserves of soldiers. This measure was quite controversial, due to the negative impact it had on the spread of the epidemic, as Civilian Health Service doctors complained. Another source of conflict between the Civilian and Military Health Services was the preventative measure of isolation. The military doctor Villalobos admitted its failure and Sierra attributed this to the fact that it had been applied less rigorously in the Civilian Health Service than in the military, due to the mildness of the first outbreak of the epidemic.[69]

The limited effectiveness shown by the preventative measures, and the speed with which influenza spread through the Spanish army in 1918, forced the army to deal swiftly with the sick soldiers. The care they received was quite uneven, especially during the second outbreak, where some had access to medical care in the different Spanish military hospitals and in civilian establishments.[70] They were studied using all the scientific resources then at the disposal of the military doctors—examination of sputum, clumping, blood cultures, inoculation of animals, autopsies, and so on.[71] In these centers, soldiers received the treatments mentioned earlier, including serums in the case of (especially pulmonary) complications, such as influenza-related bronchopneumonia. As indicated by some accounts, those treated in hospitals made better progress than the *soldados de cuota* (soldiers with reduced service) who received medical care at home, where "the poor conditions in some rooms" often aggravated their condition.[72]

The situation got out of control at the height of the first outbreak, and particularly of the second, and it was necessary to equip new premises to care for the sick soldiers.[73] Infirmaries were used and some makeshift rooms were provided in the battered barracks, though this could not satisfy all the needs. After many of the soldiers who had participated in military exercises were hit by the flu, other solutions were sought, such as the "installation of a convalescent hospital in Montjuic Castle" in Barcelona or the conversion of the ancient castle of Zamora into a makeshift infirmary.[74]

In the case of Zamora, the working-class newspaper *El Socialista* reported that "neglect by the authorities reached such an extent that the Sisters of Charity who were entrusted with the care of the patients had to pay from their own pockets for lighting, matches and candles. . . . Under these conditions some soldiers died."[75]

All these measures were inadequate for dealing with the epidemic conditions created from September onward, when reserve soldiers called up to the different barracks for training came down with influenza.[76] In some military areas the lack of space to treat all of those affected, and the need to prevent any further spread within the army, led to a decision to demobilize the newly recruited soldiers. Although Deputy Medical Inspector Valderrama believed this measure had prophylactic value within the army, as the nonmilitary doctor Gonzalo R. Lafora reported in *El Sol*, the discharge of these soldiers served to spread the epidemic to their places of origin.[77] It also caused the death of many of them who were already sick or who fell ill during the journey or soon after reaching their homes. Both *La Correspondencia Militar* and the Ministry of War refuted Lafora's antimilitarism claim.[78] Military authorities instituted legal proceedings against *El Socialista*, which had simply reproduced in its pages what *El Sol* had already published.[79]

A few weeks later Dr. Lafora replied to *La Correspondencia Militar*—again, through the pages of *El Sol*—providing detailed and well-documented information on numerous cases that had occurred in Soria, Burgos, Zamora, and Cadiz, where soldiers were discharged without fulfilling the sanitary precautions necessary to prevent the spread of the epidemic.[80] In some of the cases he cited, soldiers were already sick before arriving at the train station or became sick on the train and died on their way home. These new denunciations by Lafora were reproduced in *El Socialista* and were also presented before the military courts.[81] Lafora criticized the actions of the military authorities, denouncing them as an impediment to achieving the improvements in health promoted by the Civilian Health Service. But he did exempt military doctors from his criticism (a point *El Socialista* left up in the air, and even questioned). It is true that in the case of influenza, it would have been difficult to avoid the spread of the epidemic even if the military had followed the rules set out in the Ministry of War's circular of September 17, in which the Junta de Sanidad Militar (Military Board of Health) recommended proceeding with the discharge of soldiers.[82]

Although the strict implementation of the rules theoretically could have limited the spread of influenza to some degree and might have allowed for better care for the soldiers who were already sick or who fell ill during the journey, perhaps even preventing some deaths, the sanitary conditions of the time made it especially difficult to apply these measures correctly. To do so would have required "premises in habitable conditions" in which, according to the orders of the Junta de Sanidad Militar, "to isolate the individuals from the recruits who were healthy" for eight days, after which those soldiers who were still healthy would be discharged.[83] Although military doctors, like their civilian counterparts, were attempting to modernize and improve the Military Health Service, the Spanish army and its infrastructure had serious shortcomings and deficiencies that became more obvious during the 1918–19 flu pandemic.[84] The events surrounding the discharge of the reserve soldiers is an example of the failure of one of the preventive measures advocated by a number of military doctors and highlighted inequalities in the care and treatment Spanish army soldiers received during the pandemic.

Tensions Suffered by Spanish Military Doctors during the Pandemic

The experience of the 1918–19 influenza pandemic curtailed Spanish military doctors' confidence in the prevailing scientific paradigm of the time, provoking a feeling of professional disaster, as other authors have reported for other countries that took part in World War I.[85] Their theoretical discourse largely coincided with that of the doctors of the Civilian Health Service and that of their colleagues in other countries, as we can see in previous and subsequent chapters of this volume. But, as expected, there was greater pragmatism in the positions military doctors adopted, especially in dealing with the diagnosis of the disease, its prevention, and treatment. The tension they must have felt in their capacity as both physicians and soldiers is reflected in the example of discharging soldiers, under orders from their superiors, even if the soldiers were sick. This action perpetuated the spread of the pandemic and was strongly criticized by doctors of the Civilian Health Service. The extreme conditions imposed by the health crisis of 1918–19 also helped to highlight the tense and troubled relationship between the Military and Civil Health Services, which had characterized Spanish life ever since the reign of Isabel II (1833–68). This tension became more prominent during the first decades of the twentieth century, when some doctors, politicians, and sanitary authorities were favorable to the modernization of Spain and to the need to pay special attention to public health. Military and Civil Health Services competed for a portion of a very meager national budget.

The relationship between the 1918–19 influenza pandemic and World War I was less central in Spain than in other countries. It was limited practically to the introduction of the pandemic into Spain through Portuguese soldiers and Spanish workers returning from central Europe and France. Although the movement of Spanish soldiers contributed to the pandemic spreading, their actions were not determined by the exigencies of war but by poor Spanish military and socioeconomic conditions, an expression of Spanish backwardness.

Notes

1. Esteban Rodríguez Ocaña, "La salud pública en la España de la primera mitad del siglo XX," in *El Centro Secundario de Higiene rural de Talavera de la Reina y la sanidad española de su tiempo,* ed. Juan Atenza and José Martínez (Toledo: JCCM, 2001), 21–42; María-Isabel Porras-Gallo, *Un reto para la sociedad madrileña: La epidemia de gripe de 1918–19* (Madrid: Complutense / Comunidad Autónoma de Madrid, 1997), 107–9; Porras-Gallo, "Una ciudad en crisis: la epidemia de gripe de 1918–19 en Madrid" (PhD diss., Faculty of Medicine, Complutense University of Madrid, 1994), 373–94. Textual quotations are from the CD-ROM version: *Una ciudad en crisis: La epidemia de gripe de 1918–19 en Madrid* (Madrid: Complutense, 2002), www.ucm.es/eprints/2765/.

2. The Military Medical Service refers to the Spanish army, air force and navy. Francisco Javier Martínez Antonio, "Salud pública e imperio en la España Isabelina (1833–1869): El caso de la Sanidad Militar," *Història, Ciências, Saúde: Manguinhos* 13, no. 2 (2006): 445–51; Patrocinio Moratinos Palomero, *Algunos datos para la historia del Instituto de Medicina Preventiva "Capitán Médico Ramón y Cajal," Instituto Anatómico de Sanidad Militar* (Madrid: printed by author, 1988).

3. Charles E. Rosenberg, *Explaining Epidemics and Other Studies in the History of Medicine* (Cambridge: Cambridge University Press, 1992), 279.

4. In addition to the *Revista de Sanidad Militar*—the main professional scientific journal of the Military Health Service—we have consulted *La Correspondencia Militar* and *El Heraldo Militar,* two politico-military newspapers with a long tradition in the nineteenth century, which disappeared in the Second Republic (1931–39). María Dolores Saíz, "La prensa madrileña en torno a 1898," *Historia y Comunicación Social* 3 (1998): 195–200. We have also examined *El Liberal, El Sol, ABC,* and *El Heraldo de Madrid,* the main national daily newspapers of the time, and examples of the commercial press, which gathered strength in the first decades of the twentieth century in Spain. This selection provides a broad spectrum of opinions, from the most conservative and monarchist to the most progressive. But to broaden this spectrum, we have also reviewed *El Socialista,* the organ of the Spanish Socialist Workers' Party. More detailed information on the newspapers mentioned can be found in María Cruz Seoane and María Dolores Saíz, *El siglo XX: 1893–1936,* vol. 3 of *Historia del periodismo en España* (Madrid: Alianza, 1996).

5. Porras-Gallo, *Reto;* Porras-Gallo, *Ciudad en crisis;* María-Isabel Porras-Gallo, "La lucha contra las enfermedades 'evitables' en España y la pandemia de la gripe de 1918–19," *Dynamis* 14 (1994): 159–83; Porras-Gallo, "La profilaxis de las enfermedades infecciosas tras la pandemia gripal de 1918–19: Los seguros sociales," *Dynamis* 13 (1993): 279–93; Porras-Gallo, "Sueros y vacunas en la lucha contra la pandemia de gripe de 1918–1919 en España," *Asclepio* 60, no. 2 (2008): 261–88; Porras-Gallo, "The Place of Serums and Antibiotics in the Influenza Pandemics of 1918–1919 and 1957–1958 Respectively," in *Circulation of Antibiotics: Journeys of Drug Standards, 1930–1970,* ed. Ana Romero, Christoph Gradmann, and María Santesmases (Madrid, ESF Networking Program DRUGS, Preprint no. 1, 2010), 77–96, http://drughistory.eu/downloads/Madrid_Preprint.pdf.

6. As demonstrated in the references contained in notes 6 and 9 of Porras-Gallo, "Sueros y vacunas." In fact, in Spain the influenza pandemic of 1918–19 has

principally been studied from the perspective of historical demography and especially from the social history of medicine. Beatriz Echeverri Dávila, *La gripe española: La pandemia de 1918*–19 (Madrid: Centro de Investigaciones Sociológicas / Siglo XXI, 1993), 110–16. Echeverri Dávila has used as sources the statistics of monthly morbidity of the army, which refer only to the sick members of the rank and file who were hospitalized.

7. Alfred W. Crosby, *Epidemic and Peace, 1918* (Westport, CT: Greenwood, 1976); Crosby, *America's Forgotten Pandemic: The Influenza of 1918* (1989; repr., Cambridge: Cambridge University Press, 2003); Carol R. Byerly, *Fever of War: The Influenza Epidemic in the U.S. Army during World War I* (New York: New York University Press, 2005).

8. Howard Phillips and David Killingray, eds., *The Spanish Influenza Pandemic of 1918–1919: New Perspectives* (London: Routledge, 2003); Dorothy Pettit and Janice Bailie have also studied the 1918–19 pandemic's impact on World War I, as well as on the 1919 Paris peace conference and postwar American life. Dorothy A. Pettit and Janice Bailie, *A Cruel Wind: Pandemic Flu in America, 1918–1920* (Murfreesboro, TN: Timberlane Books, 2008).

9. Byerly, *Fever of War*, 8; italics in the original. In chapter 1 of this volume, the virologist Esteban Domingo offers an extensive explanation on this topic.

10. As Porras-Gallo and Davis and Bertucci have noted, when the flu epidemic started, physicians generally had high confidence in medicine's ability to cope with the epidemic. But when it was over, this confidence was replaced by a feeling of a professional disaster. See the introduction and chapter 2 of this volume.

11. Byerly's *Fever of War* also examines the impact of the 1918–19 epidemic on the United States army, its medical officers, and their profession through the impact of infectious disease on the American conduct of the war at home and in Europe, the government's responsibility for the health and welfare of its soldiers, and the ways in which cultural values and politics shaped medical policy and historical memory of the epidemic.

12. Thomas Robert Malthus, *An Essay on the Principle of Population* (London: J. Johnson, 1798; repr. 1998, Electronic Scholarly Publishing Project), chapter VII, http://www.esp.org/books/malthus/population/malthus.pdf.

13. From the perspective of the history of the *idea* of relating wars to epidemics, Roger Cooter examines in a stimulating article how this notion was formulated, deployed, and transformed over time. "Of War and Epidemics: Unnatural Couplings, Problematic Conceptions," *Social History of Medicine* 16, no. 2 (2003): 283–302.

14. On Spain as the point of connection, see Porras-Gallo and Davis, introd., in this volume.

15. Sobral, Lima, and Silveira e Sousa also mention the role of Portuguese workers from Spain as vectors for introducing the pandemic in Portugal. See chapter 4 in this volume.

16. Echeverri Dávila, *Gripe española*, 120–22; Porras-Gallo, *Reto*, 52–65; Porras-Gallo, *Ciudad en crisis*, 212–39.

17. José Alberto Palanca, "A propósito de la epidemia actual," *Revista de Sanidad Militar* 8, no. 9 (1918): 573.

18. Echeverri Dávila, *Gripe española*, 111–12; The Commission of the Military Hygiene Institute stressed this characteristic during the pandemic. Ángel Morales, A. Ramírez Santaló, and Emilio Pérez Noguera, "Instituto de Higiene Militar: Informe

sobre las causas de la epidemia desarrollada en esta Corte durante los meses de Mayo y Junio del corriente año," *Revista de Sanidad Militar* 8, no. 15 (1918): 487.

19. Generals and officers are not included in the rank and file. Detailed information on the incidence of influenza in the different corps of the army and Spanish military regions is available in Echeverri Dávila, *Gripe española*, 112, table 23.

20. Echeverri Dávila, *Gripe española*, 113.

21. G. Sierra, "La epidemia reinante: Sus efectos en el ejército," *Revista de Sanidad Militar* 11 (1918): 352.

22. Echeverri Dávila, *Gripe española*, 110–11.

23. Santos Rubiano, "La gripe," *Revista de Sanidad Militar* 21 (1918): 653, 655.

24. Palanca, "Propósito," 577; Rubiano, "Gripe," 652. José Alberto Palanca y Martínez Fortún (1888–1973) was a military doctor, professor of medical microbiology and hygiene at the University of Granada and later of hygiene and health at the Faculty of Medicine at the Complutense University in Madrid, member and president of the Royal National Academy of Medicine as well as of the National Medical Association, director general of health, and director general of Military Health Service. He was a member of the Spanish Parliament from 1933 until the Spanish Civil War and later *procurador* (attorney general) of Las Cortes—a decision-making organ established during Franco's regime.

25. A number of the soldiers discharged during the second outbreak died on their way home or very soon after their arrival. "Para el Ministerio de la Guerra: La gripe y las acusaciones del Doctor Lafora," *El Socialista*, November 16, 1918, 2.

26. Dr. Lafora's denunciations were echoed above all by the news dailies *El Sol* and *El Socialista* throughout the second outbreak, especially during the months of October and November. Gonzalo Rodríguez Lafora (1886–1971) was an important neurologist and psychiatrist and disciple of Santiago Ramón y Cajal and Luis Simarro, with complete international scientific training in Germany. He described the "Lafora disease" and founded the Instituto Médico-Pedagógico (Medico-Pedagogical Institute). After the Spanish Civil War he had to go into exile, cofounding the Instituto de Estudios Médicos y Biológicos (Institute of Medical and Biological Studies) in the Autonomous University of Mexico. Valentín Matilla Gómez, *202 Biografías Académicas* (Madrid: Real Academia Nacional de Medicina, 1987), accessed March 1, 2012, www.ranm.es/academicos/academicos-de-numero-anteriores/945-1933-rodriguez-lafora-gonzalo.html.

27. See chapters 2, 4, 6, and 7 of this volume.

28. The members of this committee were Maj. Dr. Ángel Morales, Lt.-Col. Dr. Alberto Ramírez Santaló, and deputy head Lt.-Col. Dr. Emilio Pérez Noguera. This committee issued a report on July 12 1918, which was published on August 1, 1918, in Morales, Ramírez, and Pérez, "Instituto de Higiene Militar."

29. Sierra, "Epidemia reinante," 349–52; Morales, Ramírez, and Pérez, "Instituto de Higiene Militar"; Rubiano, "Gripe," 653–55.

30. Porras-Gallo, *Ciudad en crisis*, 316. Bertucci studies the Brazil case in chapter 2 of this volume.

31. Manuel Martín Salazar (1854–1936), military doctor, professor of military hygiene, director of the Section of Serums and Vaccines of the Instituto de Higiene Militar (Military Institute of Hygiene), *inspector general de sanidad exterior* (general inspector of foreign health), and, later, *director general de sanidad* (director general of health), and member of the Real Academia Nacional de Medicina (Royal National

Academy of Medicine), where he played an important role in its scientific debates. Valentín Matilla Gómez, "Martín Salazar, Manuel." In *202 Biografías Académicas*, Madrid: Real Academia Nacional de Medicina, 1987 (www.ranm.es/academicos/ academicos-de-numero-anteriores/1051-1913-martin-salazar-manuel.html, accessed March 1, 2012). The role of Manuel Martín Salazar during the pandemic as *director general de sanidad* was similar to Ricardo Jorge's in Portugal. See Nunes's contribution to this volume in chapter 3.

32. Detailed information on the etiological debate and the different theories advanced both during and after the pandemic in Spain can be found in Porras-Gallo, *Ciudad en crisis*, 311–27, and in chapter 2 of this volume we can follow the same debate in Brazil.

33. Rafael Criado Cardona, "Las broncopneumonías gripales y su tratamiento," *Revista de Sanidad Militar* 23 (1918): 721–24.

34. Martín Salazar expressed this opinion not only in military medical forums, but also in the Spanish Royal Academy of Medicine. "Session of November 2, 1918," *Anales de la Real Academia de Medicina* 38 (1918): 425–30; "Session of November 9, 1918," *Anales de la Real Academia de Medicina* 38 (1918): 430–49.

35. Nicolle's research included "experiments on animals," which for Martín Salazar had "more validity than all the research based on looking for the germ and dyeing it." "Session of October 26 1918," *Anales de la Real Academia de Medicina* 38 (1918): 410.

36. Porras-Gallo, *Ciudad en crisis*, 324. As Bertucci notes in chapter 2 of this volume, this was also the position of Brazilian doctors without knowing the discovery of Nicolle.

37. Manuel Martín Salazar, "Comentarios al presupuesto de Sanidad: Los hospitales de epidemias," *Revista de Sanidad Militar* 8 (1920): 219–23; José Alberto Palanca, "El papel del Bacilo de Pfeiffer en la gripe," *Revista de Sanidad Militar* 20 (1918): 612–18.

38. Porras-Gallo, *Ciudad en crisis*, 326.

39. Palanca, "Propósito," 573. As Bertucci shows in chapter 2 of this volume, similar debate was in Brazil.

40. This situation came about at the beginning of the second outbreak of the epidemic. It was not exclusive to military doctors, but also happened in the civilian sector. Porras-Gallo, *Ciudad en crisis*, 294–311.

41. For example, see José Valderrama, "La actual epidemia," *Correspondencia Militar*, June 10, 1918, 1.

42. The disagreements between clinicians and bacteriologists became clear after the late May 1918 session, which the academy devoted to the 1918–19 influenza. "Session of May 25, 1918," *Anales de la Real Academia de Medicina* 38 (1918): 310–19; Sierra, "Epidemia reinante," 349; Rubiano, "Gripe," 653–54.

43. Palanca, "Bacilo de Pfeiffer," 614.

44. Ibid., 573. The declarations of Palanca should not lead us to believe that he eschewed the laboratory in his clinical practice. Quite the contrary: the latter was very much marked by its use, as shown by his work "Propósito."

45. Palanca, "Bacilo de Pfeiffer," 614.

46. It is worth considering chapters 3, 4, 6, and 7 of this volume to compare similarities and differences among the different prophylactic and therapeutic measures adopted during the Spanish influenza in Spain, Portugal and Brazil.

47. Morales, Ramírez, and Pérez, "Instituto de Higiene Militar," 487.

48. Valderrama, "Actual epidemia."

49. Morales, Ramírez, and Pérez, "Instituto de Higiene Militar," 487.

50. Coinciding with the first outbreak of the pandemic, Parliament was discussing the draft of a bill for military reorganization and reform, which some military doctors hoped would mean more money available for, among other things, improving the conditions of the barracks. "Dictamen de la comisión sobre el proyecto de ley dando fuerza de tal a los reales decretos relativos a reorganización del Ejército . . . ," *Diario de las Sesiones de Cortes: Congreso de los Diputados*, Madrid, May 21, 1918, app. 19–41, pp. 1–27; "Ley sancionada por S. M., dando fuerza de tal a los reales decretos relativos a reorganización del Ejército . . . ," *Diario de las Sesiones*, July 11, 1918, app. 3–74, pp. 1–29. In fact, when the act was adopted and Spain was in the middle of the second outbreak of the epidemic, the pages of *La Correspondencia Militar* urged that it was time to proceed to its application, thereby achieving a solution to the "barracks issue," which in the writer's view was "the army's fundamental problem, often denounced but without achieving any solution so far." As the newspaper went on to say, "its solution must be swift, for if not we run the serious risk of military reforms being reduced to an increase in salary and material benefits, which would be fatal to the prestige of the army." "La aplicación de las reformas militares," *Correspondencia Militar* (September 18, 1918), 1.

51. Valderrama, "Actual epidemia," 1.

52. "Session of June 28, 1918," *Anales de la Real Academia de Medicina* 38 (1918): 385.

53. "Session of November 9, 1918," 437, 448.

54. Francisco Huertas y Barrero (1847–1933), military and civilian doctor, director of the Medical Service at the General Hospital of Madrid, member of the Real Consejo de Sanidad (Royal Council of Health), and member of the Real Academia Nacional de Medicina. Valentín Matilla Gómez, "Huertas y Barrero, Francisco." In *202 Biografías Académicas* (www.ranm.es/academicos/academicos-de-numero-anteriores/1001-1904-huertas-y-barrero-francisco.html, accessed March 1, 2012).

55. José Codina Castellví (1867–1934), excellent doctor, specialist in respiratory and infectious diseases, professor of the Faculty of Medicine in Barcelona, correspondent member of the Academia de Medicina de Barcelona (Academy of Medicine of Barcelona), member of the Real Academia Nacional de Medicina. Valentín Matilla Gómez, "Codina y Castellví, José." In *202 Biografías Académicas* (www.ranm.es/academicos/academicos-de-numero-anteriores/894-1902-codina-y-castellvi-jose.html, accessed March 1, 2012).

56. Gregorio Marañón y Posadillo (1887–1960), very prestigious doctor with German postdoctoral training, member of the special governmental commission sent to France for studying the influenza pandemic, member of different academies (the Real Academia Nacional de Medicina [Royal National Academy of Medicine], the Academia de la Lengua [Language Academy], the Academia de la Historia [History Academy], the Bellas Artes [Beaux-Arts Academy], and Ciencias Exactas, Físicas, y Naturales [Exact, Physical, and Natural Sciences]), and prolific author. Marino Gómez-Santos, *Gregorio Marañón cuenta su vida* (Madrid: Aguilar, 1961); Pedro Laín Entralgo, *Gregorio Marañón: Vida, obra y persona* (Madrid: Espasa Calpe, 1969); Gómez-Santos, *Vida de Gregorio Marañón* (Madrid: Taurus, 1971); Laín

Entralgo, *Cajal, Unamuno, Marañón: Tres españoles* (Madrid: Círculo de Lectores, 1988); Enrique Cornide Ferrant, *Apasionante biografía de Gregorio Marañón: Un hombre para la historia* (A Coruña, Spain: Maxan, 1999); Gómez-Santos, *Gregorio Marañón* (Barcelona: Plaza and Janés, 2001); Juan Francisco Jiménez Borreguero, *Gregorio Marañón: El regreso del humanismo* (Madrid: Egartorre Libros, 2006); Antonio López Vega, *Gregorio Marañón: Radiografía de un liberal* (Madrid: Taurus, 2011).

57. This laboratory was among those that played the most important role during the 1918–19 influenza pandemic. Porras-Gallo, *Reto*.

58. Porras-Gallo, "Sueros y vacunas," 284. César Chicote Riego (1861–1950)—pharmacist, director of the Laboratorio Municipal de Madrid (Madrid Municipal Laboratory), member of the Real Academia Nacional de Medicina, and honorary member of the Real Academia de Farmacia (Royal Academy of Pharmacy)—played an important role in the sanitary municipal modernization during the influenza pandemic. Instituto de España, *Académicos numerarios del Instituto de España (1938–2004)* (Madrid: Instituto de España, 2005), www.ranm.es/academicos/academicos-de-numero-anteriores/889-1911-chicote-y-del-riego-cesar.html (accessed March 1, 2012).

59. In chapter 2 of this volume, Bertucci notes the same in Brazil.

60. Morales, Ramírez, and Pérez, "Instituto de Higiene Militar," 487.

61. Valderrama, "Actual epidemia," 1; "Por la salubridad del ejército: Cuestiones sanitarias," *Correspondencia Militar*, September 17, 1918, 2.

62. Porras-Gallo, *Reto*, 71–99; Porras-Gallo, *Ciudad en crisis*, 509–13.

63. Criado, "Broncopneumonías gripales," 722–24; Villalobos, "Algunas observaciones sobre el tratamiento de la epidemia reinante," *Revista de Sanidad Militar* 2 (January 15, 1919): 25–32; Valderrama, "Actual epidemia," 1. As noted in chapters 2, 4, 6, and 7 of this volume, a similar situation occurred in other countries.

64. Valderrama, "Actual epidemia," 1.

65. A detailed account of Maestre's fierce defense of antidiphtheria serum as the specific treatment for flu is to be found in Porras-Gallo, "Sueros y vacunas," 271–73. Tomás Maestre Pérez (1857–1936) was doctor of several provincial hospitals, inspector de salubridad (inspector of health) in Murcia, Spain, during the cholera epidemic of 1885, professor of forensic medicine and psychiatry at the Central University of Madrid, director of the Instituto de Medicina Legal y Toxicología (Forensic Medicine and Toxicology Institute), and member of the Real Academia Nacional de Medicina and of the Academia Anatómica Española (Spanish Anatomical Academy). Instituto de España, *Académicos numerarios del Instituto de España (1938–2004)* (Madrid: Instituto de España, 2005).

66. The Congreso and the Senado constitute the Spanish Parliament, represent the Spanish people, and exercise the legal authority of the state.

67. For information on the therapeutic resources proposed for doctors belonging to the Civilian Health Service and the debates over the validity of the different serums and, particularly, over the controversial antidiphtheria serum, see Porras-Gallo, "Sueros y vacunas," 274–71.

68. "La epidemia reinante: Adopción de medidas," *La Vanguardia*, October 9, 1918, 18.

69. Villalobos, "Algunas observaciones," 25; Sierra, "Epidemia reinante," 350–52. The truth is that, as Martín Salazar alleged in 1920, the lack of adequate civilian

hospitals in which to isolate people with infectious diseases had been the real reason why this measure could not be implemented during the 1918–19 influenza and why the health crisis had become more serious in Spain. "Comentarios," 219–21.

70. This happened to the soldiers of the Reus light infantry battalion when they were attacked by influenza during the second outbreak. Many of these soldiers were treated at the civilian hospital in Manresa. "La epidemia reinante: La guarnición de Manresa," *La Vanguardia*, October 9, 1918, 18.

71. Palanca, "Propósito"; Morales, Ramírez, and Pérez, "Instituto de Higiene Militar," 487.

72. "La epidemia reinante: La guarnición de Manresa," 18.

73. The speed with which the pandemic spread and the large number of victims meant that the service in many corps was disrupted. Such was the case with the Military Medical Corps, where the number of physicians affected was so high that, in the case of Madrid, it was necessary to call on the services of students from the Military Medical Academy. Sierra, "Epidemia reinante," 350.

74. "La epidemia reinante: Adopción de medidas," 18.

75. "Zamora," *El Socialista*, October 13, 1918, 2.

76. As some military doctors pointed out, the lack of immunity of the recently drafted men was responsible for their being affected by the influenza. Palanca, "Propósito," 577; Rubiano, "Gripe," 652.

77. Valderrama, "Actual epidemia," 1; Gonzalo R. Lafora, "Desarrollo de la epidèmia de gripe en España," *El Sol*, October 21, 1918.

78. "La actitud antimilitarista: Horrores contra la verdad," *La Correspondencia Militar*, October 22, 1918, 1; "Ministerio de la Guerra," *El Socialista*, October 24, 1918, 2.

79. "Para el Ministerio," 2. Ever since the so-called Colonial Disaster of 1898 (i.e., the Spanish-American War), and especially since the Disaster of Annual (1909), the Spanish military reacted very badly to criticism and calls for accountability for its actions. Juan Picasso González, *El expediente Picasso: Las sombras de Annual* (Madrid: Almena, 2003). Different sectors of Spanish society made these criticisms in various forums, including the general and workers' press, as occurred during the 1918–19 influenza pandemic.

80. Gonzalo R. Lafora, "Para el Ministro de la Guerra. Sobre la epidemia gripal. Realidades y no insidias," *El Sol*, November 3, 1918, 2.

81. Gonzalo R. Lafora, "Señalando responsabilidades," *El Socialista*, October 22, 1918, 1; "Para el Ministerio Guerra."

82. "Para el Ministerio."

83. "Los reclutas y la gripe," *El Socialista*, February 18, 1919; "Para el Ministerio."

84. According to Democratic Party member Francos Rodríguez, the Military Health Service was just as neglected in terms of resources as the civilian service. "Mitin Sanitario," *El Socialista*, November 3, 1918, 2.

85. Byerly, Tognotti and Witte report similar reactions. Byerly, *Fever of War*; Eugenia Tognotti, "Scientific Triumphalism and Learning from Facts: Bacteriology and the 'Spanish Flu' Challenge of 1918," *Social History of Medicine* 16, no. 1 (2003): 97–110; Wilfried Witte, "The Plague That Was Not Allowed to Happen: German Medicine and the Influenza Epidemic of 1918–19 in Baden," in Phillips and Killingray, *Spanish Influenza Pandemic*, 49–57.

Chapter Six

The Reign of the Spanish Flu

Impact and Responses to the 1918 Influenza Pandemic in Minas Gerais, Brazil

ANNY JACKELINE TORRES SILVEIRA

When the 1918 influenza pandemic irrupted onto the world, Belo Horizonte, the capital of the state of Minas Gerais, Brazil, had been in existence for only two decades. Inaugurated on December 12, 1897, the city was constructed in accordance with the scientific knowledge of engineering and other propositions considered essential for the planning and good governance of urban spaces and was therefore proclaimed young and modern. Despite harking back to the colonial period, the project to construct a new capital in Minas became effective only with the arrival of the republic in 1889.

The construction of the new capital of Minas Gerais can be understood best within the context of the economic, social, and political modernization that characterized the Brazilian nation from the 1870s onward. The abolition of slavery in 1888 and the establishment of the republican regime in 1889 would be two cornerstones in this process, which had as one of its major scenarios the space of the cities. At the turn of the nineteenth and twentieth centuries, various Brazilian cities experienced the phenomenon of urban growth and its impacts on the social and economic order. The sanitary problems brought about by urbanization reaffirmed the association between disease and dirt and influenced the views of doctors and laypeople alike, thus conditioning the public imaginary about the city and grounding the many urban interventions undertaken by the authorities of that period. Another important association existed between progress and hygiene: the salubrity of urban areas was seen as an index of modernity and civilization.[1] This ideal permeated the history of the new capital from the moment of its conception well until into the twentieth century.

Unlike the reforms seen in other Brazilian cities, which favored a particular area of the urban fabric, the project of the new capital of Minas ignored previous occupations and uses attributed by the population to the areas of the old town. The old town was completely destroyed to make room for a new city designed on paper. Buildings, squares, streets, and avenues were entirely new and predetermined, as were the activities housed in each region, with defined areas for commerce, housing, and administration. Palaces, boulevards, squares, and high-scale commerce were designed to give the new capital, bathed in fresh air and sunlight, a tone of civility and cosmopolitanism. The city also provided services essential for good hygiene—water, sewage, and a series of regulations to guide the activities and use of spaces. But if building a city in an area without taking into account what was already there was novel at the time, the principles that motivated Belo Horizonte's construction were similar to those that underpinned the major urban reforms of the nineteenth century.[2]

The unique urban history of Belo Horizonte impressed on the popular imaginary the notion that Belo Horizonte was a salubrious city par excellence. In addition, the absence of maladies—plague, yellow fever, cholera—that periodically afflicted other Brazilian cities led, in the words of a chronicler in 1918, to real indifference from the population when faced with epidemic threats. Nonetheless, despite its history, Belo Horizonte, like so many other cities, succumbed to the great influenza pandemic of 1918. As in other cities around the world, the disease caused astonishment and fear in the Belo Horizonte population and bewilderment in the public health and scientific authorities, incredulous that the manifestation of a disease as ordinary as the flu could bring so much damage and suffering.

Throughout this chapter, we explore the cultural dimensions of the 1918 influenza pandemic by examining certain aspects of the life experiences of Belo Horizonte residents.[3] Our analysis builds on historiographical thinking that identifies an epidemic as an event that is at once biological and cultural, that possesses a standard dramaturgic narrative, and that is structured by denial, recognition, action, and reflection on the epidemic experience.[4] In the first part, we discuss how the influenza contaminated both the press and the population of Belo Horizonte, even prior to the disease outbreak in the city. Uncertainty regarding the etiology of the disease, combined with mortality data at odds with what seemed to be such a familiar disease, contributed to the spread of the viewpoint that the so-called contagion of fear was responsible for the damages caused by the pandemic.[5] We also show how the acclaimed salubrity of the capital was insufficient to prevent the devastation caused by the influenza.

In the second part of the chapter, we deal with the experience of the pandemic among the city's population. If there was disbelief initially about the turmoil the disease could cause, it dissipated as soon as the influenza manifested in Minas. Given public authorities' inability to prevent the disease from spreading, it was left to the city's population to mobilize itself to tackle the repercussions of the epidemic. The Spanish flu disrupted every sphere of social life, from daily labor, the supply of merchandise, and the provision of public services to those aspects that structure and organize human experience, such as religious rites, beliefs, and sociability.[6]

News of Contagion

Even before Belo Horizonte fell prey to the influenza pandemic of 1918 in early October, news of the disease had already infected the media and popular imagination. In mid-August, a Brazilian navy division traveling from Freetown to the port of Dakar experienced the first manifestations of the disease.[7] By mid-September, around fifty-five members of the group had died.[8] News reports on the mainland of a frightening flu epidemic that had attacked the Brazilian squad while on its way to France began to appear that same month. In addition to officer airmen and the squadron of seamen, the navy division had a medical mission composed of civilians and military people bound for campaign hospitals on the European continent.[9] Among its members were two professors of the Faculty of Medicine of Belo Horizonte, two nursing assistants, and the head of the laboratory of the Santa Casa de Misericordia hospital, all of whom enjoyed a certain degree of reputation in the capital city.

The publication and rapid circulation of news reports about the sick and the dead immediately piqued public curiosity about the disease. The inclusion of prominent members of local society among victims of the disease and the controversy surrounding the nature of the flu only added to the interest. Given that the exercise of naming is also one of learning and mastering, the uncertainty surrounding the nature of the malady threatening Brazilian society could only produce apprehension and interest.[10] And despite published reports that referred to the disease as influenza, its virulence and increasing death rates prompted doctors and laypeople to doubt the diagnosis.[11]

During September the chief of the army's Corps of Health, Adm. Lopes Rodrigues, stated that it was difficult to determine the etiology of the epidemic that had struck the Brazilian squad, adding that the disease was not "the flu we know because it does not kill the same way."[12] As noted by Liane Maria Bertucci in chapter 2, the variety of symptoms and the number of casualties prompted doctors to suspect different diagnoses: dengue fever, typhus, and cholera. The press referred to it as the "plague of Dakar."[13] An example of the uncertainty that prevailed within the medical establishment is shown in the following statement from Dr. Carlos Seidl, director general of public health in Rio de Janeiro and one of the country's leading health authorities: "I only know that it is flu or malignant influenza [the nature of which], however, is still shrouded in doubt."[14]

News reports increased in frequency and length when the pandemic reached Brazil. In early October newspapers in Belo Horizonte confirmed the presence of influenza in Rio, the country's capital. The first disease cases, which erupted in Vila Militar, were significant because they called attention to the large number of people infected, not because of how virulent they were. The justice and internal affairs minister, Carlos Maximiliano Pereira dos Santos, stated that health authorities would remain vigilant "against the invasion of the malady of Dakar, not taking, however, exceptional measures [to act] in cases of the influenza that had occurred in Rio, because this malady visits us periodically in a benign form, with no serious effects, but [the same authorities would be] acting permanently against the imported cases of Dakar, which, it seems, came in a more serious form. During the following days, army officials endeavored to tackle fears surrounding the influenza cases, asserting that patients presented a mild disease. They contended that flu incursions among the troops happened every year and that October (a spring month in the southern hemisphere) was a predetermined period when the disease manifested. In view of this, had it not been for the concern about the Spanish influenza, which was raging in Europe at the time, cases in Belo Horizonte would have gone unnoticed.[15]

On October 12 the flu was reported among employees of the railway Central do Brasil, which was on the verge of having all its services suspended. Subsequent reports highlighted the multiplication of infected people and the effects produced by the disease that was spreading in Rio de Janeiro. News reports about the first victims sought to dispel fears, attributing deaths to the poor health and social conditions of people who were ill rather than to the disease itself.[16] Despite being reproduced exhaustively in the city's newspapers, however, such reports did not seem to deter the spread of terror, which increased daily among residents of the capital. While the population turned its attention to events in Rio de Janeiro, the disease emerged unnoticed in Belo Horizonte.

The Contagion of Fear

The discrepancies between the statements about the benignity of the disease found in the country and the press data being published daily, which indicated an exponential growth of notifications and fatalities, only increased the uncertainty among the general population and the medical profession. In an epoch in which science seemed to have the answers to all of society's ills, especially after the triumphs of the "bacteriological era," medicine had no explanation for such an unusual flu manifestation. Without the necessary tools to understand and respond to the biological contamination of the influenza, doctors began to discuss the contagion of fear. Frequent press statements by doctors stated that they were convinced many people were suffering as a result of alarm and disorientation produced less by the disease itself than by the "sensational news."[17] This emphasis on the consequences of the threat of the epidemic disease on social behavior was promulgated in different medical manuals of the period: "If courage does not protect against infection, it cannot be denied that terror, in the presence of an infectious agent, is a predisposing cause for an attack capable of promoting fatal termination; everything that tends to decrease an individual's vital resistance creates a morbid predisposition in epidemic times."[18]

This position was repeated exhaustively by the country's health authorities in newspaper reports published in the republic's capital and by the local press in Belo Horizonte. On October 17 the *Minas Gerais* published the advice of a renowned homeopath from Rio de Janeiro, who affirmed the need to maintain calm "and not be frightened even by the almost terrifying symptoms which sometimes can occur."[19] Two days later the newspaper highlighted the physician Teófilo Torres's declaration that the "auto-suggestion and excessive fear which had developed in people" contributed to worsening their disposition, facilitating the disease attack. Considering the disease a "very curable malady," he called on people to assist the authorities in combating it energetically through detachment and moral strength.[20]

On October 23 the *Minas Gerais* reproduced an article titled "Influenzaphobia," which pointed out the need to combat the state of panic created by the flu. The disease was considered to be harmful to patients and healthy people alike, as well as to the most essential and regular community services and activities, such as the commerce of manufactured goods. The author also noted that "disorder of the spirit causes disorder of things" and that the flu's severity, to that point, was not due to its mortality but to the fact that it "prostrates whole populations, suddenly disorganizing services and causing suffering to all." To counteract this disorganization, he called for a bit of calm and judgment to dispel the "collective madness" that had taken hold of society.[21]

The attitude of blaming the tragic and even lethal character of the disease on fear was a truth accepted outside medical circles too. On October 20 the press in Minas welcomed the measures set up by the federal government for the restoration of normality in Rio de Janeiro, which included, apart from the creation of rescue posts and the free distribution of medicines, the resolution of "not allowing alarming stories to circulate."[22] Censorship, officially established by the government in the federal capital and also observed in other cities in the country, was aimed at protecting weak minds from the "dangerous ideas" and "climate of fear" generated by the sensationalism of some newspapers.[23] This "diagnosis of fear," although mentioned by the medical and sanitary authorities of the country at the time, has its roots in the distant past when the line between truth and legend was less clear.

The Modern City versus the Influenza Pandemic

On October 19 an article titled "The Contagion of Panic" reproduced an Asian legend describing a dialogue between a muezzin—the person who summons the faithful to prayer from a minaret—and the angel of cholera. After seeing the angel with its black wings cross the skies toward the European continent, the muezzin supplicates him to save the people from that terrible scourge. The "archangel of extermination" declares he is obeying an injunction from God, who had ordered him to reap twenty thousand lives, returning to the Ganges estuary within six months. Questioned after his return about the fact that more than sixty thousand people had died, the angel replies, "I killed only twenty thousand: the others were killed by fear."[24]

The story served as a pretext for the author to justify the bleak outlook that the pandemic produced in the capital of Minas and to try to buoy up the spirits of his readers. The text makes it clear that panic is an integral aspect of epidemics and linked to the omnipresence and invisibility of danger and death. It states that all epidemics are accompanied by "two minions, lies and fear." Once a disease erupts, it leads to the "contagion of fear," which renders individuals incapable of any reasoning and, because of this, is equally or more harmful than the disease itself. This irrational fear fuels rumors, which change "small truths into an enormous nebula of vague and horrific forms."[25]

To neutralize the fear imposed by the influenza on the city's population, the author invoked the city's salubrious image. He maintained it was necessary to bear in mind that "in terms of hygiene, Belo Horizonte is an ideal city." Unlike some of world's major capitals where cholera epidemics were an important reason for reforming the precarious conditions of housing and hygiene that existed in the nineteenth century, Belo Horizonte was already salubrious at the time of its foundation, the construction of which was based on the same precepts of health interventions that occurred in cities like London and Paris. The city of Belo Horizonte had wide avenues that promoted increased air circulation and sunlight and a well-equipped public health service ready to "give a good fight to any epidemic that will visit us." In this way, the author claimed, the flu would produce a plethora of "catarrhal people and little else" and would not lead to more than "three days of fever and lack of appetite."[26]

Nonetheless, if some saw the capital's salubrity so positively, others perceived it as a real problem. Such was the opinion of Dr. Octaviano Almeida, who, after responding to two cases of influenza in people living in a guest-house in Belo Horizonte, was "seriously impressed by the lack of fear with which its inhabitants joked about the 'Spanish' flu, which seemed not to have been taken into account by anyone." Almeida felt people had not yet been concerned about the disease, believing "the flu was worth as much as having any coryza." According to him, this behavior was explained by the wide acceptance among the city's residents of a discourse that proclaimed the good hygiene conditions of the capital. Another factor supporting the belief in the capital's immunity to the flu outbreak was the absence of terrible epidemics—such as cholera, yellow fever, and plague—which had racked some of the main Brazilian cities. As a result, people let their guard down against epidemic threats. Almeida suggested that if the influenza epidemic were to disrupt the city's life, the residents' behavior could be blamed.[27]

But press reports from the latter months of 1918 reveal the capital's salubrity was not a deterrent to the outbreak and spread of the pandemic in the city. On the other hand, these reports also made it clear the city's salubrious image related only to some parts of the urban fabric: the city center and the area intended for housing state employees and the installation of public offices. A city patterned after Washington, DC—with its checkerboard layout, long highway circling the whole city, broad avenues lined with trees, well-lit and spacious streets, low buildings that provided for open space and landscaping, efficient urban services, and sanitary regulations—Belo Horizonte's modernity was nevertheless not a reality for the entire population. Underprivileged people who were ignored in the planning and construction of the new capital occupied the outskirts of the city. In this space, daily life was different, as revealed in the complaints sections published in the city's periodicals since the beginning of the twentieth century: the layout of streets was irregular, there was a lack of sanitation and drinking water, and residents were subjected to surveillance efforts by law enforcement.[28] In many ways, these areas of the city differed little from the insalubrious neighborhoods found in Rio de Janeiro, London, or Paris in the mid-nineteenth century.

Not only was Belo Horizonte's modernity accessible only to a limited segment of the population, but it was also unable to stave off the impact of the Spanish flu, the viral nature of which bacteriology had yet to reveal. The influenza was different in nature from other diseases encountered in the course of the nineteenth century, such as plague or cholera. These diseases, even if they could not be explained, were capable of being contained by quarantine, urban improvements, and other interventions founded on the theories of hygiene and environmentalism of the second half of the nineteenth century, which were aimed at eliminating the causal agent of diseases. Due to airborne transmission, urban crowding, and the growing ease of movement of people in the modern world, the flu called for a health agenda much more refined and complex, one that could be monitored and administered. In 1918 this organization did not exist anywhere in Brazil or the world.[29]

The Experience of Contagion

The first cases of the pandemic flu arrived in the capital of Minas Gerais on October 7, through an officer's family who had recently arrived from Vila Militar in Rio de Janeiro. Twenty-four hours later they were transferred in an assistance vehicle to the Hospital de Isolamento (Hospital of Isolation). The rigorous disinfection to which the house and hotel where they stayed were subjected terrified the population.[30] The director of hygiene, Samuel Libânio, stated that they were really cases of a benign flu, that the patients were in good condition, and that their discharge was expected shortly. He also said the measures taken by the board were only preventive. A week later the director of hygiene advised the population about the adoption of measures for individual prophylaxis, "which is what can profitably be applied to restrict the malady."[31] Also that same day the state government declared that the "flu," or Spanish influenza, was a disease of compulsory notification.[32] In the same act, it suspended the operation of schools for eight days and admitted the impossibility of isolating Belo Horizonte from Rio de Janeiro, from where several individuals contaminated with the malady had arrived. Despite the city's "privileged conditions for resisting invasion, it was advisable to take all preventive measures within the scope of the public authorities."[33]

On October 18 the Board of Hygiene recorded thirty-two notifications of the disease. The first death from influenza in the city occurred on October 21.[34] From that date until mid-December, the Board of Hygiene released daily bulletins to provide information about the spread of the epidemic. The official data disseminated by the authorities and published by the press showed that before the end of October, the pandemic had taken hold of the city. On October 31 there were 779 official notifications recorded. But it would not be an exaggeration to conclude that the actual number of sick people was far greater than the one divulged.[35] Despite the frightening increase of notifications, health officials continued to assert the benignity of the malady. The disparity of information about the disease and the confusion this generated in the daily life of the city caused much anguish and uncertainty.

One of the most striking aspects of the critical literature on epidemics is the information it provides about the changes in the daily lives of individuals and collectives. The experience of an epidemic, with its entourage of dead and sick people, leads to significant changes in urban life, disorganizing services, promoting escape and isolation of the population, and disrupting relationships, habits, and human beliefs. During an epidemic the images, sounds, attitudes, perceptions, and interpretations that characterize, guide, and give meaning to the city's day-to-day life are either substituted or acquire other meanings. A disease "gives new meaning," whether it is the plague of the Middle Ages, cholera in the nineteenth century, or the Spanish flu in 1918.[36]

The Pandemic and Daily Life in Belo Horizonte

The impact of the pandemic on daily life in the capital was visible as early as October 18, with the suspension of all public school activities. During the following days the doors of private education establishments; the schools of dentistry, pharmacy, veterinary, and agriculture; and the colleges of law and medicine were also closed. The latter reopened a few days later as an interim hospital in which teachers and students took turns caring for flu patients, especially poor people who, according to public authorities, had no way of observing the rules of home isolation.[37] Until that time, hospital treatment was directed to the poor and, in particular, to those who had no material resources to meet medical recommendations regarding medicines, diets, and rest. Wealthy people, on the other hand, took care of themselves at home and received attention from family members apart from daily visits by a trustworthy doctor.[38]

Like schools, commercial establishments and public offices also saw their activities profoundly altered due to the illness of owners and employees. Cinemas, clubs, and other places of entertainment were also closed. Religious, civic, and social events were postponed or canceled due to the "alarming sanitary state of the capital."[39] Streetcars circulated with few passengers. But social unrest was seen only in pharmacies, which were flooded by crowds in search of purgatives and prescriptions for the sick and convalescent. As can be seen in the local press reports, only a week after health authorities had recognized the presence of the influenza in Belo Horizonte, the movement of daily life in the city had been radically altered: "Belo Horizonte lost its bustling life during these days of epidemic. The streets are deserted. . . . All people fled from the most frequented places, and the cafés and restaurants are entirely abandoned, rarely having customers who will come in. All turned away, fearful of the contagion of evil."[40]

The expansion of the epidemic significantly increased the price of many products, including foodstuffs prescribed by doctors—milk, meat, chicken, and lemons—and medicines, most notably quinine, a supposed wonder drug recommended for all ailments.[41] The poor, who suffered most in this situation, were at the mercy of public charity. A broad plan for social mobilization led to the setting up of rescue posts to help in the distribution of medicines and diets, thereby lending moral and material comfort to patients and families from poor neighborhoods. Between the end of October and December, newspapers published daily reports on the setting up of subscription lists for donating diverse items to the poor: food, clothing, medicine, and money. Religious, literary, recreational, and sports associations mobilized their members to care for the sick too. Doctors, nurses, and pharmacists made themselves available to the authorities to attend to patients in hospitals, rescue posts, and homes. Similarly, women and nurses from the Red Cross who had recently qualified in a war-nursing course rendered assistance where possible.[42]

Jean Delumeau has said "the time of pestilence is the time of forced solitude."[43] Quarantines, deserted streets, the reclusion of families, and the escape from cities all mark the reports about the scourge of epidemics from the fourteenth to the eighteenth centuries. People's fear of both the living and the dead undermined the solidarity that traditionally bound them together.[44] But along with this sense of fear, the stories of epidemic events also identify a broad social mobilization aimed at tackling threats posed by disease and insufficient action from public authorities. If an epidemic event is a time of contrasts and extremes, and one that often poorly accommodates itself to the physical and emotional structures that organize and explain social life, then fear and solidarity are certainly examples of contradictory feelings and actions brought about by events of this nature.[45]

In the Brazilian case the network of solidarity established during the 1918 pandemic was not something unusual (see chapter 2); rather, it reinstated a recurrent practice from the nineteenth century, when health assistance involved the work of public charity, religious organizations, and municipalities.[46] The role of the state's public authorities during the nineteenth-century epidemics was limited to supplying medicines and providing medical assistance through doctors responsible for the care of patients. Medical doctors were also in charge of reporting clinical cases about patients and providing feedback on the causes and evolution of disease as well as on the therapies used to eradicate the condition.[47] The collectivization of health, that is, its transformation into a public good, is a process that began in the country only in the 1910s. The Spanish influenza, with its deadly impact, was only one of many events that helped convince Brazilian elites of the intensification of the effects of interdependence on modern societies, leading in the decade ahead to a gradual replacement of individual solutions through the formation of a public health agenda.[48] The epidemic manifestation of bubonic plague, malaria, and yellow fever in large cities and the scientific movement organized in the 1910s in defense of sanitation of the vast Brazilian territory also contributed to this awareness of the importance and interdependence of public health actions—or the collectivization process in public health.[49] It needs to be borne in mind that, regardless of this still traditional and somewhat inefficient organization, no health service would have been able to cope with the extreme situation imposed by the pandemic of 1918.[50]

The Impact of the Pandemic on Social Dynamics

Besides the provision of material relief, epidemic diseases also mobilize a broad repertoire of representations and attitudes that help to illuminate another dimension of human life: the social imaginary. In the face of fear caused by an epidemic, populations employ the most diverse means of understanding, explaining, and dealing with the threat. These means reveal a lot about the beliefs, values, and prejudices of a given society, including how it views disease, its cure, and the world itself.[51] In the case of Belo Horizonte, it is possible to perceive that people used various resources to try to explain and face the tragic episode of the influenza epidemic. Natural phenomena, plots, prayers, processions, amulets, superstitions, herbs, and other traditional healing practices were among the resources invoked by the society to explain the disease and protect itself from the danger it posed.[52] These practices reappeared in narratives about the pandemic in other urban centers and even other epidemic events.[53]

Religion became a fundamental support for people in Belo Horizonte, helping them to bear the losses and changes imposed by the pandemic, besides allowing a possibility for intervening in the course of the scourge, which seemed out of human reach.[54] The religious perception of illness attributes its existence to a divine will, a punishment that requires expiation and retaliation. In the eyes of the Catholic Church, prayer and penance could combat diseases, and the healing of the body was identified with the purification of sins.[55] Thus, on October 23, 24, and 25 the São José Church held public prayers for the cessation of the pandemic and followed the Via Crucis.[56] On October 26 two processions were scheduled, one in São José Church and another in the neighborhood of Quartel, to supplicate San Sebastian for protection and support "against the terrible evil of the epidemic of influenza." Throughout the whole of November the prayers and litany continued, with people begging for the preservation of the city against the "scourge of the plague."[57] While such practices may suggest a return to the behaviors of a distant past—such as that observed during the medieval plagues—they also show that religion still played an important role in the intermediation between humans and disease.

A mixture of tragedy, science, and fruitful imagination imbue the various explanations about the origins of the disease. Some saw the influenza as a harbinger of the Apocalypse, the end of the world marked by constant warfare, famine, and plague. Others perceived the disease as the result of a diabolical machination by Germans who had filled the world with microbe nurseries chemically preserved in the hulls of their ships, an explanation that combined conspiracy theory with the search for scapegoats and the scientific discourse popularized in the period. Some people believed the pandemic resulted from atmospheric changes due to toxic gases produced during the four long years of World War I. Toward the end of December a new explanation linked the disease to the conjunction of three comets whose routes of passage by the earth coincided that year.[58]

Even more diverse than the explanations about the origin of the disease was the repertoire of cures promoted during the pandemic. Vaccines, purges, tonics, and other allopathic remedies as well as a great variety of medicinal plants were given to the sick and healthy. One valuable hint came from France: onion juice, taken through the nose, cured influenza almost instantly, whether it was "Russian, Spanish, Italian or German, it did not matter."[59] Alcoholic beverages were considered to be privileged prophylactics, and many people used little bags that contained naphthalene around the neck.[60] A veritable flood of announcements about the most diverse remedies—powders, pills, syrups, invigorating remedies, and soaps—all of which claimed rather flamboyantly to be infallible in eliminating the germs that caused influenza and even curing it, invaded the classifieds section of the city's periodicals.[61]

The variety of therapeutic approaches to the disease can be examined from various angles. Many of the practices constitute a cultural heritage founded on beliefs and knowledge accumulated from past generations. In this regard, the contribution of society's recent experiences with such substances and practices to the formation and reaffirmation of these beliefs and knowledge cannot be neglected. For instance, a significant part of the publicity about the pharmaceutical preparations recommended against the influenza suggests a wide circulation of science-based propositions such as the theories of germs and contagion. But the list of medicinal plants published in the press also reveals a profusion of substances that made up the unofficial or domestic pharmacopoeia.[62] This variety of foundations on which treatments and explanations of the disease were built helps to clarify how beliefs and knowledge of the experience of illness were based on a complex approach that combined different rationales.

Attempts to curb the impact of the pandemic also addressed social behavior. During November one newspaper began a campaign against the "ingrained habit" of the handshake. Seen as a vehicle of dangerous contagion, the newspaper called for doing away with it as a prophylactic means to prevent the influenza, citing the authorities of science and progress. On the one hand, it stated that scientists had proven that such a greeting could facilitate the spread of the "most reprehensible" diseases. On the other hand, the habit was viewed as "old-fashioned" and capable of leading to "unnecessary waste of time amid the turmoil and the intensity of modern life," being "a hick custom that revealed a lack of absolute civility." In its place it suggested adopting a military salute, "so elegant . . . simple and fast."[63]

Apart from the flu, the capital was also invaded by various rumors in the last months of 1918, feeding the popular imaginary with truly macabre stories: suicide due to the loss of close relatives, murder to save loved ones from suffering, the sacrifice of corpses for the theft of jewelry, and the rape of recently deceased young women.[64] Rumors of this nature increased people's fear and apprehension, though authorities condemned the rumors as promoting thoughtless and misguided attitudes. Assertions about "unjustified panic" and the "irrational actions" it motivates merit reflection in their own right, though it hardly seems surprising that in the context of the 1918 epidemic, reports of this nature frightened Belo Horizonte residents. Besides, considering the real threat posed by the disease and the failure of measures recommended by public authorities and the medical profession, how can their efforts at self-preservation be dismissed as simply wrong and unreflective? Although many of the attitudes and practices reflected during the reign of the influenza were not grounded in science, it must be remembered that a society's logic of being and living extends beyond the scope of scientific rationale.[65]

The Spanish Flu Leaves the Scene

The pandemic faded quickly from public attention. As fewer references to the flu were made in the daily press, other disasters quickly replaced it. In December, for instance, the press paid particular attention to the "terrible accident" that occurred at kilometer 175 of the Central do Brasil railway. The night train that ran from the capital to Rio de Janeiro derailed, burning in the waters of the Paraíba River. "Since Saturday our city does not talk about anything else, from morning to night."[66] Some days later the death of the poet Olavo Bilac, "the great dead of yesterday," began to attract attention.[67] In 1919 and 1920 the influenza emerged once more as a threat, only to disappear quickly into oblivion.[68]

No doubt many individuals' private memories about the pandemic have refused to fade with time, like those of people who lost loved ones or those orphaned by the flu. Others must recall the disruption of daily life and the difficult days experienced toward the end of 1918. But these memories are difficult to retrieve and do not appear in many of the testimonies that preserve this past.[69] Among the few personal memories about that time, the Spanish flu remains a unique experience people would rather forget.[70] In November 1918, a sonnet published by the press predicted man would curse the Spanish flu "for life, [as] the darkest page of history."[71]

But if the catastrophic and poignant character of epidemics can be seen as an explanation for inducing oblivion among people, it is also what makes this experience a rich event for historical analysis. As the historiography of epidemics shows, epidemics are, par excellence, a vantage point capable of illuminating various aspects and levels of social life in different historical contexts. Thus, the Spanish flu of 1918 reveals many of the characteristics that marked Brazilian society in the second decade of the twentieth century: social inequalities inherited from the colonial and imperial periods, the presence of a strong Catholic imaginary, the incipient involvement of the state in the resolution of problems imposed by public health issues, and economic hardships imposed by wartime. More specifically, the influenza pandemic also provides an opportunity to critically assess how the city was laid out and what life in Belo Horizonte at the beginning of the twentieth century was like. The design of the urban layout of the new city contrasted that of the old cities of colonial times, which had grown up mostly in a random and haphazard fashion. Belo Horizonte presented itself as modern city, making use of knowledge and resources offered by the science of hygiene to avoid the problems of overcrowding and lack of planning experienced by major world capitals. It was a city seemingly blind to its poor inhabitants, relegating them to a sort of "unofficial" or "ghost" city on the outskirts that came into view only as the disease spread.

In a more general context, the influenza of 1918 suggests that scientific theories are not absolute or true propositions but contextually produced. Science is knowledge in construction and often has no clear or correct answers for the events that affect us. An example can be seen in relation to the propositions of hygiene on which the construction project of the city was founded. Although these proposals were fundamental tools for confronting the cholera epidemics that occurred in large cities in the nineteenth century, serving as the background for the health reforms of that period, they were ineffective in fighting the influenza of 1918.

The narratives of the life experiences of Belo Horizonte residents during the pandemic of 1918 point to the validity of approaching these events as "dramaturgical incidents." As noted, the impact of the disease and the social responses to it follow a narrative logic similar to that of other epidemics in other places and at different times. The occurrence of fear, the disruption of daily life, the mobilization of society for the relief of victims, and the restoration of order are all aspects of the terrible plague epidemics in medieval Europe as well as the cholera epidemics that ravaged the great cities of the West in the nineteenth century. But, as shown in this chapter, although epidemic events share certain characteristics and story lines in common, they are also framed by the specific experience of the different societies in which they occur.

Notes

1. Oswaldo P. Rocha, *A era das demolições: Cidade do Rio de Janeiro, 1870–1920* (Rio de Janeiro: Secretaria Municipal de Cultura, 1995); Jaime L. Benchimol, *Pereira Passos: Um Haussmann tropical; A renovação urbana do Rio de Janeiro no início do século XX* (Rio de Janeiro: Secretaria Municipal de Cultura, Turismo e Esportes, 1990); Sidney Chalhoub, *Cidade Febril: Cortiços e epidemias na Corte Imperial* (São Paulo: Companhia das Letras, 1996).

2. The urban reforms that occurred in the nineteenth century in London and Paris became a model for various other urban interventions and were strongly influenced by the ideals of modernization and hygiene. Cf. George Rosen, *A History of Public Health* (Baltimore: Johns Hopkins University Press, 1993); Margaret Pelling, *Chólera, Fever and English Medicine, 1825–1865* (Oxford: Oxford University Press, 1978); Richard Sennett, *O declínio do homem público: As tiranias da intimidade* (São Paulo: Companhia das Letras, 1988); Steven Johnson, *The Ghost Map: The History of London's Most Terrifying Epidemic and How It Changed Science, Cities and the Modern World* (New York: Riverhead, 2006).

3. An analysis of the cultural meanings attached to epidemic events can be found in Jean Delumeau, *História do medo no ocidente: 1300–1800* (São Paulo: Companhia das Letras, 1996); Charles E. Rosenberg, *The Cholera Years: The United States in 1832, 1849, and 1866* (Chicago: University of Chicago Press, 1987); Terence Ranger and Paul Slack, eds., *Epidemics and Ideas: Essays on the Historical Perception of Pestilence* (Cambridge: Cambridge University Press, 1992); and Richard J. Evans, *Death in Hamburg: Society and Politics in the Cholera Years, 1830–1910* (London: Penguin Books, 1987), among others.

4. Charles E. Rosenberg, *Explaining Epidemics and Other Studies in the History of Medicine* (Cambridge: Cambridge University Press, 1995).

5. As noted in chapter 10 of this volume, the contagion of fear was also present in Argentina during the Spanish flu.

6. See also chapters 7 and 9 of this volume.

7. The 1918 flu reached unprecedented levels of virulence in the three port cities of Freetown, Brest, and Boston, where the epidemic exploded at the end of August. Alfred Crosby, *America's Forgotten Pandemic: The Influenza of 1918* (Cambridge: Cambridge University Press, 1999), 19.

8. More details on the importance of this Brazilian navy division traveling from Freetown to the port of Dakar can be found in chapter 2 of this volume.

9. Carlos L. Meyer and Joaquim R. Teixeira, *A gripe epidêmica no Brasil e especialmente em São Paulo* (São Paulo: Casa Duprat, 1920).

10. On the force of naming, see Michel Foucault, *As palavras e as coisas*, 8th ed. (São Paulo: Martins Fontes, 1999). In chapter 2 of this volume, Bertucci deals extensively with the effects of the uncertainty surrounding the etiology and nature of the malady during the pandemic.

11. Initially, the disease was considered to be similar to a fulminant epidemic that had occurred in Spain between February and April 1918 and was therefore called the Spanish flu. "A influenza espanhola," *Diário de Minas*, September 24, 1918. On discussions about the origin of the name of the 1918 pandemic, see Gina Kolata, *Flu: The History of the Great Influenza Pandemic of 1918 and the Search for the Virus That*

Caused It (London: Macmillan, 2000), 8–10; and María-Isabel Porras-Gallo, *Un reto para la sociedad madrileña: La epidemia de gripe de 1918–19* (Madrid: Complutense / Comunidad Autónoma de Madrid, 1997), 41–42.

12. "Debates na Academia de Medicina," *Revista Médico-Cirúrgica do Brasil*, no. 11, 1918.

13. The term "pestilence" is often used to refer to diseases that have some of the following characteristics: high morbidity or mortality rates, sudden and uncontrollable onset, a dehumanizing or repulsive character, and an unknown nature that puts it at odds with the current medical literature at the time. The term is also used metaphorically to refer to other situations of human experience. Susan Sontag, *Doença como metáfora: AIDS e suas metáforas* (São Paulo: Companhia das Letras, 2007).

14. Carlos Seidl, "A pandemia de gripe e o ex-diretor geral de saúde pública," *Revista Médico-Cirúrgica do Brasil* 26, no. 10, 1918.

15. "A influenza no Rio," *Minas Gerais*, October 10, 1918.

16. On the blaming of victims, see María-Isabel Porras-Gallo, "Ateniéndose al consejo de los expertos: Los madrileños frente a la gripe durante las epidemias de 1889–90 y de 1918–19," in *De la responsabilidad individual a la culpabilización de la víctima: El papel del paciente en la prevención de la enfermedad*, ed. Luis Montiel and María-Isabel Porras-Gallo (Madrid: Doce Calles, 1997), 101–10.

17. "A influenza," *Minas Gerais*, October 20, 1918.

18. George M. Sternberg, *Desinfecção e profilaxia individual contra doenças infectuosas* (1889; repr., Rio de Janeiro: Laemmert e Cia, 1920), 39. George Miller Sternberg (1838–1915) was a pioneer American bacteriologist and US Army physician, distinguished by his studies of the causation and prevention of infectious diseases and by his scientific investigations of yellow fever. He published the first *Manual of Bacteriology* produced in the United States in 1892 as well as other important texts: *A Study of the Natural History of Yellow Fever* (1877), *Malaria and Malarial Diseases* (1884), *Disinfection and Individual Prophylaxis against Infectious Disease* (1886), *Etiology and Prevention of Yellow Fever* (1890), *Text Book of Bacteriology* (1892, 1896). Cf. George M. Kober, "George Miller Sternberg, M.D., LL.D.: An Appreciation," *American Journal of Public Health* 5, no. 12 (1915): 1233–37; Eugene Flaumenhaft and Carol Flaumenhaft, "Evolution of America's Pioneer Bacteriologist: George M. Sternberg's Formative Years," *Military Medicine* 158, no. 7 (1993): 448–57; and the entry for "Sternberg, George Miller" on the American Society for Microbiology's webpage, http://www. asm.org/index.php/choma3/71-membership/archives/848-sternberg-george-miller (accessed May 13, 2014).

19. "A influenza no Rio," *Minas Gerais*, October 17, 1918.

20. "A influenza," *Minas Gerais*, Ocober. 19, 1918. Teófilo Torres had replaced the former director general of public health of Rio de Janeiro, Carlos Seidl, who had been dismissed due to criticisms of his performance before the outbreak of the disease.

21. Plácido Barbosa, "Influenzaphobia" *Minas Gerais*, October 23, 1918.

22. "A influenza," *Minas Gerais*, October 20, 1918.

23. In chapter 10 Feldman relates a similar case of the "contagion of fear" and responses to it in Argentina.

24. Gustavo Pena, "The Contagion of Panic," *Minas Gerais*, October 19, 1918.

25. Ibid.

26. Ibid.

27. Ibid.

28. Letícia Julião, "Belo Horizonte: Itinerários da cidade moderna (1891–1920)" (master's thesis, Universidade Federal de Minas Gerais, 1992).

29. In the mid-twentieth century, the World Health Organization established an international early warning system to detect new outbreaks of influenza. This global network of surveillance has been greatly expanded in recent years and continues to play a leading role in preventing disease and controlling epidemics. Kolata, *Flu*, 87; William I. Beveridge, *Influenza: The Last Great Plague* (New York: Prodist, 1978), 96; João Toniolo Neto, *A história da gripe: A influenza em todos os tempos e agora* (São Paulo: Dezembro, 2001), 58.

30. "A influenza espanhola," *A Nota*, October 10, 1918.

31. "Diversas," *Minas Gerais*, October 17, 1918. On the measures for individual prophylaxis, see Porras-Gallo, "Ateniéndose al consejo."

32. Legislation on the compulsory notification of infectious diseases was introduced in England in the last decades of the nineteenth century. This measure represented one further step in the process of bureaucratization of health and increasing state intervention in medical practice, especially in the doctor-patient relationship. Cf. Dorothy Porter, *Health, Civilization and the State: A History of Public Health from Ancient to Modern Times* (Abingdon: Routledge, 1999), 135; and Linda Bryder, *Below the Magic Mountain: A Social History of Tuberculosis in Twentieth-Century Britain* (Oxford: Oxford University Press, 2002), 41.

33. "Diversas," *Minas Gerais*, October 18, 1918.

34. "A influenza espanhola," *Diário de Minas*, October 24, 1918.

35. Carlos H. M. Maletta, *A cidade e os cidadãos: Belo Horizonte; 10 anos* (Belo Horizonte, 1997). The population of Belo Horizonte was estimated at 55,700 inhabitants in 1918. Official demographic records indicate a total of 2,918 flu patients at the end of December 1918, but in late November the *Minas Gerais* newspaper suggested that there were more than 15,000 people affected by flu in the city. "A influenza," *Minas Gerais*, November, 30, 1918, 3.

36. Delumeau, *História*; Richard J. Evans, "Epidemics and Revolutions: Cholera in Nineteenth-Century Europe," in Ranger and Slack, *Epidemics and Ideas*, 149–73.

37. On the situation of poor people, see also chapter 4 for the Portuguese case and chapter 11 for the Spanish case, both in this volume.

38. Roy Porter, *Cambridge: História Ilustrada da Medicina* (Rio de Janeiro: Revinter, 2001); Lindsay Granshaw, "The Hospital," in *Companion Encyclopedia of the History of Medicine*, ed. William F. Bynum and Roy Porter, vol 2. (London: Routledge, 1997), 1180–1203.

39. "A influenza," *Minas Gerais*, November 20, 1918.

40. "A influenza," *Minas Gerais*, November 9, 1918.

41. A similar situation occurred in Portugal, as described by Sobral, Lima, and Silveira e Sousa in chapter 4 of this volume.

42. Anny Jackeline Torres Silveira, *A influenza espanhola e a cidade planejada: Belo Horizonte, 1918* (Belo Horizonte: Argvmentvm, 2007). On the role of Red Cross during the pandemic, see also chapters 2, 3, and 12 of this volume.

43. Delumeau, *História do medo*, 121–25.

44. Bernard Vincent, "La choléra en Espagne au XIXe siecle," in *Peurs et terreurs face à la contagion: Cholera, tuberculose, syphilis, XIXe–XXe siècles*, ed. Jean Pierre Bardet, Patrice Bourdelais, Pierre Guillaume, Claude Quètel, and Fançois Lebrun (Paris: Fayard, 1998), 65.

45. Evans, "Epidemics and Revolutions," 150.

46. On this topic during the Spanish influenza pandemic in Spain, see chapter 8 of this volume.

47. This form of activity is seen in the documents collected in the research coordinated by the author about the history of health in Minas Gerais during the nineteenth century, with funding from Conselho Nacional de Pesquisa and Fundação de Amparo à Pesquisa de Minas Gerais.

48. Gilberto Hochman, *A era do saneamento: As bases da saúde pública no Brasil* (São Paulo: Hucitec / ANPOCS, 1998); Luiz A. Castro Santos, "O pensamento sanitarista na Primeira República: Uma ideologia da construção da nacionalidade," *Dados: Revista de Ciências Sociais* 1, no. 1 (1985): 193–210.

49. Abram De Suann, *In Care of the State: Health Care, Education and Welfare in Europe and USA in the Modern Era* (Cambridge: Polity, 1988).

50. Crosby, *America's Forgotten Pandemic*, 19.

51. Chapter 9 of this volume offers an interesting take on this topic.

52. Similar dynamics can be observed in the case of Argentina, as Feldman points out in chapter 10 of this volume.

53. In Brazil, these practices were also reported by Janete S. Abrão, *A banalização da morte na cidade calada: A hespanhola em Porto Alegre* (Porto Alegre: EDIPCRS, 1998); Cláudio Bertolli Filho, *A gripe espanhola em São Paulo, 1918: Epidemia e sociedade* (São Paulo: Paz e Terra, 2003); Liane M. Bertucci, *Influenza: A medicina enferma* (Campinas: Universidade Estadual de Campinas, 2004); Christiane M. Cruz de Souza, *A gripe espanhola na Bahia: Saúde, política e medicina em tempos de epidemia* (Rio de Janeiro: Fundação Oswaldo Cruz, 2009); Beatriz A. Olinto, "Uma cidade em tempo de epidemia: Rio Grande e a gripe espanhola (RS–1918)" (master's thesis, Universidade Federal de Santa Catarina, 1995); and Adriana C. Goulart, "Um cenário mefistofélico: A gripe espanhola no Rio de Janeiro" (master's thesis, Universidade Federal Fluminense, 2003). For other epidemic events, see Delumeau, *História*; Evans, *Death in Hamburg*; Patrice Bourdelais and Jean-Yves Raulot, *Une peur blue: Histoire du choléra en France* (Paris: Payot, 1987).

54. On the importance of religion during the pandemic, see also chapter 7 of this volume.

55. François Lebrun, *Se soigner autrefois; médecins, saints et sorciers aux XVII et XVIII siècles* (Paris: Éditons du Seuil, 1995), 113.

56. The Via Crucis is the route penitent Christians travel, which represents the main scenes of Christ's passion. Antônio Houaiss and Mauro de S. Villar, *Dicionário Houaiss da língua portuguesa* (Rio de Janeiro: Objetiva, 2001), 2856.

57. "Serviço Religioso," *Minas Gerais*, October 23, 1918; "Serviço Religioso," *Minas Gerais*, October 24, 1918; "A influenza," Minas Gerais, October 26, 1918.

58. "Quem sabe," *Diário de Minas*, October 29, 1918; "Cosmorama," *Diário de Minas*, December 22, 1918.

59. "Influenza espanhola,"*Diario de Minas*, November 12, 1918.

60. Sylvio Miraglia, *Serra do Curral: Recordações* (Belo Horizonte: Imprensa Oficial, 1990), 178.

61. Silveira, *Influenza espanhola.* See also chapters 7 and 10 of this volume.

62. In addition to domestic therapies such as teas from various plants, other therapeutic approaches used included homeopathy, hydrotherapy, and diet therapy. Cf. Bertucci, *Influenza*; Françoise Loux, "Folk Medicine," in Bynum and Porter, *Companion Encyclopedia,* 1: 661–75.

63. "Crônica Social," *Diário de Minas,* November 6, 1918; "Crônica Social," *Diário de Minas,* November 13, 1918; "Aperto de mão," *Diário de Minas,* December 8, 1918.

64. "A influenza no Rio," *Minas Gerais,* October 17, 1918, "A influenza no Rio,"*Minas Gerais,* November 12, 1918; "A influenza espanhola," *Diário de Minas,* October 22, 1918, and December 7, 1918.

65. Ranger and Slack, *Epidemics and Ideas,* 11.

66. "Crônica Social," *Diário de Minas,* December 10, 1918.

67. "Olavo Bilac," *Minas Gerais,* December 29, 1918.

68. "A gripe vem aí," *A Noticia,* February 14, 1920.

69. In chapter 13 Belling gives some reasons for the dearth of firsthand accounts of the Spanish flu pandemic.

70. See Affonso S. Brandão, *Na vivência do meu tempo* (Belo Horizonte, 1977); Pedro Salles, *Notas sobre a história da medicina em Belo Horizonte* (Belo Horizonte: Cuatiara, 1977); Carlos Caiafa Filho, *Vida de menino antigo: Histórias da minha infância* (Belo Horizonte: Imprensa Oficial, 1986); Miraglia, *Páginas vividas* (Belo Horizonte: Ingabrás, 1975); and Beatriz B. Martins, *A vida é esta* (Belo Horizonte: Martins, 2000). Some personal recollections of the influenza pandemic have been collected as part of the Centers for Disease Control's *Pandemic Influenza Storybook,* available at www.pandemicflu.gov/storybook/index.html.

71. "Crônica Social," *Diário de Minas,* November 6, 1918.

Chapter Seven

The Spanish Flu in Bahia, Brazil

Prophylaxis and Healing Practices

CHRISTIANE MARIA CRUZ DE SOUZA

The Spanish flu was the biggest and most devastating disease of the twentieth century, infecting more than six hundred million people and killing between forty and one hundred million people worldwide in a short time span.[1] The disease first occurred in the Northern Hemisphere in March 1918. It was spring, an unusual time for flu, but the low rate of mortality did not cause excessive concern among doctors and public health officials in the countries where the outbreak occurred. But the flu returned in August of the same year, this time in a much more virulent form, spreading to other parts of the world up until 1920.[2]

It is difficult to specify the moment when the Spanish flu epidemic reached Salvador, the capital of the Brazilian state of Bahia, located on the country's eastern coast north of Rio de Janeiro. If we consider the intense movement in Salvador's port and its commercial connections with other countries, as well as the necessary time for the pathogen to infect individuals, spread through the city, and be noticed by the press and doctors, we can infer the disease was already in Bahia much earlier than mid-September, when the presence of an "unknown epidemic" was reported in the Bahian capital.[3] But the press did not report the specific presence of the "Spanish Lady" in the city up until September 23, 1918, blaming her presence on the English packet steamer *Demerara*, which had moored with infected passengers in the port of Salvador on September 11.[4] A report published later in *Diario de Noticias* stated that six deaths had occurred on the vessel while en route.[5] Two of these deaths were people whose final destination was Salvador, though Bahia's Directorate General of Public Health was unaware of this and therefore failed to record them.

In this chapter we analyze how the disease infiltrated the lives of Bahian-Salvadoran residents and its repercussions in the daily life of the city: the attitudes of the inhabitants in relation to the invasion of the disease and the threat of death, as well as their peaceful resistance to public health measures that went against cultural practices related to illness and death rites. We are interested in understanding the significance that certain social groups gave to the epidemic experience and discovering the strategies and resources used to fight it. This way, in addition to prophylactic measures, we also analyze the therapeutic approaches used not only in academic medicine but also in domestic medicine and healing practices based on religion. To create a picture of Bahia under siege by the epidemic, we use a wide range of sources, most of which have not been published previously. Newspapers from the Bahian state are valuable, as they unveil specific social and cultural values as well as the vicissitudes of daily life in the cities where the disease erupted.

Under the Impact of the Epidemic

The port of Salvador was seen as the gateway to the city for various diseases. Flu figured among the maladies that regularly visited the port without actually causing great disruption to the city. Consequently, the first rumors about the existence of a flu epidemic in Salvador did not cause alarm among doctors or political and public health authorities, who believed it was another outbreak of a benign flu, something that regularly occurred in Bahia. It therefore took a while before Bahian society officially recognized the existence of a flu epidemic in Salvador. While trying to assimilate this fact, political factions held a heated debate in the press to identify who was responsible. The opposition sought to blame the government for the invasion of the epidemic, while the government accused the opposition of using the epidemic to destabilize the group that was in power.[6] For their part, doctors sought an explanation for how a supposedly familiar and benign disease had shown such a strange virulence.[7]

The calamity, which struck many quarters of the world almost simultaneously, confused the international medical community, which began to suspect that a new disease was responsible for the situation. The different names attributed to the disease in the various countries affected by the epidemic reflect this perception: the Americans called it "three-day fever" or "purple death"; the French named it "purulent bronchitis"; the Italians, "sandfly fever"; and the Germans, "Flanders fever" or "Blitzkatarrh."[8] In Spain the flu was called "la dançarina" and, especially, the "soldado de Nápoles" (Naples soldier), while in Portugal the disease was known as a "pneumónica."[9] In other countries, it became known as "Spanish flu" or influenza.[10] Physicians were surprised by cases in which individuals who had apparently recovered would suffer serious relapses, as if their organisms were incapable of triggering immunization.[11] The complications appeared during the recurrence. Those affecting the respiratory system, such as bronchopneumonia and pneumonia, and cardiovascular complications, would lead to death within a few days. According to physicians, asphyxiation gave victims' corpses a purple hue.[12] Moreover, the inconsistency of Pfeiffer's bacillus in laboratory results, as well as the occurrence of diverse microorganisms in the blood, secretions, and body liquids of those suffering and dying from the disease contradicted the hypothesis of a specific agent and generated controversies among medical practitioners and researchers.[13]

The pressing circumstances of the epidemic compelled scientists and medical and health authorities from the countries affected by the epidemic to provide at least a provisional diagnosis of the disease and to propose an explanatory framework for understanding the set of signs bound up with it.[14] In the process, a body of knowledge that had apparently achieved a degree of stability was suddenly overturned, inaugurating a period of uncertainty, controversy, experimentation, and negotiation as efforts were made to establish a diagnosis and a correct form of treatment for the disease in question.[15]

As noted in chapter 2 of this volume, questions about the disease spilled over into the pages of newspapers: What was the Spanish Lady? Was the current illness a "meteoric catarrhal fever," dengue fever, summer fever, trench fever, three-day fever, or simply seasonal influenza or flu, more virulent this time round? Was the disease as contagious as it appeared? If it was transmitted by direct contact, how had it broken out across the world almost simultaneously? What other mechanisms accelerated its transmission? What was the etiological agent responsible for causing the affliction? The local newspapers reproduced articles published in the international press in which the most renowned European physicians issued a range of explanations concerning the disease and its causes. According to these reports, three schools of thought were prominent in the national and international community at the start of the pandemic crisis. The first believed that the flu had begun in a benign form only to assume a more serious form and become lethal. The second view accepted the flu diagnosis but remained puzzled over the anomalous circumstances and symptoms presented by the epidemic. Finally, the third group rejected the diagnosis of flu from the outset: the disease was "three-day fever" or "pappataci (sandfly) fever," provoked by an invisible and filterable etiological agent like those responsible for dengue and yellow fever.[16]

The lack of agreement among European physicians who had been dealing directly with the epidemic cases, in relation to the nature, causes, and mechanisms of the pathogen in question reinforced the disposition among health authorities to designate a team of physicians to investigate the disease and offer an informed opinion on the matter.[17] In spite of pressure from the press, Bahia's Directorate General of Public Health (DGSPB) decided to appoint a commission to study the epidemic before adopting any specific measures. The professionals chosen—Frederico Koch, Dyonisio Pereira, and Aristides Novis—became the representatives of the state's medical elite, enjoying considerable renown among their peers and Bahian society alike. As well as being members of the Health Inspectorate, a division subordinated to the DGSPB, they ran clinical practices and were professors of the local Faculty of Medicine.

For those threatened by the epidemic, the time that elapsed between the initial cases of the disease, its recognition, and the official reaction to the epidemic seemed interminable, and society demanded a response from public authorities. The press naturally criticized the public authorities' paralysis, accusing the DGSPB of inaction in relation to the disease, which had spread throughout the city, infecting half of the population, with reports of homes in which entire families had disappeared.[18] *O Imparcial* newspaper published a cartoon that satirized the situation, in which "Public Health" is shown lying in a hammock under the shade of palm trees while the Spanish Lady goes about her business of harvesting lives. The caption under the illustration reads, "While Public Health, rocked by patrician breezes, innocently sleeps, the 'Spanish lady' benefits, carrying away contingents of people every day to dwell in the necropolis."[19] Along with the image, the reprobation and irony contained in the phrase reinforces the vision of inertia and irresponsibility of Bahian authorities in relation to the baleful action of the epidemic.[20] Such was the image of the epidemic constructed in the media—an image that confirmed the role of Bahian political and public health authorities, who in trying to minimize the scope of the epidemic were characterized as negligent toward the population.

The usual benignity and seasonality of influenza offers a partial explanation for Soteropolitanos' (residents of Salvador) muted response to the epidemic. Medical and public health authorities paid more attention to diseases like the plague, smallpox, and, especially, yellow fever because they were considered far worse than the flu. But, considered from another angle, it is clear that the political and economic context played a key role in preventing the event from immediately becoming a public or political question. The political disputes that agitated Bahia at that time, the economic weakness of the state and the municipality, and the need to protect the image of cleanliness for a port that was a large agricultural exporter all combined to obscure the perception of the disease as epidemic, which subsequently hindered public health authorities from taking appropriate measures of intervention.

Further overshadowing the importance of the Spanish flu was the fact that when it reached Bahia, the population was already besieged by the presence or threat of numerous other diseases. Tuberculosis and malaria were raging in an almost epidemic fashion. The population was also suffering from yellow fever, despite Bahian authorities' claims that it had been eradicated. Figure 7.1 illustrates the situation well by showing the Spanish Lady and the yellow fever fighting over victims.

Paul Slack calls attention to the fact that past stories can mold the perceptions of the present.[21] Thus, what can make some diseases more or less feared than others are the memories they evoke. The images of influenza and cholera, crystallized in the memory of Soteropolitanos in previous epidemics also interfered with the responses to the influenza epidemic in Bahia in 1918. The threatened invasion of cholera, which could come to Bahia aboard ships traveling through the theater of World War I, concerned health authorities more than the influenza epidemic actually in progress.[22] The reaction merely to the threat of cholera, as opposed to its actual impact, can be explained by the physical horrors caused by the cholera epidemic of 1855–56 and its concomitant social impact, which killed around forty thousand persons in Bahia, causing panic, supply crises, and population escapism.[23] Despite their extreme morbidity, the flu epidemics that hit Bahia in 1890 and 1895 did not cause many deaths or great disturbances to residents. The memory of previous epidemics and the seasonal incidence of influenza, as well as the insignificant number of deaths registered during the six years prior to 1918 all contributed to the feeling of familiarity with the disease and reinforced the idea that it was benign.

Multiple factors contributed to delaying the decision-making process during the epidemic: the need to establish a diagnosis, the financial difficulties faced by the state and municipality, the bureaucratic red tape and pace characteristic of public services, and the benign image of influenza. The issue of time was also significant. The flu spread at a speed inversely proportional to the time necessary to establish a diagnosis and to take the relevant prophylactic and therapeutic measures.

Ruptures in Daily Life

At the end of September the flu was already "raging and ever more violently," shocking Soteropolitanos due to the "extraordinary number of cases."[24] The disease affected corporations, workshops, and factories, interfering in the routine of these establishments and disrupting people's daily lives.[25] Traffic on the streetcars of the Linha Circular and Trilhos Centrais companies was seriously affected, since after the onset of the disease more than two hundred streetcar employees did not show up for work.[26]

In October the flu epidemic continued to spread throughout the city, raiding houses, taking over whole blocks, emptying the barracks, and

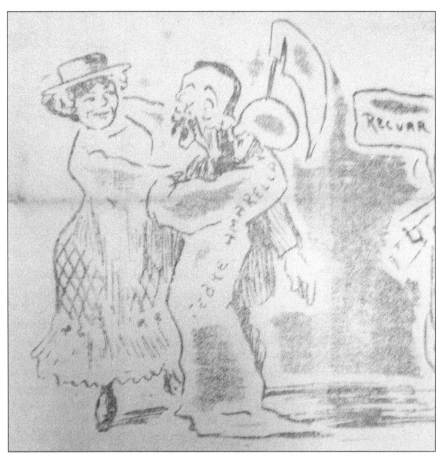

Figure 7.1. Malign harassment. *O Imparcial*, October 3, 1918, 1.

increasingly hampering the operation of services, schools, and factories.[27] In the short period of a week—from October 27 to November 2—a total of 225 people suffering from the flu resorted to the health care provided by the Directorate General of Public Health in Bahia for indigents.[28] Given this scenario, fear spread throughout the city: "there was no one . . . who did not have any fears, [or] apprehensions, given the frightening number of people killed by and suffering from the devastating pandemic."[29]

The city suddenly became sick and was obliged to deal with the assault of the Spanish Lady and the intensification of experiences of death. Figure 7.2, which appeared on the front page of *O Imparcial*, captures the general feeling of powerlessness in the face of inevitable harm. The personified figure of death characterized as the Spanish Lady harvests lives indiscriminately under the impotent gaze of the people.

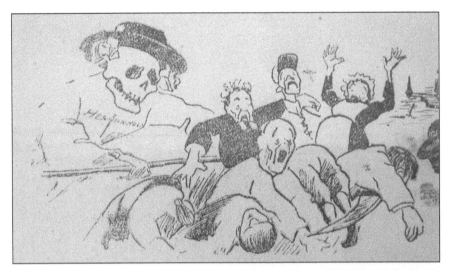

Figure 7.2. The impotence of the people against the actions of the Spanish Lady. *O Imparcial,* October 28, 1918, 1.

As a result of the epidemic, the Directorate General of Public Health in Bahia prohibited many customary activities, a common approach seen throughout the world in those areas affected by the pandemic. The military parade to commemorate the proclamation of the republic, as well as religious festivals and school trips, were suspended due to the threat of contamination they presented. To prevent contagion from outside Bahia, the Directorate General of Public Health prohibited onboard visits to ships moored in Salvador's port.[30] Onboard visits were common among Soteropolitanos, whether to say farewell to those traveling, greet those arriving, or to see the beauty, comfort, and technological advances introduced on the vessels that moored there. The arrival of a large ship in port was an attraction due to the leisure opportunities it offered and because of the sociability among the people on board. To prohibit this activity was thus to strike at the heart of Bahian social life.

Public authorities also interfered with funeral and burial rites.[31] In the event of death due to an infectious or contagious disease, people were prohibited from attending to the rites that accompanied the deceased's passage to the next life. Burials had to take place quickly and with discretion, with friends and family being prohibited from attending. Anyone who did not obey the law would be fined. Even the pilgrimage to cemeteries on All Souls' Day was forbidden.[32] To prevent people from circumventing the government's restrictions, the police patrolled all cemeteries.[33] In this way Soteropolitanos were prevented from carrying out their traditional homage to the dead.[34] Nevertheless, residents never complied fully with the stipulations of the law, as people continued to accompany the dead to their final resting place, despite the risks involved.

The measures specifically related to funeral rites were extremely unpopular, since they were contrary to a custom deep-rooted in Bahian society. The suppression of the funeral liturgy took away the sacredness of death, making it even more feared.[35] The deprivation of certain rites, which gave those who had lost loved ones some comfort, security, and identity, could not be peacefully accepted. The need to resort to political force denotes that the authorities not only feared disobedience of the law but also suspected that prohibitions could rupture the fragile equilibrium of the city.[36]

During this period Plácido Barbosa published a note in *O Imparcial* titled "Influenzaphobia," in which he sought to calm the population. He argued that citizens did not irrationally need to fear the pandemic disease affecting Salvador, because its seriousness did not result from its mortality, which was limited at that point, but because it left a large part of the population suddenly prostrate, disorganizing services and causing general suffering. Barbosa warned that panic harmed everyone—the sick and healthy alike— since "the disorder of spirits causes the disorder of things."[37] The doctor feared that panic and disorder would spread through the city since Bahians were going through a time of great tension. In addition to the threat of epidemic diseases such as the flu, yellow fever, the plague, and malaria, the population was suffering from the pressure of a housing crisis, the constant increase in the cost of basic goods and rent, and unemployment. Fortunately, Barbosa's fears were not confirmed, as the Spanish Lady's passage through Bahia did not lead to manifestations of panic like collective hysteria, fleeing from infected places, social disturbances, and so on.

Nevertheless, an article titled "A cidade doente" (The sick city) spoke of the modifications that occurred in the physiognomy of Salvador. The city was afflicted by a "bad physical feeling [that disturbed] the organism." The flu, "benign in its effects, but martyring in its outbreaks," spread to everyone in such a way that it was "a spectacle to see the population cough, cough, cough." "The air of the city, filled with the dust of summer, makes [people] sad, despite its cheerfulness," lamented the writer, describing the sickening aspect of the city and the sense of desolation that dominated the spirit of the population. For the author of the article, these "ephemeral states of morbidity" had some use, since they caused reflections about the "equality of the luck of all men in light of the natural hostilities of the world."[38] In this way, as well as evoking human fragility in the face of these natural phenomena, the writer shows the egalitarian character of the epidemic. The flu, like other contagious diseases, is not socially selective or concentrated; it therefore represents a threat that can affect everyone indiscriminately.

During this period a statement issued to the press reported that the sessions of Congress were sparsely attended, since a large number of deputies and senators were stricken with influenza.[39] Newspapers highlighted the fact that the governor of Bahia, Moniz de Aragão, and the future president of Brazil, Rodrigues Alves, had been affected by the disease.[40] In similar news, it was implied that the epidemic represented a threat to the elites, because it did not spare even the figures in local and national politics. The discourse constructed around the democracy of the disease contributed to raising awareness and alerting the elites about health problems revealed by the epidemic.

But the equality of individuals before the disease was relative, such that the newspapers sometimes reinforced its egalitarian character and at other times contradicted this view.[41] In fact, the disease affected everyone, though some individuals were more vulnerable than others. There was a higher number of deaths among those whose bodies were already weak, owing to preexisting or chronic diseases (tuberculosis, heart disease, kidney disease, etc.), to pregnancy and postpartum conditions, and to precarious conditions associated with life's basic necessities.[42]

Prophylactic Measures and Healing Practices

The tension unleashed by the epidemic crisis increased expressions of religiosity—most residents were Catholic—as people sought an explanation of and consolation for the punishment of the disease.[43] While the flu epidemic was passing though Bahia, citizens participated in masses, pilgrimages, the adoration of images, and the *beija-pé* of saints with the purpose of supplicating divine mercy.[44] Rituals brought together many of the faithful, even though public health authorities advised against gathering in the confined spaces of churches. This behavior reveals that the faithful were so assured of divine protection in these sacred spaces that they did not fear the risk of contamination. Moreover, religious rituals offered spiritual comfort and represented an effective action to deal with fear and the sense of powerlessness in the face of the disease's progression.[45]

In times of crisis, devotees from all parts of Bahian society resorted to Nosso Senhor Bonfim (Our Lord of Bonfim), praying for his miraculous intervention. Devotion to Nosso Senhor do Bonfim has a very long tradition in Bahia. It was introduced to Bahia by the Portuguese captain Theodozio Rodrigues, who brought the image from the Portuguese city of Setúbal in 1745. The image of the crucified Jesus dominates the high altar in the church constructed in the place where Rodrigues erected the first chapel in 1751 on the Itapagipe hill.[46] Since that time, when calamity strikes, Bahians appeal to Our Lord of Bonfim, asking him to placate the horrors of starvation, drought, or plague.

In times of epidemics, when no amount of prayers seemed enough, and the gravity of the moment required closer contact with the sacred, the image came down from its altar and was placed in the main chapel, bringing it closer to the adoration and supplication of the faithful. When the Spanish flu epidemic erupted, newspapers reported that the image was taken from the throne on the high altar, as had occurred during the cholera outbreak in 1855. Although the faithful wanted to be closer to the image, the administrative body responsible for its care was slow to move it. The perpetual treasurer of the brotherhood, José Eduardo Freire de Carvalho Filho, made clear their fear that moving the image could damage it, which at the time was more than two hundred years old. Moving the image would be authorized only if the epidemic worsened. Until that time, Our Lord of Bonfim would keep vigil over Bahians, alleviating their suffering from where he hung "unveiling the city and the sea."[47] Accordingly, when the epidemic worsened, Carvalho Filho moved the image to the nave of the church, where it was exposed to the adoration of the devout. Accord to a writer from *Jornal de Noticias*, the number of people who came to church was extraordinary, and they prostrated themselves before the image, kissing it and imploring Our Lord of Bonfim to stop the evil that was afflicting them.[48]

In times of epidemics, certain Catholic rituals contradict the recommendations of Western medicine, even though in the influenza pandemic, priests posed no threat to the doctors because, despite offering divine protection, they had no intention of exercising the art of healing. The same cannot be said about doctors' relations to practitioners of traditional medicine. Healers linked to traditional medicine were pejoratively labeled as charlatans and sorcerers and accused of exploiting the credulous with offers of miracle cures. Doctors in particular sought to prohibit the practices of traditional medicine, arguing that the only legitimate knowledge for health care was the knowledge acquired from the Faculty of Medicine of Bahia. Furthermore, during the second decade of the twentieth century, Bahian elites associated Catholicism with European culture, considering it to be superior to other religious manifestations. In light of this, the press waged a campaign against expressions of African culture, which were also severely repressed by the police. Victims of intolerance, members of *batuques* and practitioners of *candomblés* were prohibited from entering the city.[49]

Despite the prestige of academic medicine, traditional practices reached elites and the middle class in Bahia.[50] Forged by combining the knowledge of Indigenous, European, and African cultures mixed during the colonial period, domestic medicine offered a number of prophylactic and therapeutic practices regularly used to combat influenza. At the first symptoms of the disease—light fever, head colds, body aches, and headaches—people from various social groups resorted to domestic medicine, for example, the various teas that were immediately administered. As Hildegardes Vianna has documented, herbal teas with purgative properties, such as chicory tea, were very commonly used because it was believed at the time that "a clean intestine was the best way to cure any disease." Syrups, prepared with natural ingredients, such as ants, *folha-da-costa*, watercress, orange tree leaf, *angico*, and *carqueja* were also used as complements to the teas.[51] Generally, one or more of these ingredients were placed in alternating layers with brown sugar or *rapadura* (depending on the consistency desired) and warmed over a fire in a covered clay pan to cook in the juices produced by the mixture.[52] After being cooked, the syrup was bottled and used according to a rigorous schedule of use and abstinence. Some were administered for a period of twenty-one days, followed by seven days of no syrup. Others followed a balanced period of seven weeks on treatment and seven weeks off while waiting to observe the results. To relieve throat aches, ginger or licorice was chewed and infusions of guava leaves, a plant rich in tannin, were gargled. To loosen catarrh, the chest was massaged with chicken lard. It was applied by rubbing the skin until it was completely absorbed. After this patients were covered with a cloth (generally made of flannel) to warm them up.

In addition to the remedies mentioned, sweating was also a therapy that was much used at the time. Common sense held that toxins were expelled much more quickly through sweat. The simplest form of sweating was the *escalda-pés* (foot scalding): the feet of sick people were plunged into a bucket of very hot water, to which more hot water was constantly added to prevent the temperature from falling. When the patients began to sweat, they were given a strong tea or an alcoholic drink, and shortly afterward their feet were removed from the water and wrapped in a thick cotton or woolen fabric. Their body was then covered with layers of blankets, and they would sweat until their clothes and the bed linen became wet. Then the blankets were slowly removed to avoid a brusque change of temperature. After patients removed their sweaty clothes, their body was rubbed with camphorated alcohol, and they were dressed and then warmed with clean bed linen. After taking tepid porridge or tea, they finally went to sleep. In the case of "strong fluxes, influenzas, and similar diseases, if they were not improved with sweating, caustic or vesication was used, the type of which was most in vogue was sinapism." Sinapism was a mustard-based cataplasm capable of burning the skin and causing blisters. This was considered positive, "because everything bad would go out that way."[53]

At that time, the therapeutic treatment of diseases remained restricted to the domestic environment—people used hospitals only when they lacked family assistance or financial resources for treatment or when they endangered the people around them through contamination. Thus, whatever treatment aimed at strengthening the body and relieving the symptoms of the disease that doctors prescribed, it was administered by family members close to the patient. For this reason, during the flu epidemic in Salvador, existing hospital beds were occupied mostly by indigents or by crewmembers of vessels moored in the city.[54]

But these spaces were insufficient for dealing with all the sick who were seriously attacked by the flu. Many who died from the flu were abandoned in the streets. The news circulating in the press leads us to believe that only people integrated in some form in society—those whose names, ages, jobs, and addresses were known—obtained any sort of health care. Anonymous people, those who lived in the most absolute misery, died outdoors and were certainly not included in official statistics. For example, according to a note published in *Diario de Noticias*, "an unfortunate black women" around the age of thirty-two died a victim of the flu "in miserable abandonment" at the gate of Santa Isabel Hospital, continually exposed to bad weather.[55] The press exploited these facts to pressure the government to offer assistance to the poorest part of the population.

To make the public assistance program feasible, the city was divided into six public health zones, with a doctor responsible for each one and with registered pharmacies to distribute medicines. Although this assistance service covered the whole urban area of Salvador, a columnist in *A Tarde* complained that a single pharmacy was not sufficient to deal with the immense quantity of inhabitants in the working-class neighborhoods of Penha and Mares.[56] The journalist argued that to provide satisfactory care to the population of these factory districts, another pharmacy would have to be contracted because Penha was situated a long way from the workers' tenements where the working class lived. But this demand was never met, and the assistance post of the sixth public health zone continued to function only in the pharmacy contracted by the Directorate General of Public Health. In many ways, then, although the state offered assistance to its underprivileged residents, the reality of the matter was much less sanguine.

At the end of October the doctors designated by the Directorate General of Public Health to investigate the epidemic—Frederico Koch, Dyonisio Pereira, and Aristides Novis—confirmed the suspicion that the ongoing epidemic really was the Spanish flu. The commission decided to conduct a clinical investigation in a number of Salvador's public and private corporations and institutions where people were agglomerated—barracks, factories, asylums, schools, boarding schools, and so on. After examining more than five hundred patients, the physicians concluded that in Bahia the flu was manifested in its most common clinical form—respiratory—sometimes with mild gastrointestinal disturbances. The disease took hold quickly and generally those affected presented a temperature increase from thirty-eight to forty degrees Celsius (100 to 104 degrees Fahrenheit), inflammation of the upper airways, myalgia, headaches, and weariness. These symptoms could worsen, but under treatment they would fade, tending to disappear in three or four days.[57]

Thus the commission appointed to study the epidemic unfolding in Bahia suggested that the places or events where people were brought into close proximity should become a target of medical attention and sanitary action.[58] Places of leisure, theaters, cinemas, markets, elevators, streetcars, churches and temples, boarding schools, barracks, and so on needed to be systematically disinfected. The streets would have to be constantly irrigated to prevent dust from irritating the airways. Meetings would be discouraged. Along with these general prophylactic measures, the commission's members also recommended that people should take care of their own personal hygiene, avoid crowded and confined spaces, and, as a precaution, use disinfectants in their upper airways. They prescribed "applications of Vaseline containing menthol or gomenol in the nostrils and gargl[ing] with phenosalyl or oxygenated water."[59]

Informed of the results of clinical studies and feeling pressured by the growing numbers of sick people, the Directorate General of Public Health finally began to take the measures demanded by society at large. Aware that they were dealing with a very contagious microbial disease, doctors focused their intervention on spaces of social interaction. It was known that when infected individuals coughed or sneezed, they became disseminating agents of disease, since they expelled saliva contaminated with the microbe into the environment, which could be inhaled by those nearby. Thus work environments and confined spaces; places for entertainment or religious worship; and, above all, collective habitations, which were widespread in the capital of Bahia during that decade, became targets of medical and public health action because they were seen as important foci for the dissemination of the flu.

People infected with the flu could not personally seek out a doctor. Rather, they had to request house calls, presenting the requisite form in the registered pharmacies between eight and five o'clock.[60] Prescriptions had to be clear and precise, written on letterhead from the public assistance service and dispatched in pharmacies contracted by the government. In an article published in the newspaper *O Imparcial*, Plácido Barbosa suggested that, "strictly speaking, only the most serious forms of influenza require the presence of a doctor." In this way it was deemed convenient to use the pages of the newspaper to provide advice to the general population in terms of therapies available for the disease. For simple cases of the flu, Barbosa recommended rest "in a ventilated room, with a constant temperature and without drafts" and a light liquid diet. If those sick experienced "gases or [a] coated tongue," they should take a purgative of bitter salt, castor oil, or mercury chloride, which doctors believed could help with the disease.[61] They needed to carry out an antisepsis of the nose, mouth, and throat by gargling with mouthwash three times a day and then placing liquid Vaseline in the nostrils mixed with an antiseptic such as eucalyptol, cloretone, or salol.[62] If they were suffering from chills, measures were to be taken to relieve them and to promote a reaction, including covering them sufficiently and giving them warm drinks. In these cases Barbosa advised that febrifuges should not be abused, since "the fever of influenza does not have the same danger as in other infections and needs to be combated only when excessive." The doctor advised moderation in the use of painkillers such as antipyrin, phenacetin, and aspirin. They were to be used only when pain in the body or headaches was "strong or unbearable."[63]

Accacio Pires also prescribed one type of therapy for simple cases and another for the most complicated ones.[64] Therapies for simple cases were aimed at fortifying the body, especially the heart, and combating certain symptoms (vomiting, pain, hyperthermia, etc.). In severe and complicated cases, the medication was administered according to the nature of the disturbances, which could be nervous, circulatory, pulmonary, and gastro-intestinal. In his thesis, "A Small Contribution to the Study of the Flu," presented to the Faculty of Medicine of Bahia in 1900, Nicanor J. Ferreira spoke about the medication used in complicated cases: strychnine and glycerophosphoric were used for nervous asthenia; revulsives, expectorants, and vomitives for pulmonary complications; hydrochloride ammonia in cases of pulmonary congestion; opium, subnitrate, bismuth, salicylate, and benzonafitol for gastrointestinal disturbances; a milk medication for the symptoms of prostration, lethargy, neutralization, and toxemia; caffeine to regularize the status of the pulse and heart; and, finally, hydrotherapy for neurasthenia and weakness.[65]

Although the various therapies mentioned predate the Spanish flu pandemic, they were widely used by doctors during the illness. In an article written in 1919, Accacio Pires mentioned the same drugs, adding only a few procedures used in pulmonary complications, such as the use of a ventilator and emetine in severe cases of pneumonia with dyspnea, and hair tonic for treating alopecia that occurred after a heavy infection.[66]

When the epidemic crisis had passed, many physicians and pharmacists expressed their dissatisfaction with the therapies prescribed by medical science.[67] According to Pires, one of the drugs most used by physicians were tonics.[68] For physicians, however, the term "tonic" was not appropriate, since none of the substances had the power to invigorate the body. Rather, the tonics merely stimulated the body to use its own resources. For Pires, food constitutes the true tonic since it is the fuel the body uses to make energy. He thus criticized the misuse of tonics mainly because doctors could not reliably measure patients' strength. Quinine compounds also were shown to be inefficient, both as prophylactics and as curative agents for the Spanish flu.[69] In Bahia the popular poet Lulu Parola poked fun at quinine in a poem: "in Rio the quinine prescribed / Against the flu it did not work, / It did not take any sick person out of his bed."[70] Some alleged that the treatment applied by academic medicine differed very little or not at all from that of other curing practices—the lack of a specific medicine meant that the medication administered was restricted to relieving symptoms and to strengthening the organism so that it could resist the disease.[71]

According to Accacio Pires, even though the comforting belief prevailed that the therapeutic measures used were effective, what actually saved the population from a "hecatomb was the fact that flu is a disease that is highly contagious for men and of great mortality for chickens."[72] In other words, although people could contract the disease easily, it was (typically) only fatal to animals.

The City Survived the Scourge

The Spanish flu did not cause the same amount of public calamity in Salvador as in cities like São Paulo and Rio de Janeiro.[73] After the crisis has passed, the governor Moniz de Aragão insisted that Bahia was "one of the places in the world the influenza epidemic was more benign, less deadly, and less extensive." In a population of 320,000 inhabitants, it was estimated that about 130,000 were affected by the flu and only 386 people died from the disease.[74] Nevertheless, the pandemic caused brutal ruptures in daily life and social relations. The disease invaded homes and rapidly spread throughout the city, modifying the behavior and mood of the general population, causing isolation, and fomenting feelings characteristic of periods of epidemic crisis: sadness, dejection, restlessness, and fear borne of the natural desire for self-preservation.

Given the danger represented by the Spanish flu, people from all parts of society sought the help of supernatural forces. Bahia witnessed an intensification of religious faith, as manifested in numerous rituals: prayers, masses, adoration of images, cleansing of the body, offerings made to gods, and so on. In addition to spiritual protection, Bahians sought to strengthen and cure the body by availing themselves of the resources provided by academic medicine as well as by making use of the teachings of traditional and domestic medicine. In this sense, Bahian's efforts to mitigate the effects of the flu pandemic are marked by great eclecticism. The examination of these rituals, those informed by both scientific and religious concepts, reveals the social values of the epoch and the coexistence of beliefs and authority structures in permanent tension. In examining the response of Bahian society to the flu pandemic, I have tried to avoid establishing a hierarchy of knowledge. My purpose has been to demonstrate that each response had its own rationality, and the way people reacted to this disease is related to the social, political, economic, and cultural context of the period as well as to the collective memory of this particular disease.

Notes

1. Karl David Patterson, *Pandemic Influenza, 1700–1900: A Study in Historical Epidemiology* (Totowa: Rowman and Littlefield, 1986); Ann H. Reid, Jeffery K. Taubenberger, and Thomas G. Fanning, "The 1918 Spanish Influenza: Integrating History and Biology," *Microbes and Infection* 3, no. 1 (2001): 81–87, doi:10.1016/S1286-4579(00)01351-4.

2. Howard Phillips and David Killingray, eds., *The Spanish Influenza Pandemic of 1918–19: New Perspectives* (New York: Routledge, 2003); Fred R. Van Hartesveldt, ed., *The Pandemic of Influenza, 1918–1919: The Urban Impact in the Western World* (New York: Mellen, 1993).

3. "Mala da Europa. Chegou o 'Demerara,'" *O Imparcial*, September 23, 1918; "Uma nova epidemia está assolando a capital. Influenza? Gripe Espanhola?," *A Tarde*, September 25, 1918.

4. "Mala da Europa. Chegou o 'Demerara'"; "A influenza hespanhola espalha-se em nossos navios," *O Imparcial*, September 23 and 24, 1918. See also chapter 2 of this volume.

5. "Dos influenzados do 'Demera,' dois vieram a fallecer já nesta capital," *Diario de Noticias* October 2, 1918.

6. Christiane M. Cruz de Souza, *A gripe espanhola na Bahia: Saúde, política e medicina em tempos de epidemia* (Salvador: Editora da Universidade Federal da Bahia / Fundação Oswaldo Cruz, 2009). The political scene of Bahia was characterized by a strong personalism and incipient political party organization. The new generation of politicians, which emerged in the late nineteenth century, was more prone to the leadership of a strong personality than the command of a political party. Each group revolved around a charismatic figure, whose name was more representative than the symbol of the party. One emblematic figure of this period, José Joaquim Seabra, played a leading role in the politics of Bahia for a period of twelve years (1912–24). Seabra was a senator and minister, and he ruled the state twice. But several groups were opposed to him and his ally, Antonio F. Moniz de Aragão, who ruled the state at the time of the epidemic: *severinistas* (allies of former governor Severino Vieira), *marcelinistas* (allies of former governor José Marcelino), *vianistas* (allies of former governor Luis Vianna) and *ruistas* (supporters of Ruy Barbosa's candidacy for president). To learn more, see Eul-Soo Pang, *Coronelismo e oligarquias (1889–1934): A Bahia na República Brasileira* (Rio de Janeiro: Civilização Brasileira, 1979); Consuelo Novais Sampaio, *Os partidos políticos da Bahia na Primeira República: Uma política de acomodação* (Salvador: Editora da Universidade Federal da Bahia, 1999); and Israel de Oliveira Pinheiro, "A política na Bahia: Atraso e personalismos," *Ideação, Feira de Santana* 4 (jul./dez. 1999), 49–78.

7. Bertucci gives more details on this in chapter 2 of this volume.

8. Alfred W. Crosby, *America's Forgotten Pandemic: The Influenza of 1918* (New York: Cambridge University Press, 1989).

9. On the significance of the "soldado de Nápoles" name, see Ryan A. Davis, "Don Juan versus Bacteriology: Competing Narrative Explanations of the 1918–19 'Spanish' Flu Epidemic in Spain," *Ometeca* 16 (2011): 171–89. For the Portuguese case, see chapters 3 and 4 of this volume.

10. "A 'influenza hespanhola.' Victimas brasileiras," *Diario de Noticias*, September 23, 1918. At the time, Pacífico Pereira stated to the *Diario da Bahia* that the name

derived from "Spain's neutrality in the great world conflagration," which had provided the flu with easier access to the Iberian Peninsula, "from where it left to invade Africa, Brazil and probably the whole of South America." "A epidemia reinante," October 29, 1918. Porras-Gallo and Davis discuss the origins of the name "Spanish" flu in the introduction to this volume.

11. Ribeiro da Silva, "Grippe pandemica e grippe nostras," *Brazil-Medico* 33 (1919): 44.

12. "A gripe hespanhola o que ella é – como agir," *Diario de Noticias*, October 5, 1918.

13. Bertucci deals extensively with this issue in chapter 2 of this volume.

14. The various researchers investigating the etiology of influenza during the pandemic of 1918–19 include Henri Violle, Charles Nicolle, and Charles Lebailly from France; H. Selter from Germany; and T. Yamanouchi, S. Iwashima, and K. Sakakami from Japan. Olympio da Fonseca Filho, *A Escola de Manguinhos: Contribuição para o estudo do desenvolvimento da medicina experimental no Brasil*, vol. 2 (São Paulo: Oswaldo Cruz Monumenta Histórica, 1974); María-Isabel Porras-Gallo, *Un reto para la sociedad madrileña: La epidemia de gripe de 1918–19* (Madrid: Complutense / Comunidad Autónoma de Madrid, 1997). The investigation of both the French and Japanese teams sought to prove that an invisible and filterable agent caused this illness. In Brazil Henrique Aragão, Ulysses Paranhos, Arthur Moses, and the team formed by Aristides Marques da Cunha, Olympio da Fonseca Filho, and Octavio de Magalhães conducted similar research on the etiology of the disease independently of their French and Japanese counterparts. See Henrique de B. Aragão, "A proposito da grippe," *Brazil-Medico* 32, no. 45 (1918): 353–6; Bowman C. Crowell, "Exposição dos resultados de estudos sobre anathomia patológica da gripe," *Boletim da Academia de Medicina*, November 21, 1918, 668–75; Aristides Marques da Cunha, Octavio de Magalhães, and O. Fonseca, "Estudos experimentais sobre a influenza pandêmica," *Brazil-Medico* 32, no. 48 (1918): 174–91; Arthur Moses, "Exposição dos resultados de estudos sobre a etiologia da gripe," *Boletim da Academia de Medicina*, November 21, 1918, 681–6; Arthur Moses, "Bacteriologia da gripe," *Brazil-Medico* 33, no. 5 (1919): 37–39; Ulysses Paranhos, "Ensaios da esputo-vacinação anti-grippal," *Brazil-Medico* 33, no. 3 (1919): 20–21. This subject is discussed in more detail in Christiane M. Cruz de Souza, "The Spanish Flu Epidemic: A Challenge to Bahian Medicine," *História, Ciências, Saúde: Manguinhos* 15 (2008): 945–72.

15. Souza, "The Spanish Flu Epidemic," 945–72.

16. "A Influenza hespanhola é 'febre dos tres dias' (mal dos papatases)," *Diário da Bahia*, September 26, 1918; n/a "O que diz o dr. Carlos Seidl sobre a epidemia," *Diario de Noticias*, October 1, 1918. Pappataci fever is a disease caused by an invisible and filterable agent, like that of dengue or yellow fever. It is transmitted through the bite of the female of the mosquito species *Phlebotomus papatassi*. Since the final years of the nineteenth century, various research studies had shown or investigated the possibility of diseases being transmitted by insects, either in mechanical form or as intermediary hosts for microorganisms, including those then described as viruses invisible to optical microscopes and capable of passing through filters that retained the smallest bacteria. Jaime Larry Benchimol, *Dos micróbiosaos mosquitos: Febre amarela e a revolução pasteuriana no Brasil* (Rio de Janeiro: Fundação Oswaldo Cruz / Universidade Federal do Rio de Janeiro, 1999), 396; María-Isabel Porras-Gallo,

"Una ciudad en crisis: La epidemia de gripe de 1918–1919 en Madrid" (PhD diss., Universidad Complutense de Madrid, 1994), 323.

17. To learn more about the subject, see chapter 2 of this volume; and Souza, "The Spanish Flu Epidemic." See also Janete Silveira Abrão, *Banalização da morte na cidade calada: A hespanhola em Porto Alegre, 1918* (Porto Alegre: EDIPCRS, 1998); Cláudio Bertolli Filho, *A gripe espanhola em São Paulo, 1918: Epidemia e sociedade* (São Paulo: Paz e Terra, 2003); Liane Maria Bertucci, "Entre doutores e para os leigos: Fragmentos do discurso médico na influenza de 1918," *História, Ciências, Saúde: Manguinhos* 12, no. 1 (2005): 143–57; Bertucci, *Influenza, a medicina enferma: Ciência e práticas de cura na época da gripe espanhola em São Paulo* (Campinas: Universidade Estadual de Campinas, 2004); William I. B. Beveridge, *Influenza: The Last Great Plague: An Unfinished Story of Discovery* (New York: Prodist, 1977); Crosby, *America's Forgotten Pandemic*; Adriana da Costa Goulart, "Um cenário mefistofélico: A gripe espanhola no Rio de Janeiro" (PhD diss., Universidade Federal Fluminense, 2003); Gina Kolata, *Gripe: A história da pandemia de 1918* (Rio de Janeiro: Record, 2002); Porras-Gallo, *Reto*; Anny J. Torres Silveira, "A medicina e a influenza espanhola de 1918," *Tempo: Revista do Departamento de História da UFF* 10, no. 19 (2005): 91–105; and Eugenia Tognotti, "Scientific Triumphalism and Learning from Facts: Bacteriology and the 'Spanish Flu' Challenge of 1918," *Social History of Medicine* 16, no. 1 (2003): 97–110.

18. "Grippe," *Diario da Bahia*, October 3, 1918.

19. "A Semana d'O Imparcial," *O Imparcial*, October 15, 1918.

20. As Feldman notes in chapter 10, similar reactions were seen in Argentina during the pandemic.

21. Paul Slack, Introduction to *Epidemics and Ideas: Essays on Historical Perception of Pestilence*, ed., Terence Ranger and Paul Slack (New York: Cambridge University Press, 1992), 8–9.

22. The Bahia state had trade relations with European countries involved in the conflict. In addition, the Brazilian troops were part of a military medical mission sent to war to support allied forces. See "Ainda o terrivel mal que victimou os marujos nacionaes, nas costas africanas," *Diário de Notícias*, October 2, 1918, and "A influenza alarma a cidade. Benigna porém epidêmica," *O Imparcial*, September 26, 1918.

23. To learn more about the cholera epidemic, see Johildo Lopes de Athayde, *Salvador e a grande epidemia de 1855* (Salvador: Universidade Federal da Bahia, Centro de Estudos Baianos, 1985); Cleide de Lima Chaves, "'Fluxo e refluxo' do cólera na Bahia e no Prata," *Anais Eletrônicos do IV Encontro da ANPHLAC* (Salvador, 2000); Anna Amélia Vieira Nascimento, "O cólera morbus como fator de involução populacional da cidade do Salvador," *Anais do Arquivo Público da Bahia* 45 (1981): 263–89; and Onildo Reis David, *O inimigo invisível: Epidemia na Bahia no século XIX* (Salvador: Editora da Universidade Federal da Bahia, 1996). For in-depth studies of the social impact of cholera, see also Steven Johnson, *O mapa fantasma: Como a luta de dois homens contra o cólera mudou o destino de nossas metrópoles* (Rio de Janeiro: Zahar, 2008); and Richard J. Evans, "Epidemics and Revolutions: Cholera in Nineteenth-Century Europe," in Ranger and Slack, *Epidemics and Ideas*, 149–73.

24. "A grippe impressiona pelo extraordinário número de casos," *O Imparcial*, September 30, 1918.

25. "Uma nova epidemia está assolando a capital. Influenza? Gripe Espanhola?," *A Tarde*, September 25, 1918; "A influenza na cidade. As providencias da Hygiene (Dr. Alberto Muylaert)," *O Imparcial*, September 29, 1918.

26. "A grippe na Bahia," *A Tarde*, September 30, 1918; "A grippe impressiona pelo extraordinário número de casos," *O Imparcial*, September 30, 1918.

27. "A grippe prossegue na sua derrocada," *O Imparcial*, October 16, 1918.

28. "Directoria Geral da Saude Publica da Bahia," *O Democrata*, November 10, 1918.

29. "Socorrei o povo!," *O Imparcial*, October 23, 1918.

30. "Ainda a 'influenza,'" *Diario de Noticias*, October 25, 1918; n/a "Directoria Geral da Saude Publica da Bahia," *O Democrata*, October 25, 1918.

31. See also chapters 6 and 9 of this volume.

32. "A 'influenza' na Bahia. Conselhos e providencias," *Diario de Noticias*, October 28, 1918.

33. "Por causa da epidemia. Este anno não haverá romaria aos cemitérios," *O Imparcial*, October 27, 1918; "Directoria Geral da Saude Publica da Bahia. Aviso," *A Tarde*, November 1, 1918.

34. João José Reis (1991) has studied representations of death and the meaning of transformations in funeral rites in Bahia during the nineteenth century. As noted in chapter 9 of this volume, similar reactions occurred in Spain during the pandemic.

35. Jean Delumeau, *História do medo no Ocidente: 1300–1800, uma cidade sitiada* (São Paulo: Companhia das Letras, 1989).

36. In 1835 a revolt exploded in Bahia—the Cemiterada—when public health authorities imposed alterations in funeral rites. Cf. João José Reis, *A morte é uma festa: Ritos fúnebres e revolta popular no Brasil do século XIX* (São Paulo: Companhia das Letras, 1991).

37. Plácido Barbosa, "Influenzaphobia," *O Imparcial*, October 24, 1918.

38. "A Nota. A cidade doente (The Sick City)," *Jornal de Noticias*, October 8, 1918.

39. "O senador Luiz Vianna de gripe," *O Imparcial*, October 22, 1918.

40. "O estado de saude do futuro presidente da República," *Diário de Notícias*, October 28, 1918.

41. Patrick Zylberman states, "The virus might well have behaved 'democratically,' but the society it attacked was hardly egalitarian," "The Holocaust in a Holocaust: The Great War and the 1918 "Spanish" Influenza Epidemic in France," in Phillips and Killingray, *Spanish Influenza Pandemic*, 199. In the chapter about the epidemic in Rio de Janeiro, Sam Adamo highlights the disastrous consequences of the disease among blacks and mulattos, which resulted from poor living conditions observed in this layer of society in the thirty years following the abolition of slavery. "Rio de Janeiro," in Van Hartesveldt, *Pandemic of Influenza*, 185–200. In *Gripe espanhola* Bertolli Filho discusses the myth of democratic mortality, showing that, in São Paulo, most deaths from influenza occurred among the poorest strata of society. See also Beatriz Anselmo Olinto, "Uma cidade em tempo de epidemia: Rio Grande e a gripe Espanhola (RS–1918)" (master's thesis, Universidade Federal de Santa Catarina, 1996); and Souza, *A Gripe espanhola na Bahia*. Sobral, Lima, and Silveira e Sousa also discuss this topic in chapter 4 of this volume.

42. A comparison of information from the sources consulted leads us to conclude that most flu victims in Bahia were Brazilian, unmarried, male workers between

twenty and forty years of age—farmers, soldiers, civil servants, and trade workers—subject to an exhaustive system of work and living in extreme poverty due to low salaries (at a time when food prices and housing costs were high). Cruz de Souza, *Gripe espanhola na Bahia.*

43. On increasing expressions of Catholic religiosity during the pandemic, see also chapters 4 and 12 of this volume.

44. *Beija-pé,* or "kissing of feet," is a ritual in which the faithful prostrate themselves before the image of the saint to kiss his feet or the hem of his clothes in an attitude of supplication and humility.

45. According to Slack, "From the plague of Athens onwards, people . . . [have] sought solace in religious practices," which held out the promise of effective action, even if (in gathering people together) such rites conflicted with other assumptions about the kinds of defense responses called for by epidemics. Paul Slack, Introduction to *Epidemics and Ideas,* 4.

46. Pierre Verger, *Notícias da Bahia: 1850* (Salvador: Corrupio, 1999).

47. "Senhor do Bonfim não vae descer. Do alto Elle velará por nós," *Jornal de Noticias,* October 6, 1918.

48. "A fé não more: O Senhor do Bonfim já desceu," *Jornal de Noticias,* October 29, 1918.

49. *Candomblés* is an animistic religion originating from Nigeria and what is today called Benin. Captured Africans brought it to Brazil during the slave trade. Its adherents hold public and private ceremonies in which they embody the forces of nature and the spirit of the ancestors. Antônio Houaiss, ed., *Dicionário eletrônico Houaiss da língua portuguesa* (Rio de Janeiro: Objetiva, 2001), CD-ROM, Versão 1.0.

50. Jaqueline de Andrade Pereira, "Práticas mágicas e cura popular na Bahia (1890–1940)" (PhD diss., Universidade Federal da Bahia, 1998).

51. Hildegardes Vianna, *Antigamente era assim* (Salvador: Fundação Cultural do Estado da Bahia, 1994), 213–18. According to Vianna, "the syrup made from leaf-cutting ants prevents the lung from being affected during bronchitis." *Antigamente era assim,* 213. Folha-da-costa (*Kalanchoe brasiliensis*) is a succulent plant. In traditional medicine, *Kalanchoe* species have been used to treat ailments such as infections, rheumatism and inflammation." The angico (*Anadenanthera colubrina*) is a medicinal plant. A syrup of the bark and resin is used to treat upper respiratory infections and angina pectoris. See Houaiss, *Dicionário eletrônico Houaiss da língua portuguesa.* Leaf of *carqueja* (*Baccharistrimera*) is used to treat gastrointestinal and respiratory infections, fever, and rheumatism. Patrícia Shima Luize, Tatiana Shioji Tiuman, Luis Gustavo Morello, Paloma Korehiza Maza, Tânia Ueda-Nakamura, Benedito Prado Dias Filho, Diógenes Aparício Garcia Cortez, João Carlos Palazzo de Mello, and Celso Vataru Nakamura, "Effects of Medicinal Plant Extracts on Growth of Leishmania (L.) amazonensis and Trypanosoma cruzi," *Revista Brasileira de Ciências Farmacêuticas* 41, no. 1 (2005): 85–94.

52. Vianna, *Antigamente era assim,* 213, 214, 221. *Rapadura* is a traditional food from northeastern Brazil made from boiled sugarcane juice, molded, and then dried in small blocks. Some recipes added macerated *aguardente* (spirits). After being bottled, the mixture was left outdoors or buried upside down.

53. Ibid., 224–26. The *sabugueiro* (European elder) was often used in cases of measles. *Tília* (linden) was used for coughs and for mucus of the lungs and the bronchial tubes.

54. See Antônio Ferrão Moniz de Aragão, *Mensagem apresentada à Assembléia Geral Legislativa do Estado da Bahia na abertura da 1a sessãoordinária da 15a legislatura pelo Dr. Antônio Ferrão Moniz de Aragão, governador do estado* (Bahia: Imprensa Oficial do Estado, 1919); Santa Casa de Misericórdia da Bahia, *Atos da Provedoria,* Livro 2°, B/2ª/159, 1917–31; "Diretoria do Hospital Santa Izabel," *Relatório do Serviço do Hospital Santa Izabel durante o anno de 1918* 1919: 129–31.

55. "E a grippe dizima," *Diario de Noticias,* October 24, 1918.

56. "Não haja ilusões," *A Tarde,* October 31, 1918.

57. Frederico Koch, Dionísio Pereira, and Aristides Novis, "A epidemia de gripe: Parecer da comissãonomeada pelo diretor da saúde publica da Bahia," *Gazeta Médica da Bahia* 50 (1918): 150–51.

58. A similar conclusion was reached in Spain. See chapters 9 and 11 of this volume.

59. Koch, Pereira, and Novis, "Epidemia de gripe," 153.

60. "Directoria Geral da Saude Publica da Bahia," *O Democrata,* October 25, 1918.

61. Plácido Barbosa, "Influenzaphobia," *O Imparcial,* October 24, 1918, 1.

62. Barbosa ("Influenzaphobia") advised washing the mouth and throat with carbolic water at a 1 percent concentration or with water and salicylic acid at 1 per mil, though another antiseptic could also be used. At the beginning of the twentieth century, Ferreira recommended that antisepsis and asepsis of the mouth and nose be carried out using substances such as Van Switen's liquor in half a glass of water and that a formol, menthol, or carbolic solution be used for gargling and washing the mouth. See Nicanor José Ferreira, *Ligeira contribuição para o estudo da grippe: Tese inaugural apresentada à Faculdade de Medicina da Bahia* (Salvador: Typographia d'Estandarte Catholico, 1900).

63. Barbosa, "Influenzaphobia." Antipyrin was used to relieve pain and lower the temperature. Accacio Pires, "A gripe e a therapeutica," *Saúde: Orgão da Liga Pro-Saneamento do Brazil; Mensário de hygiene e de assumptos soceaes e econômicos* 2 (January–February 1919): 3–4. But Ferreira warned that this substance should not be abused, "since it has the property of reducing renal excretion, which is inconvenient, because the organism cannot get rid of the toxins that it itself has prepared." Ferreira, *Ligeira contribuição,* 21–22.

64. Pires, "A Gripe e a therapeutica," 4.

65. Other sources also mention the use of other purgatives, such as calomel and anidiol. See Antonio Contreiras, *Cartas recebidas pelo diretor do serviço sanitário sobre ataques de gripe e outros asuntos,* Arquivo Público do Estado da Bahia. Seção Republicana. Secretaria do Interior e da Justiça. Diretoria Geral da Saúde Pública. Datas limite: 1912–18, caixa: 3697, maço: 1032, 19.10. 1918; and Pires, "A Gripe e a therapeutica," 6.

66. Pires, "A Gripe e a therapeutica," 6.

67. According to Lori Loeb, similar problems occurred in England. Patients self-medicated, doctors considered many remedies and treatments quackery, and many drugs prescribed by doctors were similar to those they condemned. "Beating the Flu: Orthodox and Commercial Responses to Influenza in Britain, 1889–1919," *Social History of Medicine* 18, no. 2 (2005): 203–24, doi:10.1093/sochis/hki030.

68. The author classifies tonics as general (alcohol, cola, cinnamon, and quinine); cardiac (camphor oil, caffeine, sparteine, and digitalis); and "nervines" (strychnine, glycerol phosphoric, and arsenic). Pires, "A Gripe e a therapeutica," 4.

69. In 1900 Nicanor J. Ferreira had already emphasized that flu scholars were unanimous in stating there was no proper treatment for influenza. According to the author, some doctors insisted on using quinine as a specific remedy for flu, believing that the presence of substance in the blood became a medium unfavorable to the Pfeifer bacillus. But Ferreira emphasized that the therapeutic action of this substance was a controversial issue, considering that this bacillus was not found, except in exceptional conditions, in the blood of those suffering from the disease. See Ferreira, *Ligeira contribuição*.

70. Lulu Parola, "Cantando e rindo," *Jornal de Noticias*, October 25, 1918.

71. According to Lori Loeb similar problems occurred in England. Patients self-medicated, doctors considered many remedies and treatments as quackery, and many drugs prescribed by doctors were similar to those they condemned, "Beating the Flu," 203–24.

72. Pires, "A Gripe e a therapeutica," 6.

73. See chapter 6 of this volume.

74. Moniz de Aragão, *Mensagem apresentada*.

Chapter Eight

A Collaborative Experience: The Mutual Benefit Societies' Responses to the 1918–19 Influenza Pandemic in Pamplona, Spain

PILAR LEÓN-SANZ

The influenza pandemic that wreaked havoc in Europe in 1918 was an ordeal for the societies it affected, as evidenced by governments' efforts to fight it, health professionals' responses to it, and the general population's behavior.[1] Scholarly attention to these issues has expanded our understanding of the epidemic beyond what we learn from morbimortality data, which are important in their own right. Nevertheless, relatively little work has been done on nongovernmental and not-for-profit organizations during the 1918–19 epidemic, despite current broader interest in the provision of welfare services "outside the purview of the State" from individuals, families, mutual-aid associations, and private charities.[2] This chapter examines the pandemic from the point of view of the mutual benefit societies (MBSs) in Spain—whose work became vital for the attention received at the time by workers and their families—to shed light on the history of these societies and their relationship with the state system and other public administrations as well as on the 1918–19 influenza pandemic.

We look specifically at the effort of the physicians employed by these societies in Pamplona, Spain. As a general rule, these societies were linked to the social hygiene movement that became prominent in Europe at the beginning of the twentieth century as a means to social reform.[3] They were known for assisting authorities in fostering health care practices, and they played a leading educational role in the improvement of health among the inhabitants of Pamplona during the first two decades of the twentieth century.[4] In this period Spanish activists and physicians, frequently funded by private charity with hardly any support from public authorities, organized medical-social campaigns to improve the public health of society.[5]

At the time of the influenza epidemic, Pamplona had the same medical health care systems as the rest of Spain. At the turn of the twentieth century the Spanish sanitary structure were based on nineteenth-century models, which had shifted from the social assistance characteristic of the Ancien Régime to a humanitarian model more in keeping with the liberal state.[6] Particularly from the 1880s the reformist and social hygiene movements, statutory provisions, and socioeconomic conditions brought about changes in the organization and provision of public health assistance. These reforms were also due to the fact that the liberal public care model left much of the population unprotected, as it covered only families on the dole. Furthermore, the development of social protection in Spain was connected to worker associationism and the movements that arose from the social doctrine of the Catholic Church, promoted by Pope Leon XIII's 1891 encyclical on social justice, *Rerum novarum.*

The development of social protection in Spain was clearly inspired by its practice in other European countries. Initially the debate focused on the Bismarckian mandatory insurance system, but when the Instituto Nacional de Previsión (National Institute of Social Protection) project was being designed, between 1903 and 1906, it also took into account the Italian and Belgian systems, which were based on collaborations with private initiatives, particularly with the *cajas de ahorro* (savings banks). In the end, the Instituto Nacional de Previsión, inaugurated in 1908, maintained its subsidiary relationship with the state in the promotion of social security.[7]

The first projects for social protection legislation led to the passing of the Ley de Accidentes de Trabajo (Law on Labor Accidents) in 1900 and the regulation of working conditions for women and children. Moreover, in 1919 the Retiro Obrero (Workers' Obligatory Retirement)—which protected the elderly and disabled—was approved, the first insurance system of its kind. Until the 1940s, when Spain introduced obligatory health insurance, about 60 percent of workers and their families entrusted their health care to diverse mutual assistance societies and mutual insurance associations. The generalized workers' crisis and the social conflicts in Spain in this period were not as active in the province of Pamplona as in others. Nonetheless, in the first few years of the twentieth century Pamplona also suffered a serious social problem because of a high rate of unemployment.[8] For this reason, an analysis of the assistance offered by MBSs during periods of ill health—like the 1918–19 influenza pandemic—provides an interesting perspective on the history of medical care.

The MBSs were not-for-profit collectives that worked outside the auspices of the state to provide a form of welfare to workers and their families.

Members often participated in their management and administration. Some of these societies had their roots in the old guilds, but the majority were new, promoted by the Ley de Asociaciones (Associations Act) of 1887. Workers' subscriptions, contributions from employers and patron-members, and other donations covered the expenditures. In general, these organizations reflected the ideological inspiration of their sponsors.[9] To date, the role of the MBSs during the influenza pandemic has not been explored in detail, perhaps because of the difficulty in finding information about these organizations. But it is interesting to analyze the repercussions of the pandemic using the societies, as they gave medical care to a significant portion of Spanish society. In the case of Pamplona, MBSs provided medical assistance to over one-third of the city's population, at the time some thirty thousand people.

Several studies have analyzed the situation of medical and social associations in Navarre in the period under consideration, but in Navarre Catholic inspiration lay behind many of the workmen's institutions.[10] Such is the case with La Conciliación (Conciliation Society), an MBS founded in 1902 to provide labor mediation, medical-pharmaceutical care (with a medical staff of four physicians—Pedro Subelza, Ramón Sanz, Sergio Lazcano, and Saturnino Lizarraga—who had a protagonist role during the pandemic, as we will see), and monetary aid to 1,400 male workers and their families.[11] Until 1920 La Conciliación was the most important MBS in the city. Until 1920 a so-called Mixed Board—composed of eighteen members, six from each group of workers, employers, and patrons or donors)—governed La Conciliación. Any tradesman or employee living within a ten-kilometer radius of Pamplona could belong to the society.[12] A host of other aid associations, workers' associations, and trade unions also provided assistance. These included the Sociedad de Artesanos (Craftsmen's Guilds), which dates from the mid-nineteenth century; the Unión Productora (Producers' Union), with some 488 members plus their families; the Hermandad de la Pasión (Brotherhood of the Passion), a workers' society with 127 members plus their families; Federación Local de las Sociedades de Trabajadores (Local Federation of Workmen's Societies), started in 1902; and the Sindicato Católico Libre (Free Catholic Union), created in 1915.[13]

Using the minutes of these MBSs, local news reports, and the archives of the Navarrese and Pamplona public administration offices, I analyze the associations' perceptions of the epidemic. These documents reveal a spirit of complementarity in their varied responses to the emergency. Especially noteworthy is the role of the organizations' physicians who, in mediating this response, successfully integrated the aid organizations into the broader medical health care network in the city. I also discuss the effects of the influenza outbreak on these societies, noting how the rise in the number of sick leaves modified working procedures, which in turn influenced the relationship between the organizations, their members, and physicians. The increase in the number of the people affected by the epidemic, and who therefore needed assistance, exceeded the economic calculations of the MBSs, which became a serious problem since these societies were basically maintained by their members' financial contributions. To overcome this critical situation, they were forced to seek financial aid (which they were granted) from local and provincial governments.

The Epidemic as Experienced by the Pamplona Mutual Benefit Societies

Navarre and, in particular, Pamplona, its capital city, was one of the areas in Spain most gravely affected by the second wave of the 1918–19 influenza epidemic.[14] Pamplona's population remained largely unchanged in the first two decades of the twentieth century. Its scant demographic growth was due in part to the fact that it was a walled town and, particularly, to the slow process of industrialization, which was hampered by the negative effects of the Carlist Wars.[15] Moreover, between 1900 and 1920 Navarre experienced negative net migration because of the large number of Navarrese who moved to surrounding areas such as Vizcaya or Guipuzcoa and to foreign countries.[16] These key concerns of Navarrese society were reflected in various population studies including the comparative analyses of deaths, births, and marriages, as well as the search for the causes of high death rates. Not surprisingly, these studies influenced the actions of physicians, including those employed by MBSs. For instance, Agustín Lazcano, who was on the medical staff of La Conciliación, drew up new bylaws to organize the municipal registry of births and deaths that was begun in 1902. He compared the health statistics and demography of Pamplona with those of other places and countries and expressed concern about the mortality figures in Pamplona at the time.

An analysis of the illness rates during the influenza pandemic reveals a steady rise in both the illness rate and sick leave for respiratory disease that actually stretches back to 1915. This led to increased control over sick leave as societies sought to minimize its negative economic consequences. Despite this general increase, during the first epidemic wave in May 1918, the minutes of La Conciliación show no significant increase in sick leaves, with the exception of a moderate peak in illness rates for the week of June 26 (63 sick leaves). As a result of the minimal impact of the first epidemic wave, the city went ahead with its plans to celebrate the festival of its patron saint, San Fermín, in July. By August 1918, however, La Conciliación's minutes resounded with the "terrifying" onset of the disease.

Indeed, the data on the illness rates from La Conciliación show that the epidemic broke out suddenly in the second fortnight of September. A routine number of sick leaves was recorded on September 16 (24), but this almost doubled within a week (40) and remained constant (and constantly high) for ten weeks, until the second fortnight in November. Although data from the MBSs show that the epidemic continued during the first three weeks of November—data later supported by the official figures published in the *Boletín Mensual de Estadística Demográfico-Sanitaria* (Demographic-Health Statistics Bulletin, 1918)[17]—the press reported that the exceptional measures that had been adopted in the first few days of the month to curb the spread of the epidemic had been discontinued. The motives for the divergence between the decisions of the public authorities and the sick leave figures remain unexplained.

The month of October and the first fortnight of November registered the highest number of victims, peaking from October 14–28, 1918. After November 25 the illness rate began to drop and soon returned to average levels (fig. 8.1). The data from other MBSs reveal a similar pattern.

According to the deaths recorded at the Registry Office in Pamplona, 216 people died during the autumn influenza period: 215 between September 17 and November 17, and 1 on December 1.[18] Table 8.1 provides information on the 27 fatalities among the members of the different MBSs, calculated from the postmortem subsidies paid by the MBSs to the families. The morbidity rates recorded in the archives of La Conciliación and in the *Boletín Mensual de Estadística Demográfico-Sanitaria* attest to a relative mildness of the third epidemic wave, which took place from mid-February to the end of March 1919.

The Reaction of the Mutual Benefit Societies

In Pamplona, the municipal and provincial organizations coordinated relief efforts—including the administration of medical attention and the provision of basic foodstuffs—with nongovernmental MBSs. This was combined with the MBSs' efforts to obtain funds to fulfill their commitment to the affected members and to maintain solvency. The public health resources used against the epidemic were those typical of the time: isolation, street cleaning, disinfection of business premises, and immediate removal of corpses.[19] Throughout the epidemic, city hall maintained "brigades" with atomizers for cleansing and disinfecting courtyards, doorways, and staircases, and by the end of the epidemic they had effectively cleaned all the houses in the city several times.[20] They also closed schools.[21]

In addition to the specific measures taken, an intense public health education campaign was waged in the press and through city hall proclamations—that is, the distribution of leaflets containing the city bylaws on public health and "sheets reproduced by the Provincial Health Inspector with measures

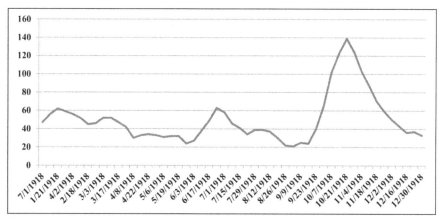

Figure 8.1. La Conciliación, illness rate, 1918. León-Sanz's elaboration (dates: day/ month/year). La Conciliación, *Books of Minutes*, 1918, Archive University of Navarra.

Table 8.1. Postmortem allowances, September–November 1918

Society	Postmortem benefit		
	Number	Amount (in pesetas)	Period
La Conciliación	10	800	September 15–October 29
Unión Productora	1	40	September 15–November 3
Unión Obrera	11	760	September 20–October 25
Artesanos	5	300	September 15–October 30
Total	27	1,900	

Source: La Conciliación, *Books of Minutes*, 1918, Archive University of Navarra; Hygiene Section, 1918, Municipal Archive of Pamplona.

to be taken by individuals to avoid the spread of the grippe."[22] Physicians recommended the consumption of milk, lemons, and eggs. In some cases they also prescribed "sudatory medications, abundant beverages, diuretics, theobromine, and antidiphtheric serum if the infection is very striking."[23] Similar medical practices were adopted in other places.[24]

Because of the effects of World War I, Pamplona was at that time in the midst of a serious provision problem, which deteriorated further with the onset of the epidemic. The market price of milk and other basic staples needed for the treatment of patients kept rising. In response, the MBSs and workers' associations demanded the intervention of the government and the city council. They held meetings with the civil governor on September 28, 1918, and with the mayor on October 15, 1918: "The representatives of Asociación de Empleados, La Conciliación, La Federación Obrera, La Unión Obrera, and Sindicato de Obreros, on 30th September last, request that, in view of the abnormal circumstances the city is undergoing, the taxes on basic subsistence foodstuffs be controlled."[25] The demand was met as the city council adopted an interventionist policy that established fixed prices for food.[26] As a result, "the reduction in the cost of bread from the Vínculo bakery is agreed upon, even if this means [financial] losses." The sale of milk and its derivatives was also centralized and a fixed price of sixty cents per liter was established. Moreover, the city council distributed vouchers through the MBSs that could be redeemed for milk, eggs, fish, meat, and coal.[27] Later rice, potatoes, and beans were added to the list of products one could obtain with a voucher. La Conciliación, which had managed a cooperative for its members since 1912, participated in the municipal interventionist policy of discounting food.

Consequences for the Societies' Medical Staff

MBSs offered general medical care through its doctors-office consultations and medical home care. At the beginning of the epidemic, the physicians used press releases to recommend that that those affected by influenza should visit the doctor immediately: "Inform him: if there are to be complications, he can prevent them and will treat them efficiently and appropriately."[28] As a consequence of this advice, doctors' home visits increased to the point that La Conciliación physicians complained they were unable to attend to so many people.[29] In Pamplona the number of patients admitted to hospitals did not rise, a fact that suggests physicians doing house calls bore the brunt of the increased demand for medical attention occasioned by the epidemic.[30] To make matters worse, Dr. Lizarraga fell ill in mid-October. Dr. Sergio Lazcano renounced his salary on the grounds he could not carry out his work, a decision accepted by the society's Mixed Board, contingent on his finding a substitute. Unable to do so, he continued to attend to patients himself. The physicians postponed paperwork—including illness reports—and administrative tasks because of the overwhelming number of patients needing attention.[31]

To lighten the load on the doctors, the Mixed Board of La Conciliación sent an official note to the president of the newly established Official Medical College of Navarre, asking him to request the use of official city council automobiles for physicians' house calls. This was speedily arranged, and La Conciliación physicians S. Lizarraga and Sergio Lazcano, as well as the physicians from the Beneficencia, were granted use of the vehicles. Moreover, on October 7 the city council, using its powers to "marshal the health care services of those who practiced health care professions" during epidemics decreed that there should be a physician on call at night, from nine at night to seven in the morning, to allow the remaining twenty-two physicians in the city to get a good night's rest.[32] The person appointed was the Pamplona forensic surgeon, though the service was discontinued in early November.[33]

On Sunday, October 20, the mayor summoned the city physicians, including those belonging to the MBSs, to coordinate aid distribution to poor patients, whether they depended on municipal charity or not. After Dr. Sergio Lazcano announced the plan at a society meeting, the city council sent foodstuffs directly to La Conciliación for their distribution by the physicians. The following note from La Conciliación serves as an example of the minutes dedicated to this issue: "The Council has sent tins of condensed milk. They are being sent to Pedro Subelza as the senior physician."[34]

When the epidemic ended, both the authorities and the press expressed their gratitude to the physicians for their labor in attending to the sick. On November 7, 1918, the *Diario de Navarra* published a statement from the mayor to the Official Medical College, praising the valuable work carried out by the Pamplona physicians during the epidemic. He profusely thanked all of them for their generous support and collaboration with the city council's arrangements. The newspaper added, "We find this praise to be deserved and join in [thanking the physicians] most sincerely."[35]

The rise in morbidity rates among worker-members of the MBSs was connected to profound changes in the structuring of the work of medical professionals.[36] The most notable of these was giving the members of La Conciliación the right to choose their own physician, an issue that at the time constituted part of a broader argument regarding the defense of the professional model and the new demands for responsibility that society demanded of its physicians.[37] In practice, in La Conciliación, sick notes had to be signed by a physician belonging to the association. But from 1915 onward, coinciding with an increase in sick leave, the Mixed Guild requested that members be permitted to visit physicians who did not belong to La Conciliación, noting that the members would pay the corresponding fees, but that the society would admit both the prescriptions and sick notes drawn up by these physicians. Surveillance to avoid abuse of the system was entrusted from early on to the workers' guilds, the society physicians, and an inspector employed for this task. Physicians were repeatedly reminded to be punctual in writing sick leave notes and discharges and, in this manner, collaborate in the management of sick leave situations. In 1916 they were urged to draw up sick leave notes at La Conciliación's headquarters and were subsequently obliged to visit members on sick leave every three days to reduce their period of convalescence. Thus, after the physician Ramón Sanz reported finding a society member supposed to be at home on sick leave absent from his home on January 14, 15, and 16, 1918, the board cut the member's benefits.[38]

Crisis in the Mutual Benefit Societies

As we have seen, the structure of income and expense was similar across the MBSs. Income came from member dues, from donations from patron-members or private individuals, and from grants solicited from public entities. Illness benefits constituted the lion's share of their expenses (about 60 percent). Other costs—which varied depending on the particular association—included medical care, pharmaceutical services, aid for the chronically ill or the unemployed, postmortem allowances for a deceased member's family, and administrative costs. During the 1918–19 influenza pandemic, the increase in the morbidity rate threw the budgets of these societies into disarray, due to the substantial rise in the subsidies paid to ill members. In the case of La Conciliación, worker-members paid dues of 25 cents per week, while the benefit amount paid out remained at 1.50 pesetas per day between 1902 and May 1928. Membership fees became a very important part of financing the society since sick leave costs from the second decade of the century on absorbed about 60 percent of them.[39]

Dated October 29, 1918, an official note from the president of the Mixed Board of La Conciliación describes the movements of its funds between September 15 and October 29, 1918. It states that the deficit on October 27 was 896.19 pesetas and also includes the data reflected in table 8.2. A perusal of the society's financial documents reveals that from September 23 to November 29, La Conciliación paid out far more in aid than it collected in income from members' dues.

To deal with its precarious financial situation, La Conciliación solicited help from the general public beginning in September. On October 5 the press published an article announcing the opening of an account to collect funds for the society. It also described the workers' woeful situation because of rising prices, the depressed postwar economy, and the absence of wages when they fell ill. Donations began to arrive immediately and, with additional help from the patron-members, the society was able to weather the storm, proof of the social support it had.[40] Much of the support it received was garnered through the personal contacts of the patron-members. Some, apart from having held political posts, had influential professional careers.[41]

Moreover, as I have noted, La Conciliación became more cautious in granting sick leave and subsidies. Prior to the pandemic, it would subsidize each illness (per member) for up to six months. But during the pandemic, it essentially grouped all respiratory illnesses together with influenza,

Table 8.2. The accounts of La Conciliación during the influenza epidemic

Expenses	Pesetas	Income guilds	Pesetas
Illness benefit			
September 16	240.00	September 15	373.95
September 23	372.00	September 22	396.00
September 30	664.00	September 29	403.00
October 6	1,058.25	October 6	579.95
October 13	1,240.50	October 13	380.00
October 20	1,335.75	October 20	342.70
October 27	1,182.00	October 27	394.60
Postmortem aids	800.00		
Total	6,892.50	Total	2,870.20
Deficit	-4,022.30		

Source: La Conciliación, *Books of Minutes,* 1918, University of Navarra Archive.

which meant members could now receive a total of only six months' worth of subsidy for all respiratory illnesses combined. Moreover, workers found to have misused the system were immediately expelled from the association with no possibility of being readmitted.[42]

The Accounts of the Other Societies

The Unión Productora, a related MBS, was also forced to appeal for financial assistance. Its 488 members were divided into three groups, depending on the type of subsidy they received: family medical-pharmaceutical assistance (92), individual medical-pharmaceutical assistance (9), and, most frequently, family medical-pharmaceutical assistance plus financial aid for members who were ill (387). Its extra expenses during the influenza epidemic (September–October 1918) came from pharmaceutical expenses (215.00 pesetas); 225 doctors' visits (252.00 pesetas); one postmortem allowance (40.00 pesetas); and, especially, the subsidies that were paid to ill patients (2,521.00 pesetas). The final tally of funds distributed by the Unión Productora amounted to a grand total of 3,028.00 pesetas, yielding a deficit of 1,626.80 pesetas. Thus, the president of the Unión Productora sent an official note to the city council on November 3 requesting support, stating, "the figures speak for themselves."[43]

Between September 15 and October 30, the Hermandad de la Pasión incurred a deficit of 354.50 pesetas due to the rise in illness among its members, paying out 545.00 pesetas in aid (471.00 pesetas plus the usual monthly expenditure in subsidies of 74.00 pesetas). At the time, the organization had 127 members, an average monthly income of 190.50 pesetas (dues of 1.00 peseta per month), and the aforementioned monthly expenditure of 74.00 pesetas. The Sociedad de Artesanos showed a deficit of 636.00 pesetas in September and 1,626.80 pesetas in October. The difference between the two months was due to the increase in financial aid paid out in October (1,512.50 pesetas) and the employment of a medical locum (499.50 pesetas). The Unión Obrera (Workers Union) did not cover medical assistance and provided only financial aid to its sick members. At the end of October, it had a deficit of 3,617.86 pesetas. We have less data on the other trade unions. On October 31, 1918, Sindicato Católico de Obreros Libres (Free Workers' Catholic Union) stated that it had five ill members to whom it was paying 1.50 pesetas per day in aid, and another fifteen members without aid, due to lack of funds.

Public Aid

La Conciliación and the other MBSs were managed by people with significant political and social influence.[44] Their representatives on the commissions set up by the city council and the regional government were thus ideally situated to address public health and social problems, as well as to seek financial assistance from the Spanish government.[45] During the influenza epidemic, the first and most urgent demand came from the Unión Obrera. Its lack of funds threatened the society's very existence, despite having reduced by half the aid given to each patient. In this "needy state" it asked the city council for an economic subsidy to survive and pay its expenses: "The Mutual Benefit Society Unión Obrera, writing on 15th October expresses that, in view of the abnormal circumstances and the rise in the number of ill members, and the precarious situation of the society, which is under threat of disappearing since it has no funds and has been forced to reduce by half the assistance it offered in normal times, finds itself in the position of appealing to the Most Honorable City Council to request an annual subsidy in the form and quantity which the Council considers convenient."[46]

The Unión Obrera's call for help provoked a political debate. Some councilors queried the petition because it meant aid would also have to be granted to other societies, if they so demanded. This was the opinion of the councilor, Dr. Javier Gortari, a physician who had been linked to La Conciliación in an early period: "The Council should sympathize with the needs of said Society but must remember that there are other Societies such as La Conciliación and *Artesanos* that will feel they have the same right to claim subsidies." Conversely, Councilor Francisco Lorda categorically supported the concession of aid requested by the Unión Obrera. After recounting the history of the society since its foundation, he stated that "the imbalance in its monetary situation has been caused by the current epidemic and that rather than allowing a Society like this to disappear it is preferable that the City Council make some sacrifices and that the Commission for the Exchequer should, when preparing the budget for the following year, 1919, take the situation of this Society into account by assigning it a subsidy."[47] At the following meeting, Lorda insisted "that the petition of the Unión Obrera should be decided today because their pressing need did not allow for delay and the Commission for the Exchequer has taken its decision on the matter."[48]

As was foreseeable, requests for financial aid arrived from the remaining societies: Sociedad de Artesanos, Hermandad de la Pasión, La Conciliación, Federación Obrera, Sindicato Católico de Obreros Libres, and the Asociación de Empleados. For example, "The Mixed Board of the Workers' Protection Society La Conciliación—alerted by friends on the Council—on October 21, requests the granting of a subsidy to cover the expenses of aiding those members who are suffering from the prevailing disease."[49] These petitions led to arguments among the councilors, as reflected in the minutes of the municipal meetings of October 16 and 23. For example, on October 23, we read,

> After lengthy discussion on several points about this proposal from the Commission for the Exchequer, in which Messrs. Gortari, Lipúzcoa, Aldaz (D. Fulgencio), Gorostiza and Martínez Azagra intervene[d]: it is agreed that said subsidies proposed by the Commission for the Exchequer be granted by the Mayor's Office and charged to the balance of the provincial rates account; and that the document from the Mixed Board of the Workers' Protection Society La Conciliación, which has motivated this debate, be passed to the Mayor's Office to be decided.[50]

The debate evinces the support each organization had in the city hall. Just as Councilor Lorda lobbied for the Unión Obrera, Gortari and Lipúzcoa defended La Conciliación; the latter was a patron-member of this society and was on its Mixed Board.[51]

Finally, at the council meeting on November 20 it was again agreed that "an extraordinary budget of twenty thousand pesetas has been approved . . . both to grant these subsidies and to cover other pressing needs caused by the current state of health of the City due to the prevailing disease, and that when the new budget is decided said sum will be allocated to cover extraordinary expenses of this kind."[52] The total granted to the MBSs amounted to 2,425.00 pesetas distributed, as shown in table 8.3.

Table 8.3. Distribution of the subsidies given to the MBSs during the influenza epidemic

Organization	Subsidy (in pesetas)
La Conciliación	700
Unión Obrera	500
Unión Productora	285
Artesanos	275
Sindicato de Obreros Libres	215
Sociedades Obreras	200
Hermandad de la Pasión	150
Solidaridad de Socorros Mutuos among workers at the Compañía Navarra de Abonos Químicos	100
Total	2,425

Source: Hygiene section, Box Hygiene 1918, Municipal Archive of Pamplona.

The total amount spent by the city council to cover the needs of the sick, however, was 19,385.39 pesetas. The city council paid most of this expense through public subscriptions opened to help with the epidemic. The City Council Archives contains a dossier titled "Subscription to Assist the Poor and Ill during the Grippe Epidemic," which lists the donations received and the letters of acknowledgment written to the donors. The first on the list is the Count of Guenduláin, who donated 1,000.00 pesetas, as did the Irati Railway Society, on October 19, 1918. The Sociedad la Vasconia (Vasconia Society, an insurance company) donated 250.00 pesetas on October 31, 1918, and smaller donations came from companies such as *El Pueblo Navarro* (a newspaper), which donated 10.00 pesetas. In any case, the municipal aid to the MBSs, although significant for the times, was insufficient to cover the organizations' deficits. As we saw with La Conciliación, they were subsequently forced to ask for donations from private individuals.

The Unión Obrera's urgent demand for help from the Pamplona City Council led to a revision of the official policy on subsidies for the societies and benefit organizations. After the influenza epidemic, the Pamplona MBSs demanded subsidies regularly and not only in exceptional circumstances. Even before the pandemic ended, on November 18, 1918, Amalio Lasheras sent the following note to the city council: "the Mutual Aid Society Unión Obrera . . . acknowledges its gratitude for the aid donated to said Society and begs the Most Excellent City Council to study if it were possible for this bonus to be made annually in future years."

Apart from direct subventions, these entities also received additional aid because the municipal government paid for pharmaceutical treatments. As of the second fortnight in October, city hall financed the pharmaceutical expenses authorized by all the physicians in the city, whether they were in private practice or worked for the MBSs or other charitable organizations: "The Mayor announces that, as of tomorrow, the poor and ill will be given vouchers to exchange for drugs in the pharmacies, as has been done with milk vouchers."[53] These drug vouchers, which were grouped by pharmacy, listed the patient's name, the prescription, and the price. For example, La Conciliación physician Sergio Lazcano frequently prescribed eucalyptus syrup, sodium bromide, potassium bromide, antipyretics, caffeine citrate, and so on, to be dispensed by the Negrillos pharmacy. Another La Conciliación physician signed prescriptions for laudanum balm, chloroform, and ammonium chlorate or perchlorate to be prepared by the Viuda de Iribarren pharmacy. Interestingly, neither of these pharmacies was under contract to La Conciliación, although both had worked with the society at earlier dates. Clearly, since city hall was footing the bill, the physicians did not feel obliged to use the society's pharmacy.

A Case of Mutual Reliance:
Benefit Societies and Public Administration

An analysis of the impact of the 1918–19 influenza pandemic on the MBSs and related associations in Pamplona, Spain, allows us to draw a more complete picture of both the pandemic and the framework of social and medical assistance at the time. The increase in the morbimortality rate from influenza and other respiratory diseases in the years preceding the pandemic, specifically since 1915, is particularly noteworthy. Also of interest is the discrepancy between the morbidity rate caused by the epidemic and the measures taken by the public authorities. In the case of La Conciliación, the most important MBS of the city, issues surrounding attention during the pandemic were leveraged to argue for worker-members' right to choose their own physician. In other words, the high morbimortality rate revealed the need for greater flexibility in the provision of medical care. In this sense, the influenza epidemic was part of a broader context in which the rise in morbimortality changed the way the MBSs functioned by modifying the patient-physician relationship. The epidemic circumstances also revealed the narrow economic margin of these entities as they realized that the safeguards put in place to guarantee their solvency proved insufficient, and if not for the timely intervention of public and private donors, the pandemic likely would have bankrupted them. In fact, the pandemic helped to usher in a postpandemic period when external support for MBSs through subventions and donations would become the norm, permanently augmenting member dues.

The analysis of the MBSs' responses to the 1918–19 influenza pandemic in Pamplona unveils the relations between power and associationism and the interconnected interests of the associations, social groups, and public entities. That these rival organizations worked so well together is somewhat surprising given that, as they espoused similar ideologies and provided the same kind of care, they competed for membership from the local population. Yet their cooperation was not limited to the extraordinary circumstances of the pandemic; they generally collaborated effectively even under ordinary conditions while networking with public offices.[54] The personal relationships among their directors certainly go a long way in explaining this attitude of cooperation. In this sense, it sheds light on the social and institutional backing they received.

In particular we should note the significance of the close contact between the town council and the local societies, as La Conciliación and other associations were generally run by local politicians and other prominent members of society. These entities depended on public support for their organization and the development of its social health care programs throughout the city. Reading the narratives of the pandemic offers valuable insights on the situation of Spanish health care management and progress in the early years of the twentieth century.

Notes

I would like to thank to my colleagues in the Department of Biomedical Humanities, Professors Juan Antonio Paniagua† and Pedro Gil-Sotres, for their input and advice. This chapter is part of the research project "La Sociedad de Obreros La Conciliación: Escenario de prácticas médicas (1902–1977)," granted by the Plan de Investigación Universidad de Navarra, 2007–9. A summary was presented at the International Seminar "Health and Welfare: Diversity and Convergence in Policy and Practice," Athens, February 19–22, 2009, organized by University of Athens and the UE Socrates Project PHOENIX.

1. Niall Johnson and Juergen Mueller, "Updating the Accounts: Global Mortality of the 1918–1920 'Spanish' Influenza Pandemic," *Bulletin of the History of Medicine* 76, no. 1 (2002): 105–15.

2. Bernard Harris, ed., *Welfare and Old Age in Europe and North America: The Development of Social Insurance* (London: Pickering and Chatto, 2012); Bernard Harris and Paul Bridgen, eds., *Charity and Mutual Aid in Europe and North America since 1800* (New York: Routledge, 2007); Ole Peter Grell, Andrew Cunningham, and Bernd Roeck., eds., *Health Care and Poor Relief in 18th and 19th Century Southern Europe* (Aldershot, England: Ashgate, 2005); Martin Gorsky and Sally Sheard, eds., *Financing Medicine: The British Experience since 1750* (New York: Routledge, 2006).

3. Esteban Rodríguez Ocaña, *Por la salud de las naciones: Higiene, microbiología y medicina social* (Madrid: Akal, 1992).

4. Pilar León-Sanz, "Networking and Interaction between a Mutual Assistance Association and Other Agencies (Pamplona, 1902–1919)," *Hygiea internationalis* 8, no. 1 (2009): 31–50.

5. Esteban Rodríguez Ocaña, *Salud pública en España: Ciencia, profesión y política, siglos XVIII–XX* (Granada: Universidad de Granada, 2005).

6. Pilar León-Sanz, "Professional Responsibility and the Welfare System in Spain at the Turn of the 19th Century," *Hygiea Internationalis* 5, no. 1 (2006): 75–90.

7. Feliciano Montero García, "El debate sobre el intervencionismo y el nacimiento del Instituto Nacional de Previsión (INP)," in *La previsión social en la historia: Actas del VI Congreso de Historia Social de España*, ed. Santiago Castillo and Rafael Ruzafa (Madrid: Siglo XXI de España, 2009), 171–96.

8. Ángel García-Sanz Marcotegui, "El ayuntamiento de Pamplona ante la 'crisis obrera,'" *Gerónimo de Uztariz: Boletín* 3 (1989): 26–39.

9. León-Sanz, "Professional Responsibility," 75–90; Feliciano Montero García and M. Esteban de Vega, "Aproximación tipológica al mutualismo popular y obrero en España: El mutualismo asistencial," in *La historia social en España: Actualidad y perspectivas; Actas del I Congreso de la Asociación de Historia Social*, ed. Santiago Castillo (Madrid: Siglo Veintiuno de España, 1991), 457–69; Francesc Andreu Martínez Gállego and Rafael Ruzafa, "Los socorros mutuos y la cooperación en la España del siglo XIX: Actitudes de los poderes públicos y soluciones populares," in Castillo and Ruzafa, *Previsión social*, 101–35.

10. José Andrés-Gallego, *Historia de la acción social de la iglesia* (Madrid: Espasa Calpe, 1984); Manuel Ferrer Muñoz, "Panorama asociativo de Navarra entre 1887 y 1936," in *Congreso de Historia de Euskal Herria* (Vitoria: Servicio Central de Publicaciones del Gobierno Vasco, 1988), 6:49–65; Javier M. Pejenaute Goñi, "Las Sociedades de Socorros Mutuos en Navarra (finales del siglo XIX–comienzos del XX)," in *Euskal Herria*, 6:273–87.

11. Pilar León-Sanz, "La concertación de la asistencia en la enfermedad en 'La Sociedad de Obreros la Conciliación' (1902–1919)," in *Navarra: Memoria e Imagen*, ed. Mercedes Galán Lorda, María del Mar Larraza Micheltorena, Luis Eduardo Oslé Guerendiain, and SEHN (Pamplona: Eunate, 2006), 2:97–108.

12. About "La Sociedad de Obreros La Conciliación," see Pilar León-Sanz, "Medical Assistance Provided by la Conciliación, a Pamplona Mutual Assistance Association (1902–84)," in Harris, *Welfare and Old Age*, 137–66.

13. On the Local Federation of Workmen's Societies, see Juan José Virto Ibáñez, "La UGT de Navarra: Algunas aportaciones al estudio del socialismo navarro," *Príncipe de Viana* 50, no. 187 (1989): 395–429. On the Free Catholic Union, see José Goñi Gaztambide, *Historia de los obispos de Pamplona*, vol. 10 (Pamplona: Eunsa, 1999).

14. There are numerous studies on the Spanish influenza pandemic. For a global perspective, see Howard Phillips and David Killingray, eds., *The Spanish Influenza Pandemic of 1918–19: New Perspectives* (New York: Routledge, 2003). See also Alfred Crosby's seminal study *America's Forgotten Pandemic: The Influenza of 1918* (New York: Cambridge, 2003); and John M. Barry, *The Great Influenza: The Epic Story of the Deadliest Plague in History* (New York: Viking, 2004). For Spain, see Beatriz Echeverri Dávila, *La gripe española: La pandemia de 1918–1919* (Madrid: Centro de Investigaciones

Sociológicas / Siglo XXI, 1993); and Echeverri Dávila, "Spanish Influenza Sees from Spain," in Phillips and Killingray, *Spanish Influenza Pandemic*, 173–90. The Spanish influenza pandemic in Pamplona has been studied by Jesús Ramos Martínez in "La pandemia de gripe de 1918 en Pamplona," in *II Congreso de Historia de Navarra de los Siglos XVIII–XIX y XX* (Pamplona: Institución Príncipe de Viana, 1992), 109–29.

15. In the nineteenth century Spain experienced three civil wars, the Carlist Wars, that pitted Carlists (absolutists), who supported Carlos María Isidro de Borbón and his descendants' claim to the Spanish throne, against Liberals, who supported Isabel II, who finally became the Spanish queen. The demographic changes are studied by Sagrario Anaut Bravo in *Cambio demográfico y mortalidad en Pamplona (1880–1935)* (Pamplona: Universidad Pública de Navarra, 1998).

16. Alfonso García Barbancho, *Las migraciones interiores españolas* (Madrid: Escuela Nacional de Administración Pública, 1967).

17. *Boletín Mensual de Estadística Demográfico-Sanitaria: Inspección General de Sanidad Exterior*. Madrid: Ministerio de Gobernación, 1918.

18. A total of 67 percent of the fatalities (forty-nine deaths) were patients in Pamplona's psychiatric asylum. See Echeverri Dávila, *Gripe española*, 139; Ramos Martínez, "Pandemia de gripe," 113.

19. María-Isabel Porras-Gallo, *Un reto para la sociedad madrileña: La epidemia de gripe de 1918–19* (Madrid: Complutense / Comunidad Autónoma de Madrid, 1997). The MBSs' physicians knew these measures well. Prior to the pandemic, Dr. Lazcano had published two books—*Higiene y salubridad pública en Pamplona* (Hygiene and public health in Pamplona) in 1903 and *Plan general de higienización de las viviendas de Pamplona y medios de realizarlo en la práctica* (General plan and practical measures for home hygiene), in 1909—popularizing the idea of disinfection, which "includes a series of measures to destroy the germs or microbes that threaten our health," including the use of disinfection stoves. Other issues included nutrition, alcohol consumption, and improvements in housing.

20. On these measures, see also chapters 9 and 11 of this volume.

21. *Book of Minutes*, Municipal Archive, October 4, 1918, 205–7.

22. *Book of Minutes*, Municipal Archive, October 4, 1918.

23. Emilio Gil Sastre, "El tifus efímero," *Diario de Navarra: Periódico independiente* (Pamplona), June 29, 1918.

24. María-Isabel Porras-Gallo, "Sueros y vacunas en la lucha contra la pandemia de gripe de 1918–1919 en España," *Asclepio* 60, no. 2 (2008): 261–88. The Navarrese physicians debated the nature of the illness within the bacteriological paradigm, as noted in an article published in the *Diario de Navarra* with the expressive, dramatic subheading: "The Ephemeral Typhus." In this, their actions mirrored those adopted by physicians in other countries and other Spanish cities. On physicians' actions in other countries, see Niall Johnson, *Britain and the 1918–19 Influenza Pandemic: A Dark Epilogue* (New York: Routledge, 2006); Antoine Nebel, *La gripe española: Su naturaleza, su tratamiento curativo y preventivo; Medidas profilácticas* (Valencia: Mínima, 2006); and Paul Kupperberg, *The Influenza Pandemic of 1918–1919* (New York: Chelsea House, 2008). On other Spanish cities, see Porras-Gallo, *Reto*. A *Diario de Navarra* article (Emilio Gil Sastre, "El tifus efímero," June 29, 1918) referred to "the reports of the Madrid Municipal Laboratory, those of the Alfonso XIII Institute, and of other centers committed to microbiological study, [which] could not reach a consensus as they

did not find a microbe in the affected individuals which could be responsible for the infection." What was clear was that it was "a disease with such a definite and characteristic cycle that it should be considered as of particular, distinct, individualized and classifiable nosological significance . . . [and] serious in itself or because of its associated complications."

25. La Conciliación, *Book of Minutes: Pro manuscript*, bk. 7 (Pamplona, 1918), 309; *Book of Minutes*, Municipal Archive, October 15, 1918.

26. Similar measures were taken in other cities. Porras-Gallo, *Reto*; Esteban Rodríguez Ocaña, "La grip a Barcelona: un greu problema esporàdic de salut publica. Epidèmies de 1889–90 i 1918–19," in *Cent anys de Salut Pública a Barcelona* Antoni Roca Rosell, coord. (Barcelona: Institut Municipal de la Salut, 1991), 131–56; Josep Bernabeu-Mestre, ed., in collaboration with Andreu Nolasco Bonmatí, Marisa Bardisa Escuder, Vicente Bartual Méndez, José María Gutiérrez Rubio, Luis López Penabad, and José Miguel Mataix Piñero, *La ciutat davant el contagi: Alacant i la grip de 1918–1919* (Valencia: Conselleria de Sanitat i Consum, Generalitat Valenciana, 1991).

27. *Book of Minutes*, Municipal Archive, October 23, 1918.

28. Emilio Gil Sastre, "El tifus efímero," *Diario de Navarra*, June 29, 1918.

29. La Conciliación, *Book of Minutes*, bk. 7 (1918), 296. The impact of the epidemic disease complicated the problems that resulted from the low number of physicians per inhabitant at the time in Spain. As Sobral, Lima, and Silveira e Sousa note in chapter 4 of this volume, this same situation occurred in Portugal during the pandemic.

30. Ramos Martínez, "Pandemia de gripe."

31. La Conciliación, *Book of Minutes*, bk. 7 (1918), 302–8.

32. Instrucción General de Sanidad de 1904, art. 155. Real Decreto aprobando con carácter definitivo la Instrucción General de sanidad pública. Ministerio de la Gobernación. *Gaceta* de Madrid 22, January 22, 1904, 273–75.

33. *Book of Minutes*, Municipal Archive, October 4, 1918.

34. La Conciliación, *Book of Minutes*, bk. 7 (1918), 316, 309.

35. "La epidemia reinante: La grippe en Navarra," *Diario de Navarra*, October 24, 1918; n/a "Cosas de casa. La salud pública," *Diario de Navarra*, November 7, 1918.

36. This type of change in the structuring of work is also described in other situations, like that of American military physicians. Carol R. Byerly, *Fever of War: The Influenza Epidemic in the U.S. Army during World War I* (New York: New York University Press, 2005).

37. León-Sanz, "Professional Responsibility," 75–90.

38. La Conciliación, *Book of Minutes*, bk. 5 (1914), 147–49; bk. 6 (1916), 36; bk. 7 (1918), 140.

39. León-Sanz, "Concertación de la asistencia," 97–108.

40. La Conciliación, *Book of Minutes*, bk. 7 (1918), 293, 322.

41. Andrés-Gallego, *Historia de la acción*; Pilar León-Sanz, "Private Initiatives against Social Inequalities and Health Vulnerabilities: The Case of la Conciliación (Pamplona, 1902–1920)," in *Vulnerabilities, Social Inequalities and Health*, ed. Patrice Bourdelais and John Chircop (Évora: Ediçoes Colibri, 2010), 93–108.

42. La Conciliación, *Book of Minutes*, bk. 7 (1918), 323–34.

43. Letter by president of the Unión Productora, Municipal Archive, November 3, 1918.

44. Pilar León-Sanz, "The Strategies of Interrelations between Assistance Associations and Other Agencies in Pamplona, 1902–1936," in *Health Institutions at the Origin of the Welfare Systems in Europe,* ed. Pilar León-Sanz (Pamplona: Eunsa, 2010), 167–92.

45. Navarre had a special administrative autonomy from the central government: the "foral" regime. This regime established that the Diputación Foral de Navarra was an executive group that depended on the parliament or the legislative body. The Diputación was directly responsible for matters relating to the social welfare of the region. In the early part of the twentieth century, there was a majority of conservative parties in both the local and regional government. José Andrés-Gallego, *Historia contemporánea de Navarra* (Pamplona: Ediciones y Libros, 1982); I. Olabarri Gortazar, "Notas sobre la implantación, la estructura organizativa y el ideario de los partidos del Turno en Navarra, 1901–1923," *Príncipe de Viana: Anejo* 10 (1988): 317–29.

46. *Book of Minutes,* Municipal Archive, October 16, 1918, 223–25.

47. Ibid., 223, 224.

48. *Book of Minutes,* Municipal Archive, October 23, 1918, 230.

49. La Conciliación, *Book of Minutes,* bk. 7 (1918), 312.

50. *Book of Minutes,* Municipal Archive, October 23, 1918, 234.

51. León-Sanz, "Private Initiatives," 93–108.

52. *Book of Minutes,* Municipal Archive, November 20, 1918, 297.

53. *Book of Minutes,* Municipal Archive, October 16, 1918.

54. León-Sanz, "Private Initiatives," 93–108.

Part Three

Interpreting the Epidemic

Sociocultural Dynamics and Perspectives

Chapter Nine

A Tale of Two Spains

Narrating the Nation during the 1918–19 Influenza Epidemic

RYAN A. DAVIS

Here lies half of Spain, it died of the other half.
—Mariano José de Larra, "El dia de difuntos de 1836"
(The day of the dead 1836)

Medicine is a social science, and politics is nothing else but medicine on a large scale.
—Rudolf Virchow, *Die Medizinische Reform* (Medical reform)

Although Spain remains nominally connected to the 1918–19 Spanish influenza epidemic, scholars often seek to minimize the connection between the country and the disease, preferring instead to emphasize its international scope. Thus Beatriz Echeverri, one of the few who has written on Spain's experience of the epidemic to a broader scholarly audience, states categorically, "Spanish flu had nothing 'Spanish' about it."[1] Considering that the Spanish flu neither originated in Spain, nor was it confined only to the country, she is right. Yet, in the rush to reduce Spain's relation to the disease to a function of the name the country and the disease share in common, something of Spain's unique contribution to the social history of the epidemic has been lost. If, from an epidemiological standpoint, the Spanish flu had nothing to do with Spain, the same cannot be said of it from a discursive standpoint.

It is now widely accepted that the Spanish flu gets its name from the news coverage the epidemic received in Spain. In contrast to its counterparts in countries embroiled in World War I, the Spanish press, as a result of the nation's neutrality, reported on the epidemic early and extensively.[2] This source of documentary material thus constitutes one of the richest archives for accessing period responses to the epidemic. Nevertheless, though most scholars of the Spanish flu can probably point to this news coverage as the source of the epidemic's name, very few have studied it. Moreover, those who have tend to use it as a means of recreating the epidemic events as they occurred—retracing what narratologists would call the *story* of the epidemic.[3] In this, they resemble examples of what Howard Phillips calls the "first wave" of Spanish flu scholarship, namely, studies that have "paid particular attention to exploring the spread and deadly impact of the disease and getting it recognized as a topic worthy of serious study by historians."[4] By contrast, my analysis builds on this foundational scholarship by turning the focus to issues not of the story of the Spanish flu but of its *discourse,* or the manner in which epidemic events were represented.[5] In this sense, my contribution falls into what Phillips calls the "second wave" of Spanish flu scholarship.[6]

A discursive analysis of the daily news coverage of the epidemic reveals that the Spanish press implicitly distinguishes between an "epidemic Spain" and a "sanitary Spain." The struggle of the latter against the former constitutes the central agon, or conflict, that structures the news of the epidemic into what we might call the emerging narrative about it.[7] In other words, if "reading a newspaper is like reading a novel whose author has abandoned any thought of a coherent plot," as Benedict Anderson has suggested, then this conflict provides precisely this plot, placing the otherwise chaotic occurrences of the epidemic into coherent relationships that would subsequently make sense to Spaniards.[8] In what follows, I trace the discursive evolution from the epidemic Spain to the sanitary Spain through three distinct phases, all of which pertain to the second epidemic wave. The first corresponds to the outbreak of the second wave, when Spaniards first acknowledged the flu as a legitimate threat to the nation.[9] In response to the perceived threat, they closed ranks as a body politic, labeling foreigners who traversed their national borders (in this case, Portuguese laborers) as dirty others.[10] The news daily *El Liberal* initiated the second phase with its call for the establishment of a sanitary dictatorship (*dictadura sanitaria*) to forcefully carry out not just the interventions called for in light of the epidemic but, through these, the necessary reforms to Spain's beleaguered public health infrastructure.[11] These measures would form the foundation of the new sanitary Spain, and their implementation constitutes the third phase of the discursive evolution toward the sanitary Spain.

National Borders and Foreign Bodies

Initial news reports about the outbreak of the second epidemic wave display two characteristics. First, they note various disease foci inside the country, beginning with Murcia and Valencia on September 8 and including various others within a week.[12] Second, they speculate a great deal about what disease or diseases were manifesting: dysentery, the flu, cholera, exanthematic typhus.[13] By September 15, however, it had been officially determined and generally accepted that, in fact, it was the flu that had returned, this time with a vengeance.[14] Although the etiology of the disease was unclear, the Spanish press soon associated the epidemic threat with Portuguese laborers who at the time of the second wave were returning home from France through Spain.[15] The inability of microbiology to isolate (i.e., identify) the pathogenic agent responsible for the flu did not diffuse the social pressure to do so. Thus, although "we live in a society that is poorly defined by national boundaries," as Paul Farmer has argued, at least in terms of how things like disease articulate real, material bonds between people, the psychological appeal of blaming often proves too much to overcome.[16] Indeed, as Charles Rosenberg reminds us, when it comes to explaining epidemics, framing and blaming are "inextricably mingled," and although the meanings we impose on an epidemic may vary, "the need to impose them does not."[17]

By September 25 the Spanish government had articulated a six-point protocol for transporting sick Portuguese laborers from the French to the Portuguese border. Only those workers with a certified visa issued by a Spanish consulate that stipulated they were not proceeding from an infected town were granted access to the country. When they arrived at the border, they were submitted to medical examinations and detained unless absolutely healthy. In a gesture that reflects both precaution and fear, those allowed to pass were directed to special train cars where they traveled incommunicado and "without any possible relation with other passengers." Once the passengers were on their way, the governors of each of the provinces through which they would pass were notified to ensure that the appropriate medical authorities were present to verify the "complete isolation [*incomunicación*] of the cars."[18] When the travelers arrived in Medina del Campo, a city just south of Valladolid and the final stop before the Portuguese border, their train car was separated from the rest and placed on an isolated track until coupled with the train that would take them the rest of the way. While waiting, the workers were not allowed to get out of the car, nor could they change cars. When they finally arrived at the border, the train cars were disinfected again.[19]

One of the clearest examples of stigmatization of the Portuguese laborers comes in a letter from the physician of Pozal de Gallinas (a small village just east of Medina del Campo), who was incensed by the failure to fully isolate some of the Portuguese. His remarks, published in the conservative newspaper *ABC*, reveal just how contagious the metaphor of contagion—and the psychological mechanism of blaming—can be: "They get off [the trains] and

spend the night in the waiting areas, which are converted into veritable infirmaries, where, piled on top of one another, many of whom are sick, they stay
for various hours; and the saddest part is that nobody bothers to disinfect
those places, since in that station the simplest measures of disinfection are
completely abandoned."[20] By their mere presence, the Portuguese convert
the waiting room of the train station into an infirmary, even though not all
of them are sick. Moreover, there is a suggestive tension between movement
and stasis, since they end up converting a space normally marked by travelers' momentary presence into one of permanence; the phrase "they stay for
various hours" is translated from the verb *permanecer*, which comes from the
Latin root meaning permanent. For the Portuguese workers who were sick,
it would seem that the Spanish flu proved to be, as Susan Sontag has said of
illness in general, a "more onerous citizenship."[21] In contrast, for their compatriots who were not sick, it was actually their Portuguese citizenship that
proved to be the more onerous illness.

Although Portuguese laborers were hardly unique in their susceptibility
to the flu (nor were they alone in crossing the border into Spain), they were
characterized by the Spanish press in a far more pejorative fashion than
were Spaniards. Whereas the Portuguese were labeled quite literally as dirty
others—some of the trains that transported them were affixed with a sign
that read "infested"—Spaniards were seen simply as victims in need of help
from their compatriots.[22] In this sense, the Barcelona-based *La Vanguardia*
referred to one group as "repatriated Spanish workers."[23] Ultimately, what
this differential treatment of the two groups demonstrates is that in the context of the epidemic crisis, outsiders were considered a threat to the national
body, whereas insiders merely evidenced functional problems with(in) that
body. Outsiders were to be expelled, while insiders needed to be integrated
more effectively.

In referring to the national body of Spain, I purposefully invoke the
organic conceptualization of the nation current at the time of the epidemic. In *Membranes: Metaphors of Invasion in Nineteenth-Century Literature,
Science, and Politics*, Laura Otis has shown how this corporal metaphor
for the nation was "supported" by advancements in fields such as cellular
pathology.[24] Nations, or national bodies, became as much a medical and
public health concern as a social and political phenomenon in the latter
half of the nineteenth century and the early part of the twentieth. Their
borders were the regulatory organ that distinguished between (national)
self and (foreign) other.[25] Nowhere is the relevance of the metaphor of
body and borders more apparent than in figure 9.1, published in *ABC* on
the same day Spain's government issued a royal decree blaming the poor
state of Spanish health on its neighbors.[26]

The artist, Sileno (pen name of Pedro Antonio Villahermosa), depicts
a man reading the "instructions to combat the flu" issued by the Board of

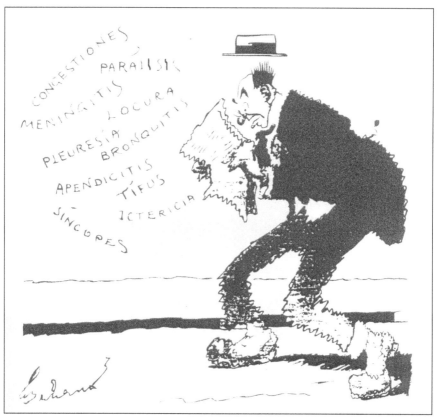

Figure 9.1. Sileno (Pedro Antonio Villahermosa), "Instrucciones para combatir la gripe," *ABC*, no. 4.848, October 3, 1918. Reproduced with permission from Museo ABC, Madrid.

Public Health. The words to his left are a list of symptoms and diseases associated with the epidemic: congestion, paralysis, meningitis, insanity, pleurisy, bronchitis, appendicitis, typhus, jaundice, and syncope. The caption gives voice to his reaction to the board's instructions: "Holy smokes! The first [instruction is] don't read the alarming [instructions] from the Board of Public Health." The thrust of the cartoon revolves around the act of reading. In its instructions the board warns of the possible consequences of the epidemic (in the image, the list of symptoms and diseases). The effect of portraying the consequences as though they were floating in the air endows them with a rhetorical unruliness that contrasts the well-ordered words of the caption, as though the rules that govern language and writing were unable to control the symptoms and diseases the words represent. Moreover, it is through the act of reading these unruly words that the man's bodily integrity—the border of his body—is jeopardized. The squiggly outline of the man's figure recalls Sander Gilman's assertion that "it is the fear of collapse, the sense of dissolution, which contaminates the Western image of all diseases."[27] In short, not only do the Spanish flu and its sequelae disrupt language's attempt to order them—to explain and therefore contain them—but also they threaten to dissolve the (reading) subject who is exposed to them.[28]

The connection between the dissolution of this particular reading subject and the Spanish nation rests on the recognition that the subject is a metonymy for the nation. That is, the subject's body stands in for the body politic of Spain. In narratological terms, the man represents the implied reader, the everyman who, it is assumed, resembles actual readers. Moreover, as a metonymy for the nation, this implied reader of Spanish flu discourse is also the visual expression of the paradigmatic Spanish subject.[29] In his seminal study on nationalism, Anderson posited the act of reading as central to and constitutive of national subjectivity. Referring to the exercise of reading the morning paper ("newspaper-as-fiction"), he writes, "The significance of this mass ceremony . . . is paradoxical. It is performed in silent privacy, in the lair of the skull. Yet each communicant is well aware that the ceremony he performs is being replicated simultaneously by thousands (or millions) of others. . . . What more vivid figure for the secular, historically clocked, imagined community can be envisioned?"[30] For Anderson, citizens process the individual act of reading the newspaper as a collective exercise, one that binds readers together as members of a shared community, the "imagined community" of the nation. In Sileno's cartoon, the reading subject's crisis actually reflects Spain's national crisis in the face of the influenza epidemic.

This point is further reinforced by Sileno's use of the artistic device known as mise en abyme.[31] Brian McHale notes that although long treated as "uncanny disruptions, fatally compromising fiction's world-modeling function," en abyme structures actually "hold a mirror up to . . . [the world], providing the reader with a kind of schematic diagram of it, or a user's manual for its proper operation." The effect of en abyme structures is thus to connect fictional worlds with the real world. Or, in Anderson's terms, "[to fuse] the world inside the novel [or in this case, the newspaper] with the world outside."[32] Spaniards reading about the epidemic in *ABC* would likely have come across figure 9.1, causing them to identify with the reading subject of the image. In this regard, the figure would have shaped Spaniards' understanding of the epidemic experience as both a national and an individual crisis, and in this way it lays the rhetorical groundwork for transitioning to a sanitary Spain, something the press did by calling for a sanitary dictatorship.

Toward a Public Health Dictatorship

The day before Sileno published his editorial cartoon on October 3, depicting the flu epidemic as a national crisis, *El Liberal* issued its call for a sanitary dictatorship.[33] The dictatorship was to have two branches: one that dealt with the nature and flow of information (i.e., how the epidemic was represented) and one that dealt with the application of and compliance with measures aimed at curbing the epidemic: "The accurate reflection of the situation should be supported by a grave severity in the sanitary measures dictated. Extreme care [should be taken] in announcing what works in stopping the progress of the sickness [*mal*] and avoiding [its] diffusion. And . . . [support should come in the form of] a veritable sanitary dictatorship—to demand that the proposed measures be carried out, without tolerating infractions or weaknesses that can have incalculable transcendence for public health." *El Liberal's* use of the term *mal* conflates biology and sociology in rhetorically reinforcing the notion that the epidemic was both an ill and an evil. All Spaniards were expected to join the fight against this common enemy. The news daily grounded its argument on the principle that "public health . . . is above [i.e., a higher priority than] any particular individual convenience."[34] Indeed, this principle of privileging the collective interest over individual interests is what made the dictatorship "perfectly excusable." Ironically, even as it called for an "accurate reflection" of epidemic conditions, *El Liberal* admitted to having censored information previously: "Until today, to avoid alarm, we have felt it prudent to retain information that we had concerning the havoc the sickness [*mal*] was causing in some provinces. We believe that from this point on, this type of reservation can be harmful."[35]

Given the historical trend away from dictatorial regimes, it is surprising to note the enthusiasm with which the Spanish government responded to the call for a sanitary dictatorship.[36] The undersecretary to the minister of the interior put it this way: "In reality, the conduct observed by the Minister of the Interior can and should be described as a dictatorship, not just since the existence of flu foci in different points in Spain was made known, but long before that. It has taken a labor of perseverance of many years to create a potent sanitary organization that makes us safe from every contingency, and thus, when the first epidemic symptoms were noted, not just in Spain, but in neighboring countries, the government has been able to utilize the worthy functions entrusted to the Body of Civil Health and make use of the necessary technical supplies." In his rhetorically florid description, the undersecretary portrays the government in the most positive light possible: "We have obviously arrived in these days at extremes in sanitary rigor, which, superficially judged, could be branded as exaggerated; but faced with the imminence of the [epidemic] danger, the government has not hesitated for an instance in appealing to every type of means, understanding that elevated considerations of humanity should take precedence over every other stimulus. . . . Nothing, not even the respect for private interests, will convince the government to depart from its current course of action."[37]

The question that arises is why the undersecretary would have voiced enthusiasm for such a polemical political form. The accelerated disintegration of the official *turnismo* system and the widespread concern over the "social question" had produced a moment rife with revolutionary fervor. Francisco J. Romero Salvadó has drawn attention to the "anarchy and indiscipline [that] appeared to be the order of the day."[38] The liberalizing trend of the Spanish press as an alternative sphere for political debate only augmented frustration over Spain's social and political circumstances. Not surprisingly, then, the day before *ABC* reported the undersecretary's enthusiasm for a sanitary dictatorship, *El Liberal* cautioned that such a dictatorship was "the only dictatorship that can be admitted in our times."[39] Such a caveat was, tellingly, absent from the undersecretary's remarks. The reason probably has to do with how the undersecretary framed the issue. The government had acted as a dictatorship only with the understanding that lofty, humanistic concerns should take precedence over other issues.[40] In other words, the government put a human(itarian) face on the epidemic and then sought to portray itself as successfully discharging its responsibilities vis-à-vis the Spanish people. In doing so, the undersecretary's actions followed an established precedent. In reference to the relationship between Spanish workers and the regency press, David Ortiz Jr. has argued that "the incorporation of the working class was at the heart of the social question, and the Regency press gave the dispute a human face. Understood as a human crisis, it required peaceful resolution."[41] Mutatis mutandis, the undersecretary's enthusiasm for the sanitary dictatorship can be read as an attempt to simultaneously win over public opinion and preserve order—all by publicizing the government's efforts to mitigate the epidemic.

Despite the difficulty of sealing off Spain from an external epidemic attack, the flu found its way into the nation. But the inside-outside dynamic that grounded the approach of the sanitary dictatorship, rather than disappearing, was focused internally. Everybody's movement became suspect if they came from somewhere known to be, or suspected of being, infected with the flu. Thus, in an editorial for the *Gaceta de Tenerife*, V. Sierra Ruiz spoke of the "mortiferous effects of the epidemic that is *getting inside of us* [*se nos adentra*]."[42] Border towns were no longer the only ones preoccupied with external threats. On September 23 the Provincial Board of Health of the centrally located Ciudad Real took measures to "avoid contagion from travelers coming from places where the epidemic has been declared, since in this capital not a single case of flu has been registered."[43] Similarly, Toledo's Board of Public Health adopted "important agreements to avoid the invasion of the sickness in the province, which is currently enjoying good health."[44] As late as October 15 Madrid's mayor Luis Silvela y Casado felt justified in claiming the epidemic had not yet reached the Spanish capital. But fear that it might prompted him to post an edict outlining the measures the local government was taking just in case. The first was the disinfection of travelers.[45] The breach of (primarily) the national border and the concomitant threat this posed to the national body justified in many ways the mobilization of the necessary resources to bring about the change from an epidemic Spain to a sanitary Spain.

From Epidemic to Sanitary State

In referring to Spain as either an epidemic or sanitary state, the polyvalence of the term *state* is key. On one hand, Spain found itself in epidemic conditions. On the other, the central political authority was in charge of responding to these conditions, which manifested at every level of individual and social life, disrupting even the most sacrosanct of local and national rituals.[46] The press registers both senses of the term in discursively tracing the evolution of the sanitary Spain. In addition to the border issues that arose, transatlantic trips were canceled because "passenger boarding has been prohibited in light of the current circumstances."[47] In Huesca (in northeastern Spain) elections were suspended.[48] In Barcelona so many post office employees became sick that residents were asked not to mail anything that was not urgent.[49] *El Sol* reported that in Ciudad Real the request was made to suspend trials by jury.[50] Schools at every level were closed down, the Ministry of Public Education ultimately issuing a royal edict granting university rectors the right to postpone the academic year "without previous consultation with this ministry."[51] In Madrid virtually every type of venue dedicated to public leisure was subjected to closure if it failed to prove it met sanitary conditions: "[Be it known] that proprietors, directors, administrators, etcetera, etc., of private teaching institutions, as well as of cafés, bars, taverns . . . food and drink establishments, theaters, circuses, jai alai courts, concert halls, dance halls, movie theaters, concert cafés, etc., etc., [must] present in the Provincial Health Inspector's offices, within fifteen days, documentation that their respective establishments meet the hygienic conditions called for by existing regulations."[52]

In Valladolid the Board of Public Health even went so far as to prohibit playing games in cafés, a measure that provoked protests.[53] At the national level, the Ministry of Public Works, headed by Francisco de Asís Cambó, published a royal edict limiting the liability of insurance companies because of the epidemic: "Following a request filed with the Commissioner of Insurance for general managers of several life insurance companies, and given the circumstances facing public health in Spain . . . the insertion of a clause in the interim policy has been approved, which holds that if the insured dies before the end of ninety days from the date of the contract, the insurer's liability will be limited to a refund of the premiums charged."[54] In Guipuzcoa, the mayor ordered the temporary cessation of butter production so the milk could be given to those recovering from the flu.[55]

The epidemic also forced various organizations to cancel meetings. In Almería (on the southeastern coast of Spain), the Commission of the Consumers' League, which had organized a banquet aimed at resolving a strike, was asked to cancel the event and donate the collected funds to victims of the epidemic, a request to which they acquiesced.[56] In Madrid the Board of the Government and Patronage of Rural Physicians canceled its assembly, as did the National Fishing Assembly in La Coruña (in northwestern Spain).[57] Perhaps most notably, however, was the rescheduling of the third National Conference on Civil Health and the first National Conference on Medicine.[58] In reference to the former, *Heraldo de Madrid* reported, "that conference has as its primary purpose to lobby the government for an effective reorganization of health services and the payment of rural doctors (*médicos titulares*) by the state."[59]

Another area of cultural life impacted by the epidemic included the fiestas of various towns, which were canceled, though not always without controversy. In places like Castellón, Las Palmas, and Toledo, Columbus Day celebrations were put on hold.[60] In Zaragoza the Provincial Board of Health voted not to declare the epidemic officially, though it did recommend "the suspension of fiestas in Pilar [in places] where the public tends to congregate," thus impacting events like religious celebrations and bull fights. The board's report—which was the "object of lively and contradictory comments"—caused various businessmen and *feriantes* (those who attend a feria to buy or sell) a significant amount of anxiety as they waited to see what concrete steps would be taken.[61]

Religious life, too, was disrupted by the flu epidemic.[62] One Mr. Laffite, a town councilman in San Sebastián, requested "the use of holy water in churches be suspended."[63] Similarly, in Zaragoza the municipal subcommittee on public health made plans to ask the archbishop to disinfect the basins that held the holy water.[64] In Villar de Cañas (Cuenca), residents died without receiving final rites because the local priest was one of the first victims of the epidemic. The mayor of Ugíjar (Granada) was reprimanded because he locked up the parish priest for having rendered assistance to those sick with the flu.[65]

Rituals associated with the cemetery were perhaps the religious ceremonies most affected by the epidemic.[66] There were reports of wood shortages that led to a lack of sufficient coffins.[67] *ABC* reported examples of doubling up on coffins in areas that lacked enough burial plots.[68] Processions from churches to the cemetery were prohibited.[69] The number of deaths was such that the horses that pulled the carts "were exhausted from excessive work." In Vigo the mayor's office ordered the "absolute prohibition of funeral cortèges."[70] In the province of Barcelona one bishop objected to nighttime burials because they were frightening the population.[71] *El Liberal* reported that, in Cartagena, carrying cadavers over the shoulder was prohibited.[72] Many places like Almería, Madrid, Córdoba, Toledo, and Bilbao also forbade cemetery visitations on the first two days of November—All Saints' Day and All Souls' Day. Those in Barcelona wishing to leave flowers on the graves of loved ones were stopped at the entrance and informed that "[flowers] will be given at the entrance of the cemetery to one of the employees designated for the purpose of placing them on the indicated mausoleums or tombs." *ABC* referred to these employees as "vigilantes," thereby associating their function with that of the police. Similarly, artistic rituals associated with the dead were also affected by the epidemic. In Alicante the governor banned representations of the play, *Don Juan Tenorio*, the viewing of which was part of the yearly ritual that included cemetery visits.[73]

In Barcelona the company contracted to provide funeral services failed to meet burial demands, which caused no small stir in the city. At six o'clock in the evening on October 13, a group of fifty people marched to the town hall to present their complaints against the company to Mayor Morales Pareja.[74] In a private conversation Morales informed three representatives of the ad hoc commission of neighbors that he had already taken up the matter with the company a number of times. He also told the representatives that not all the complaints made about the company were accurate. Three days later the issue was taken up by the city council where, after some debate, a resolution to strip the company of its contract with the city was defeated. In its place, however, it was decided that a "file to relieve [the company] of its responsibilities" would be opened. If the company was found to be delinquent in its contractual obligations, the contract would be voided.[75] For their part, company leaders were in a difficult position. In a letter to *La Vanguardia* published on October 17, they lamented the fact that despite maintaining in circulation "five cars and six backups," the number of bodies to bury—up to 370 on some days—was simply overwhelming.[76]

Notwithstanding the logistical challenges faced by the company, Barcelona residents remained displeased. When the widow of one José María Perís received a phone call from the company informing her that there was no coffin available for her husband's burial, "this incensed the neighborhood."[77] A group of some four hundred neighbors marched all the way to Civil Governor González Rothwos's office to voice their complaints. Some time later, two more "neighborhood commissions" arrived at town hall for similar reasons. As evidenced by this episode involving Barcelona's funeral services company, no area of Spanish life was unaffected by the flu epidemic, including the sacrosanct ritual of burying the dead.

In response to these conditions that constituted the epidemic Spain, numerous steps were taken to establish the sanitary Spain, including the issuance of authoritative pronouncements, the prescription and proscription of specific behavioral practices, and the application of penalties by regulatory bodies. Through these measures, the sanitary dictatorship called for by *El Liberal* became in many ways a reality. One of the most visually striking features of this dictatorship may be the use of specific public agents to maintain (public health) order. Not only was the Civil Guard used in border-sensitive regions, but police officers also accompanied doctors on house visits: "Doctors will begin to make house calls accompanied by municipal guards who will watch to see that the regulations issued by the mayor's office are followed, with the purpose of taking in the very act the necessary measures to get rid of all filth that could constitute a focus of infection."[78] In an interview with the *Gaceta de Tenerife*, the provincial director of foreign health (*director de sanidad exterior*) referred to these agents as "sanitary police."[79] Similarly, a Mr. Llopis chided Barcelona's Health Commission for its weak efforts in combating the epidemic, suggesting that "the gravity of the case requires energetic regulations, proceeding *manu militari*, rather than the city council just formulating proposals. . . . What residents are calling for and what the distressing circumstances demand is that a veritable sanitary dictatorship take over."[80] For Llopis, the call for military might, dictator style, was evidently justified both by the epidemic circumstances and the will of the people.[81]

Part of this heavy-handed approach included the formation of brigades charged with disinfecting public and private spaces.[82] Madrid actually had a regular brigade that did house calls and a special brigade for those areas where "the agglomeration of people or other motives demands the adoption of such [disinfection] measures."[83] In Murcia the governor organized youth into surveillance juntas "charged with denouncing the deficiencies they observe in the population."[84] Similarly, the governor of Barcelona encouraged neighbors to join in the effort to combat the epidemic "denouncing as quickly as possible every fault and infraction of which they are aware."[85] Along the highways leading into Málaga, the governor mandated the installation of "sanitary posts for examining pedestrians."[86]

Although less visible than whitewashing brigades and sanitary police, other official institutions and individuals were also busy behind the scenes, responding to conditions brought on by the flu epidemic. In myriad places the health boards were permanently in session, and their resolutions touched on matters both tangible and intangible. Examples of tangible matters include the opening or closing of schools, the prohibition of consecutive shows in theaters to permit "renewing the air and . . . fumigating the locale," and the cancellation of "live masses in the homes of dead people."[87] An example of an intangible matter involves Madrid's Provincial Board of

Health, which voted to "uphold the prestige of the health authorities for their conduct in the current circumstances and for the titanic battle they have to sustain."[88] Foremost among these authorities was Manuel Martín Salazar, the inspector general of public health, who received an explicit vote of solidarity from the board, which looked favorably on his efforts during the epidemic.[89]

The consequences for ignoring the dictated health measures served to reinforce the power of the sanitary dictatorship. For instance, the civil governor of Palma de Mallorca fined the mayor and physicians from Inca "for having infringed upon the sanitary regulations."[90] The provincial health inspector in Badajoz was fined for not declaring the existence of the epidemic.[91] In Vigo the mayor received a telegram from the provincial governor of Pontevedra, threatening him with a 500-peseta fine, "without fear of imposing upon him the disciplinary actions signaled in the Health law."[92] Barcelona's mayor required all those who owned farms within the city limits to cover their wells and to keep their chickens cooped up," reminding the owners that the Provincial Board of Health had the power to issue fines much more substantial than the 50-peseta limit of his own office.[93] Fines, however, hardly constituted the only penalty for disobeying dictatorial injunctions. Residents of Madrid could not receive certifications of good conduct or of residency without first documenting that they had received their vaccinations.[94] Although the vaccine in question was not a flu vaccine, the penalty associated with not receiving it highlights the extent to which Spain had become a sanitary state.[95]

The ad hoc development of the sanitary Spain invariably impinged on the concept of the Spanish state as constituted at the time of the epidemic.[96] As a result, it both called into question the various policies and practices of the Spanish state and, ultimately, posited a new concept of it. I cite just two examples. The first comes from the Medical College of Madrid. In a meeting presided over by Ortega Morejón, the four hundred participants arrived at three conclusions, each of which can be read as specifying how physicians would establish their hegemony as something of a modern-day guild vis-à-vis the social order. The first conclusion stipulated that the widows and orphans of those doctors who had died during the epidemic be included as beneficiaries of the Epidemics Law.[97] The second called for the creation of a Ministry of Public Health, which would operate independently of all other ministerial departments. The final conclusion amounted to an "energetic protest . . . against the low pay with which some had pretended to recompense the physicians who had volunteered at the Ministry of the Interior to go to infected places [to render service]." During the meeting, it was also agreed that doctors should become functionaries of the state, a move that would counteract their having been "relegated to oblivion and subjected to the nefarious 'illiterate cacique politics.'"[98] Moreover, the group threatened that if their demands were not met in a timely fashion, "the measures they would take would be extremely radical, since they would absolutely break off ties with the government."[99] The revolutionary force of the Medical College's rhetoric could not have been clearer, and in demonstration of their resolve all four hundred participants at the meeting carried their demands to Manuel García Prieto himself, the president of Spain at the time.

The second example of the changing relationship between Spanish doctors and the Spanish state comes from Gustavo Pittaluga, one of Spain's foremost physicians.[100] In an opinion piece titled "Con motivo de la epidemia de gripe" (Concerning the flu epidemic), he wrote, "When everybody recognizes the importance of public health, the payment of general practitioners by the state will become a reality, and the passive resistance of politicians, who . . . don't want to establish . . . the inevitable hegemony of physicians over mayors, will fall like one of so many fictions that uphold the most supreme fiction that is our current political order."[101]

Pittaluga clearly sees politicians and physicians as antagonists. Moreover, he believes the latter will inevitably replace the former in Spanish public life, overshadowing them in terms of social position and prestige. From this it will naturally follow that the state will assume the payment of their salary. As Pittaluga's editorial and the college's rhetoric demonstrate, the discourse on the transformation of Spain from an epidemic to a sanitary state carried with it revolutionary overtones. The new sanitary Spain threatened to replace the old epidemic Spain, in which the political system known as the "pacific turn," plagued as it was by *caciquismo*, was unable to adequately respond to the needs of the nation.

Conclusion: Yearning for Answers

One of the underappreciated aspects of the Spanish flu has to do with the cognitive pressure it must have exerted on those who experienced it. For if the need to impose meaning on an epidemic is universal, as Charles Rosenberg has suggested, then the 1918–19 flu was especially problematic (if in an intellectually intriguing way). Although I have not addressed the diagnosis of the epidemic disease here, the inability of the medical profession to conclusively demonstrate that the pathogenic agent of the epidemic was, in fact, the flu must have heightened Spaniards' desire for an explanation even as it ultimately frustrated that desire.[102] Not only does understanding the narrative of the two Spains give us greater and more nuanced historical knowledge about the epidemic, but it should also encourage scholars to appreciate more fully the role of narrative in explaining seemingly inexplicable events. At least in Spain, it was narrative that finally aided Spaniards in taming, at least discursively, the unruly epidemic that would come to bear their name.

Notes

The research for this chapter was made possible by various funding sources, which I would like to acknowledge here: Emory University's Laney Graduate School for pre-dissertation and dissertation grants; Illinois State University's New Faculty Initiative Grant and Pretenure Faculty Initiative Grant; and Spain's Ministry of Culture for a grant through the Program for Cultural Cooperation between Spain's Ministry of Culture and United States Universities. Portions of this chapter are drawn from Ryan A. Davis, *The Spanish Flu: Narrative and Cultural Identity in Spain, 1918* (New York: Palgrave Macmillan, 2013), and are reproduced with permission of Palgrave Macmillan.

1. Beatriz Echeverri Dávila, "Spanish Influenza Seen from Spain," in *The Spanish Influenza Pandemic of 1918–19: New Perspectives*, eds. Howard Phillips and David Killingray (London: Routledge, 2003), 173.

2. For more details, see the introduction to this volume.

3. See Beatriz Echeverri Dávila, *La gripe española: La pandemia de 1918–1919* (Madrid: Centro de Investigaciones Sociológicas / Siglo XXI, 1993); María-Isabel Porras-Gallo, "Una ciudad en crisis: La epidemia de gripe de 1918–1919 en Madrid" (PhD diss., Universidad Complutense de Madrid, 1994); Porras-Gallo, *Un reto para la sociedad madrileña: La epidemia de gripe de 1918–19* (Madrid: Complutense / Comunidad Autónoma de Madrid, 1997); Josep Bernabeu-Mestre, ed., in collaboration with Andreu Nolasco Bonmatí, Marisa Bardisa Escuder, Vicente Bartual Méndez, José María Gutiérrez Rubio, Luis López Penabad, and José Miguel Mataix Piñero, *La ciutat davant el contagi: Alacant i la grip de 1918–19* (Valencia: Conselleria de Sanitat i Consum, Generalitat Valenciana, 1991); and Manuel Martínez, *València al límit: La ciutat davant l'epidemia de grip de 1918* (Simat de la Valldigna: La Xara, 1999).

4. Howard Phillips, review of *Influenza 1918: Disease, Death, and Struggle in Winnipeg*, by Esyllt W. Jones, *Bulletin of the History of Medicine* 83, no. 1 (2009): 226.

5. My analysis is based on careful examination of daily news coverage of the epidemic in *El Liberal, La Vanguardia, El Sol, ABC*, and *El Socialista*. The first four were the most widely distributed news sources in Spain at the time of the epidemic and represent both conservative and liberal political leanings as well as different regional sentiments. *El Socialista* was a smaller scale newspaper, though important for its ideological connection to the working class. On the relation between epidemics and narrative, see Charles Rosenberg, *Explaining Epidemics and Other Studies in the History of Medicine* (New York: Cambridge University Press, 1992); and Priscilla Wald, *Contagious: Culture, Carriers, and the Outbreak Narrative* (Durham, NC: Duke University Press, 2008).

6. Phillips distinguishes between first- and second-wave scholarship (he uses the term "histories") in his review of Esyllt W. Jones's *Influenza 1918: Disease, Death, and Struggle in Winnipeg*, which emphasizes the role of gender in history. If first-wave scholarship establishes the foundation of what exactly happened during the epidemic, that of the second wave builds on this "by putting particular aspects of the pandemic under lenses reflecting the authors' own fields of interest." My distinction between the story and discourse of the epidemic roughly corresponds to the distinction Phillips makes between the two waves of Spanish flu scholarship. *Bulletin of the History of Medicine* 83, no. 1 (2009): 226.

7. By emerging narrative, I mean one that develops according to "the collision between expectations and unfolding events." Cheryl Mattingly, *Healing Dramas and Clinical Plots: The Narrative Structure of Experience* (New York: Cambridge University Press, 1998), 44. The Spanish flu did not come with a predetermined script; the story of it evolved in relation to what Spaniards thought would happen and what, in fact, actually did happen.

8. Benedict Anderson, *Imagined Communities: Reflections on the Origin and Spread of Nationalism* (London: Verso, 2006), 33n54. In distinguishing between an "epidemic" and a "sanitary" Spain, I purposefully invoke the familiar trope of the two Spains in Spanish history and historiography. Since the early nineteenth century, intellectuals, politicians, scholars, and litterateurs have sought to explain the nation's sui generis place in the modern world by articulating the complexities and peculiarities of its history, society, and politics as a "metahistorical tale" of two Spains. Santos Juliá, *Historia de las dos Españas* (Madrid: Taurus, 2004), 148. One was traditional, Catholic, and conservative, the other liberal and secular. The epigraph by Larra (at the beginning of this chapter), Spain's most well-known Romantic prose writer, captures the conflictive nature of the relationship between these two Spains, which culminated in many ways with the tragedy of the Spanish civil war (1936–39). For more on the two Spains trope, see José María García Escudero, *Historia breve de las dos Españas* (Madrid: Rioduero, 1980); Santos Juliá, *Historia*; and José Alvarez Junco, *Mater dolorosa: La idea de España en el siglo XIX* (Madrid: Taurus, 2001), 383–431.

9. The narrative of the two Spains I am tracing here is particular to the second epidemic wave, so my analysis focuses on press coverage from this period (i.e., the fall of 1918). Narrowing my focus in this fashion, however, obscures the fact that, at least in Spain, contemporary views of the epidemic were more ambivalent than those of today. For instance, the WHO has recently called the Spanish flu "the most deadly disease event in the history of humanity." *Avian Influenza and Human Health: Report by Secretariat* (Geneva, Switzerland: World Health Organization, 2004), 1. For a more complete treatment of the discursive nuances of Spain's press coverage of the epidemic, see Davis, *Spanish Flu.*

10. The role of Portuguese soldiers also figures in chapters 4 and 5 of this volume.

11. Porras-Gallo, *Reto*, 71–109.

12. "Otra vez la gripe," *El Liberal*, September 8, 1918.

13. Similar speculation about the epidemic disease occurred in Brazil. See chapters 2, 4, 6, and 7 of this volume.

14. "La epidemia reinante: Sólo hay casos de gripe," *El Liberal*, September 15, 1918.

15. On the scientific and medical debates in Spain at the time, see Porras-Gallo, *Reto*, 103–7; Porras-Gallo, *Ciudad en crisis*, 294–352; and Echeverri Dávila, *Gripe española*. For more recent information on the subject, see Jeffery K. Taubenberger and David M. Morens, "1918 Influenza: The Mother of All Pandemics," *Emerging Infectious Diseases* 12, no. 1 (2006): 15–22.

16. Paul Farmer, *Infections and Inequalities: The Modern Plagues* (Berkeley: University of California Press, 2001), 11. Oddly enough, the verbal stigmatization of the Portuguese has no visual counterpart. In the sources I have consulted, I did not find any editorial cartoons or photographs depicting them.

17. Rosenberg, *Explaining Epidemics*, 287. See also Howard Markel, *When Germs Travel: Six Major Epidemics That Have Invaded America* (New York: Pantheon, 2004).

18. "La salud pública: La gripe empieza a decrecer," *ABC*, September 25, 1918.

19. In fairness, Spaniards were not alone in their treatment of foreigners. In response to their actions along the border, the French also demanded, "every Spaniard who penetrates into French territory be subjected to medical examination." "La salud pública," *El Sol*, September 22, 1918.

20. "La gripe: La salud pública," *ABC*, September 29, 1918.

21. Susan Sontag, *Illness as Metaphor and AIDS and Its Metaphors* (New York: Picador, 2001), 3.

22. "El estado sanitario de España: S. M. el Rey padece escarlatina," *El Sol*, October 4, 1918; emphasis added.

23. "El estado sanitario: La epidemia reinante," *La Vanguardia*, October 14, 1918.

24. Laura Otis, *Membranes: Metaphors of Invasion in Nineteenth-Century Literature, Science, and Politics* (Baltimore: Johns Hopkins University Press, 2000).

25. In addition to Otis's work, see Alison Bashford, *Imperial Hygiene: A Critical History of Colonialism, Nationalism and Public Health* (New York: Palgrave Macmillan, 2004); Gabriela Nouzeille, *Ficciones somáticas naturalismo, nacionalismo y políticas médicas del cuerpo (Argentina 1880–1910)* (Buenos Aires: Viterbo, 2000); and Pamela Gilbert, *Cholera and Nation: Doctoring the Social Body in Victorian England* (Albany: SUNY Press, 2008).

26. Sileno (Pedro Antonio Villahermosa), "Instrucciones para combatir la gripe," *ABC*, October 3, 1918.

27. Sander Gilman, *Disease and Representation: Images of Illness from Madness to AIDS* (Ithaca, NY: Cornell University Press, 1988), 1.

28. Rita Charon eloquently treats the relationship between the body and the self in *Narrative Medicine: Honoring the Stories of Illness* (New York: Oxford University Press, 2006), 85–104.

29. That the paradigm of Spanish subjectivity, or national identity, is an upper-class, white male is not without its consequences. See chapter 5 of Davis, *Spanish Flu*.

30. Anderson, *Imagined Communities*, 35.

31. French for "placed into the abyss," mise en abyme refers to the embedding of a smaller version of (typically) a work of art into the larger work of art itself, as when Don Quixote comes across his own story in the second part of Cervantes' novel. In the case of Sileno's cartoon, it refers to the act of reading the newspaper being embedded, or depicted in, the newspaper that Spanish readers would have read.

32. Brian McHale, "En Abyme: Internal Models and Cognitive Mapping," in *A Sense of the World: Essays on Fiction, Narrative, and Knowledge*, eds. John Gibson, Wolfgang Huemer, and Luca Pocci (New York: Routledge, 2007), 202; Anderson, *Imagined Communities*, 30.

33. From a narrative standpoint, the nearly simultaneous publication of Sileno's image and the call for a sanitary dictatorship is hardly coincidental. It highlights the relation between sequence and causality. José Angel García Landa and Susana Onega define narrative as "the semiotic representation of a sequence of events, meaningfully connected in a temporal and causal way." *Narratology: An Introduction* (New York: Longman, 1996), 3. The sequential representation of the epidemic as national crisis, followed by the call for a sanitary dictatorship, carries the weight of

narrative causality. The call for a sanitary dictatorship was also sounded in local news sources. Cf. Josep Bernabeu-Mestre and Mercedes Pascual Artiaga's chapter in this collection (chapter 11).

34. "La salud pública en España. Progresos de la epidemia," *El Liberal*, October 2, 1918.

35. "La salud pública en España. Los estragos de la epidemia," *El Liberal*, October 3, 1918. *El Liberal*'s admission of censorship is tinged with irony not just because of the daily's name but also because it was the supposed lack of censorship in Spain that allowed the press to cover the epidemic and that ultimately led to naming the flu "Spanish."

36. In the Glorious Revolution of 1868, liberals and republicans deposed Spain's monarch, Isabel II. After the restoration of the monarchy a few years later, a system known as the "peaceful turn" (*turno pacífico*) was set up to ensure that neither conservatives nor liberals dominated the political landscape. Although the *turno pacífico* was in its death throes by 1918, in theory it was still ensuring the diffusion of political power. In this context, perhaps the most significant political variable to come on the scene was that of the masses. Power was increasingly being wielded from the bottom up. For an overview of this historical period in Spain, see Raymond Carr, "Liberalism and Reaction: 1833–1931," in *Spain: A History*, ed. Raymond Carr (New York: Oxford University Press, 2001); Carr, *Modern Spain, 1875–1980* (New York: Oxford University Press, 1981); Carlos Seco Serrano, *La España de Alfonso XIII* (Madrid: Espasa-Calpe, 2002); and Helen Graham and Jo Labanyi, eds., *Spanish Cultural Studies: An Introduction; The Struggle for Modernity* (New York: Oxford University Press, 1995). José Ortega y Gasset addresses the relationship between the masses and the elites in *La rebelión de las masas*, ed. Thomas Mermall (Madrid: Castalia, 1998). As the title of his text makes clear, there was significant blowback against top-down governments.

37. "La gripe. La salud pública," *ABC*, October 3, 1918.

38. Francisco J. Romero Salvadó, *Spain, 1914–1918: Between War and Revolution* (London: Routledge, 1999), 100.

39. "La salud pública en España," *El Liberal*, October 2, 1918.

40. "La gripe: La salud pública," *ABC*, October 3, 1918.

41. David Ortiz Jr., *Paper Liberals: Press and Politics in Restoration Spain* (Westport, CT: Greenwood, 2000), 79.

42. V. Sierra Ruiz "En vísperas de una epidemia," *Gaceta de Tenerife*, October 6, 1918; emphasis added.

43. "Capítulo de calamidades," *El Sol*, September 24, 1918.

44. "La salud pública: Cómo se desarrolla la epidemia," *El Sol*, September 25, 1918.

45. "La salud pública: Aumenta considerablemente la epidemia gripal," *ABC*, October 15, 1918.

46. In 1918 Spain still had no Ministry of Health and the infrastructure in place fell under the purview of the Ministry of the Interior. In fact, Porras-Gallo has argued that the 1918–19 influenza epidemic—specifically the shortcomings it revealed in the Spanish public health system—was parlayed by public health professionals into evidence of the need for a Ministry of Health. See *Reto*, 107–14.

47. "La gripe," *El Sol*, October 15, 1918.

48. "La salud pública: La gripe sigue causando numerosas víctimas," *ABC*, October 23, 1918.

49. "La salud en España," *ABC*, October 25, 1918.

50. "El estado sanitario," *El Sol*, October 15, 1918.

51. "La cuestión sanitaria en España," *El Sol*, October 5, 1918.

52. "Noticias de la epidemia en Madrid," *El Sol*, October 23, 1918.

53. "La salud pública en España," *El Liberal*, October 21, 1918.

54. "La salud pública," *El Liberal*, November 2, 1918.

55. "La salud pública: La epidemia gripal sigue haciendo numerosas víctimas," *ABC*, October 22, 1918.

56. "La epidemia de gripe," *El Sol*, October 3, 1918.

57. "La salud pública: La epidemia gripal," *ABC*, October 7, 1918; "La salud pública en España," *El Liberal*, October 11, 1918.

58. As Nunes has noted in chapter 3, the epidemic negatively impacted Portuguese participation in the National Conference on Medicine.

59. "Otro congreso aplazado. El de sanidad civil," *Heraldo de Madrid*, September 30, 1918.

60. "La salud pública," *El Liberal*, September 29, 1918; "La salud pública," *ABC*, October 9, 1918.

61. "La salud pública: La epidemia gripal," *ABC*, October 7, 1918.

62. On the impact of the epidemic on religion in Bahia, Brazil, see Cruz de Souza's chapter in this collection (chapter 7).

63. "Epidemia de gripe," *El Sol*, October 3, 1918.

64. "La salud pública: No decrece la epidemia gripal que invade toda España," *ABC*, October 18, 1918.

65. "La salud en España," *ABC*, October 26, 1918.

66. Chapter 7 of this volume offers information on this subject in relation to Brazil.

67. "El estado sanitario. Nuevas noticias acerca de la epidemia," *El Sol*, November 8, 1918.

68. "La salud pública: En Murcia y en otras provincias aumentan los casos de gripe," *ABC*, October 21, 1918.

69. "El estado sanitario. Los estragos de la epidemia," *El Sol*, October 10, 1918.

70. "El estado sanitario. La epidemia aumenta en algunas provincias," *El Sol*, October 24, 1918.

71. "Estado sanitario. Los estragos de la epidemia," *El Sol*, October 10, 1918.

72. "La salud pública," *El Liberal*, October 25, 1918.

73. "La salud en España," *ABC*, October 30, 1918.

74. "El estado sanitario. La epidemia reinante," *La Vanguardia*, October 14, 1918.

75. "Crónica general. Informaciones de Barcelona," *La Vanguardia*, October 17, 1918.

76. "El estado sanitario. La epidemia reinante," *La Vanguardia*, October 17, 1918.

77. "El estado sanitario. La epidemia reinante," *La Vanguardia*, October 18, 1918.

78. "La salud pública en la provincia," *La Voz de Galicia*, October 6, 1918.

79. "Ante el peligro de una epidemia," *Gaceta de Tenerife*, October 7, 1918.

80. "Crónica general. Informaciones de Barcelona," *La Vanguardia*, October 17, 1918.

81. I should add that military metaphors were not unique to the Spanish influenza epidemic but were an integral part of the development of public health as

a discipline and have a long history of association with disease. Deborah Lupton, *Medicine as Culture: Illness, Disease and the Body in Western Societies* (London: Sage, 2003), 65–68.

82. On this topic, see also chapter 11 of this volume.

83. "El estado sanitario. La epidemia, en vez de decrecer, aumenta," *El Sol*, October 9, 1918.

84. "La salud pública en España. La epidemia, estacionaria," *El Liberal*, October 20, 1918.

85. "El estado sanitario. La epidemia reinante," *La Vanguardia*, October 15, 1918. This style of surveillance was hardly an academic affair, as the residents of 4 Ribera de Curtidores in Madrid found out—their unsanitary home was censured in the pages of *El Liberal.* "La salud pública en España," October 22, 1918.

86. "Los estragos de la epidemia. En Barcelona hubo anteayer 297 defunciones," *El Sol*, October 25, 1918.

87. On school closings, see "La salud pública," *ABC*, September 28, 1918. On the cancellation of masses and the prohibition of shows, see "La salud pública: La gripe empieza a decrecer," *ABC*, September 25, 1918; "La gripe. Los estragos aumentan," *Heraldo de Madrid*, October 17, 1918.

88. "Noticias de la epidemia en Madrid," *El Sol*, October 25, 1918.

89. The role of Manuel Martín Salazar in Spain was similar to that of Ricardo Jorge's in Portugal. Nunes deals extensively with Ricardo Jorge in chapter 3 of this volume.

90. "La salud en España. Noticias sobre la epidemia," *El Sol*, October 22, 1918.

91. "Estado sanitario de España: S. M. El rey padece escarlatina," *El Sol*, October 4, 1918.

92. "Estado sanitario. La epidemia aumenta en algunas provincias," *El Sol*, October 24, 1918.

93. "El estado sanitario. La epidemia de grippe," *La Vanguardia*, October 6, 1918.

94. "La salud en España. Noticias sobre la epidemia," *El Sol*, October 22, 1918.

95. The vaccine was for smallpox, an epidemic of which coincided with the outbreak of the second wave of the influenza epidemic. Further information is available from Porras-Gallo, "La lucha contra las enfermedades 'evitables' en España y la pandemia de gripe de 1918–19," *Dynamis* 14 (1994): 159–83. On the related themes of vaccination and citizenship in the context of nationalism, see Bashford, *Imperial Hygiene.*

96. The dynamics of the epidemic were also bound up with those of politics in Portugal, as discussed in chapters 3 and 4.

97. "La salud pública: La gripe sigue causando numerosas víctimas," *ABC*, October 23, 1918. More details on the Epidemic Law figures in María-Isabel Porras-Gallo, "La lucha contra las enfermedades 'evitables' en España y la pandemia de la gripe de 1918–19," *Dynamis* 14 (1994): 159–83.

98. "La salud pública: La gripe sigue causando numerosas víctimas," *ABC*, October 23, 1918. For more details on the various positions taken by physicians, see chapter 5 of Porras-Gallo, *Reto.*

99. "La salud pública: La gripe sigue causando numerosas víctimas," *ABC*, October 23, 1918.

100. An Italian by origin, Pittaluga became a Spanish citizen in 1904. He studied medicine at the University of Rome and would focus on the areas of hematology and parasitology. His most significant contributions to medicine deal with malaria. At the beginning of the second wave of the 1918 influenza epidemic, the Spanish government sent him as part of a three-man commission—which included Gregorio Marañón and Antonio Ruiz Falcó—to study the Spanish flu in France.

101. Gustavo Pittaluga, "Con motivo de la epidemia de gripe: La cuestión sanitaria," *El Sol*, October 15, 1918.

102. Eugenia Tognotti deals with the challenge the Spanish flu posed to the medical and scientific professions in "Scientific Triumphalism and Learning from the Facts: Bacteriology and the 'Spanish Flu' Challenge of 1918," *Social History of Medicine* 16, no. 1 (2003): 97–110.

Chapter Ten

The Spanish Flu in Argentina

An Alarming Hostage

HERNÁN FELDMAN

After more than three decades of presidents affiliated with a closely knit aristocratic circle, in 1912 the Argentine Congress implemented more transparent electoral laws that allowed the Radical Party led by popular caudillo Hipólito Yrigoyen to seize political power in 1916. The leader of the Radical Party generally cultivated an austere and mysterious style, was rarely seen in public, handled a myriad of matters personally, and believed in old-fashioned ways. He and his cadres consistently ignored criticisms expressed by the press and the opposition. At a time in which the Argentine press vociferously demanded that the country abandon neutrality and join the Allied Powers, the Yrigoyen administration did not even flinch. In October 1918, however, the particulars of World War I in the Argentine press started to share its prominence with accounts of the flu epidemic in Spain.[1]

Throughout October and early November the Argentine press would forge a series of narratives, first, in response to the spread of the flu in Spain and Argentina's neighboring countries and, second, in response to the reaction of Yrigoyen's administration in the face of the local development of the disease. As the spread of the flu in the beginning of October was negligible, the Argentine press began its coverage by jesting about the importance of the disease. When the flu started to take its toll in neighboring countries, however, the jokes receded, and the Argentine press started to suspect that the aparent minimal impact of the disease in Argentina owed its existence more to the lack of verifiable statistics than to pure and simple good luck. As the dearth of reliable information and germane measures on the government's part seemed to remain unchanged, the reaction began to mount in major newspapers and magazines. If the purpose of this course of action was to avoid public alarm, the press denounced the fallacy of following the trail of fear instead of assessing the true impact of the flu in the country.[2] But when the government decided to undertake multiple measures, the press accused the Yrigoyen administration of fueling public alarm without having any reliable information at hand. By the end of October, confronted with the false dilemma of addressing either panic or the disease, various narratives sought to accomplish an integration of these two extremes under the conceptual umbrella of prophylaxis.

The Spanish Flu in the Argentine Press

On October 4, for example, the magazine *El Hogar* published a current affairs editorial titled "Dangerous Guest," which reflects the increasing importance attributed to the subject of the Spanish flu in Argentina. The author questions whether Argentina's characteristic hospitality might be counterproductive, since "for some time now, we have been expecting the arrival of a guest whose visit is a cruel joke on us all." The article goes on to suggest that even closing Argentina's borders would hardly provide a concrete solution, because "although we try scowling at him and closing off the entrance, the impolite guest is capable of sneaking in unannounced, without us noticing his presence among us, until he makes us aware of him in a troublesome way." The Argentines, "who are so fond of all things Spanish," would be unable to avoid offending the "*madre patria*" in these circumstances, as the epidemic was already making itself known in Rio de Janeiro, "and this is the moment in which we all anxiously ask ourselves if the worrisome illness will traverse the borders of Brazil and wreak the same havoc in our country as in the country of origin."[3]

At this time the Argentine press was intent on focusing its attention on the development of the illness in Spain, its perceived point of origin; and in Brazil, its troubling destination, which was so nearby that the spread of the epidemic into Argentina seemed likely.[4] While the government in Barcelona ordered the disinfection of streetcars and railroads and shut down theaters, Rio de Janeiro was hosting the Eighth South American Medical Conference, a convention in which the calm of participating professionals would give way to the voice of alarm in less than four days. Thus, although on October 12 the newspaper *La Nación* described physicians at the conference joking about trying different prophylactic methods against the flu, by October 16 the same paper was reporting that sources from the Brazilian government had admitted that the expansion of the disease in the country was reaching alarming levels.[5]

In response to the escalation of the epidemic in Brazil, public high schools and theaters were closed like those in Barcelona, newspapers reduced the number of typographers, and pharmacies suspended their services for lack of medicine. The carefree attitude that the doctors displayed at the Eighth Conference in Rio de Janeiro would progressively recede in the face of the deaths of doctor Alberto Salema and health inspector Gensérico Riteiro, sent to Spain by the Brazilian government to study the epidemic.[6] This change of heart is exemplified by an incident that reveals the public's growing concern over the shortage of quinine. *La Nación* reported that a Brazilian doctor, infuriated by the exorbitant price of quinine, reacted by hitting the pharmacist dispensing the medicine on the head with his cane.[7] From this point on, although the Argentine press would continue to focus its attention on the development of the epidemic outside of the country, it would also devote equal energy to examining the extent of internal alarm concerning the medical resources at the country's disposal for confronting the flu problem.

The liberties taken by the socialist newspaper *La Vanguardia* in an article titled "A New Plague: The Radical 'Flu'" are particularly noteworthy.[8] In contrast to the representation of the epidemic as a foreign phenomenon, the Socialist newspaper maintained that, within the country, there were locusts in the north, malaria in other areas, and the seven plagues of Egypt represented by the Radical Party and the disastrous Yrigoyen administration. As a result, it was not surprising to the author of the editorial that the first case of the flu appeared at the central post office, where the majority of employees had connections to the party. On this note, *La Vanguardia* contended that "the virulent microbe is not entirely imported; it has, at least, its citizenship papers. It is, undoubtedly, an eminently radical 'flu.'"[9]

On October 9 *La Nación* published an editorial below the heading "The Defense of Public Health" in its Gossip of the Day section. The author urges the government authorities to abandon their indolence in the face of the country's sanitary conditions: "Perhaps the war has created a favorable environment for the outbreak of epidemics, as a result of the devastation, or perhaps the phenomenon is a simple chance coincidence; what is certain is that the current information on the state of public health in European countries may cause justified alarm among those in communication with them."[10] The author of the editorial also emphasizes the decisive attitude of the Brazilian government in contrast to the apathy of the Argentine governing class. While the neighboring nation sent doctors to Spain to study the illness to protect their compatriots (which directly led to the death of some), the administration of President Yrigoyen left the Departamento de Higiene (Department of Hygiene) under the precarious leadership of an inexperienced interim director and demonstrated no immediate intention of replacing him with a qualified permanent director. But if the aforementioned article considers communication with Europe the sufficient element for igniting a justified alarm, the column "The Boogeyman of the Moment," published in the same paper, would qualify this justification less than a week later: "It is well known that, in dealing with the masses, nothing is so easily communicated as panic."[11]

In this way, the author of "The Boogeyman of the Moment" concentrates less on the public health danger derived from the disease itself and focuses instead on the contagiousness of fear within densely populated areas.[12] "One lives today, in effect, seeing in each moment the specter of the 'flu' [*grippe*] and forgetting that, with the more common name of influenza [*trancazo*], we have had this disease in every time and in every era." The author adds that "the mildest symptoms of common influenza are taken as a grave omen" of a fatal ending. In other words, what in other circumstances would not have generated any apprehension "now sounds a powerful alarm." The sobering interpretation of the columnist thus suggests that current cases of the flu caused by changes in temperature would be seen, in the midst of such circumstances, as the sign of a sanitary catastrophe. "And yesterday, the announcement that the epidemic had broken out in a certain government office and left behind it a long line of infected people led in many places to the belief that the familiar fear—albeit hitherto vague and latent—would develop into an intense alarm."[13]

Thus, according to the author of "The Boogeyman," it seemed as if the "masses" possessed a rare talent to create states of alarm based on information that was not necessarily alarming. Hence, the author appeals to the opinion of medical specialists, calling for them to refute the viability of the epidemic and to alert against the dangerousness of predictions generated by the "popular imagination."[14] In the same vein, *La Vanguardia* published a column on October 16 titled "Dangerous Alarms," in which it condemned the persistence of harmful fear mongering. "The popular imagination embraces the most sensationalist statements, and fear seizes many faint-hearted people, predisposing them, therefore, to the same infection that they so deeply fear."[15]

What's in a Name?

In an October 16 article titled "The 'Flu' Should Not Cause Alarm: Its Benign Presentation," *La Nación* took up once again the idea that the name of the epidemic, which was nothing more than "common influenza," appeared to be derived from motives that were not entirely scientific, motives that, in turn, revealed once again the contagiousness of fear more than considerations based on medical evidence. The anonymous author claims that every time an epidemic arises, "the popular imagination" searches for a name with which to designate it. "Influenza or 'flu,' epidemic, common cold, pious fever, Chinese, Russian, Japanese, Chilean, Spanish, etc. influenza, and an infinity of names that reveal the character or the origin of the epidemic."[16]

Similarly, on October 26, the magazine *Caras y Caretas* published an article in which the author comments on how an illness "that threatens to extend itself throughout the entire world has been baptized with various and capricious names: 'barracks influenza,' 'Spanish influenza,' 'infectious flu,' 'Hun's germ,' etc."[17]

El Hogar, too, referenced the illness's numerous names in a brief review titled "The Flu" on October 25. According to the author, it was known in France as "'coqueluche,' 'tac,' and 'petit courrier.' The name 'coqueluche' comes from the practice in which those infected wear a cap called a 'coqueluchon.' In Italy, it received the name 'influenza' in 1702 in Milán."[18] In reference to the 1918–19 epidemic, the author indicates that, "according to what we can read in the telegrams of our newspapers, it is called 'Spanish flu.' The Spanish, who, as we all know, are clever people of good humor, have baptized it, according to the time period, with the names 'dengue' and '*trancazo*,' and recently, they called it 'The Song of Forgetting' and 'The Soldier of Naples.'"[19] The great diversity of names, in addition to their creativity, seems to suggest a total lack of certainty in regard to the identity of the illness in question. It is not surprising, thus, that *Caras y Caretas* and *El Hogar* both maintained that no one knew with scientific certainty what kind of disease was actually wreaking havoc in Europe. This assessment (from two of the most preeminent sources of the popular press) was later confirmed by the Argentine scientific community in the March 1919 edition of the National Department of Hygiene's *Revista del Instituto Bacteriológico*.

Beyond the multiplicity of names associated with the epidemic concerns of the moment, *La Nación* attempted to dispel this uninformed apprehension, presenting the flu not as a foreign phenomenon but as a familiar one among the many others that occur in modern society and in a world traversed by a growing level of intercommunication. Consequently, the author of the editorial column maintained that these types of epidemics are inevitable, and that prophylactic measures are useless. Moreover, he held that the throngs of recruits in barracks and ships as well as the lack of fresh food were responsible for the seriousness of the illness in Europe. Argentina, according to this view, had nothing to fear in this regard. The climate, the excellent sanitary conditions, the abundance of fresh food, and the fast approaching summer were all factors that ensured the innocuousness of the epidemic in the country, even when in Brazil the illness was presenting epidemic characteristics.[20] "The telegrams from Brazil should not alarm us either," *La Nación* stated, "since in previous epidemics our neighbor has been hit much harder than our country, which is understandable, since there are different climatic and social conditions."[21]

In an article titled "The Sanitary Defense" that appears on the same page, *La Nación* presented an in-depth case against the alarmism derived from the seriousness of the illness in Spain, Italy, and Switzerland.

Although in Europe the epidemic presented itself as an agent of devasta-tion, *La Nación* claimed that the auspicious data that the Argentine gov-ernment was releasing regarding the development of the disease should suffice to dismiss the "gloomy predictions, overwrought with the exagger-ation that is inevitable in these cases." While *La Nación* considered "the useless alarms harmful and counterproductive," it nevertheless judged it necessary "to use all means of precaution necessary to prepare the defense of the country against the possible advances of the plague."[22] In this regard, *La Nación* warned the public about the danger of three factors that it labeled as indeed alarming. First, in a country ill-equipped to face sanitary disasters, Argentine government officials bragged with "ingenu-ous boastfulness" about the innocuousness of the disease. Second, lead-ership was lacking at the National Department of Hygiene, then under the management of an interim director. Third, renowned physicians such as Dr. Pascual Palma and Dr. Gregorio Aráoz Alfaro stepped down from their posts at critical health divisions after discovering that, in exchange for political favors, high-ranking government officials systematically filled vacant positions with personnel lacking any medical experstise.

While *La Nación* and *La Vanguardia* took advantage of the tenor of alarm over the flu to forge analogies with the political terrain, *El Hogar* carried out a similar operation in its October 18 editorial, "Contagions." "Ever since the European people have found themselves contaminated with alarming dis-eases, a serious concern has seized our public health authorities, fearing the possibilities for contagion to our country." Although the author feels that the government's concerns in this area are reasonable, he nevertheless contends that, "it is other contagions that escape all preventative measures and bring their influence to spheres worthy of healthier fates."[23] The author then pro-ceeds to condemn the recent events that led to the famous university reform initiated in the city of Córdoba, given that it seemed to have resulted in the inoculation of electoral politics in the university classrooms.[24] "Hence, we have," *El Hogar* warns, "university institutions contaminated with all the vices that characterize the atrabilious, unruly and superficial nature of the cult of personality that prevails in domestic politics." Indeed, diverse politi-cal factions now loomed in the universities. Elections and candidacies—ele-ments long foreign to academic formation—had infiltrated the university to interfere, according to this vision, with its educating mission. "And even if these contagions do not seemingly threaten public health," the author con-cludes, "they are no less dangerous or serious, because they disturb the soul of the youth, robbing it of the guidance of order, serenity, independence and justice that should reign exclusively in those spheres in which spiritual nourishment is harvested."[25] The author, consequently, denounces that the case of the university is a sample that indicates to what extent politics is becoming the dominant factor interfering with a previous state of affairs. In a similar vein, various opinions would condemn how political reasons come to occlude those necessary epidemiological facts that are crucial to deal with the defense against the flu.

The Disease versus the Alarm

By mid-October the Argentine press displayed daily information dealing with the spread of the flu in neighboring countries. Around October 18 the Uruguayan newswires reported that the illness was benign and that there was "no existing reason to become alarmed."[26] Conversely, the information arriving from Chile warned that the epidemic was expanding dramatically; hospitals were unable to treat all the ill, and the confirmed deaths, on occasion, reached 11 people per day. In an editorial titled "The 'Flu': Its Harmlessness Prevails," published in *La Nación*, the author states that at least 150,000 people in Buenos Aires had contracted the disease, "without one serious case having occurred to date." "The panic that at first was caused mainly by the indecisive attitude and contradictory actions of the sanitary authorities has already disappeared, and the public, following the example of Paris (which in a similar circumstance a century ago also exacted vengeance by disseminating picaresque and spiritual 'couplets'), begins to joke about the illness of the day and its effects."[27] The negligence of the Argentine political class once again became the primary cause for alarm, while the concrete evidence allowed the public to resume treating the illness with humor. In this vein, an article titled "The Topic of the 'Flu': Victims and Victimizers," from the October 19 issue of *La Nación*, begins with a letter that an employee had sent to his boss explaining his absence from work:

> Dear Boss, I regret very much having to miss work today. I am a victim of the prevailing epidemic. I spent an atrocious night, consumed by fever. The doctor is ordering me to stay in bed and observe a strict antiseptic regimen of my mouth, nostrils, and pharynx. I will be condemned for three days, at least, to *salipirina*, quinine, and calomel. Take pity on me. Sending my sincerest wishes that you do not also pay tribute to the terrible scourge that strikes us, taking my leave of you, etc. etc.

The author of the article explains that analogous versions of this letter would soon arrive at any of the offices that did not deduct a day's pay for sick leaves. "Especially on Thursdays, the day of the horse races," the author adds with obvious sarcasm, "the terrible 'flu' epidemic wreaked havoc." Meanwhile, those honestly convinced of the danger of the contagion stormed the pharmacies, sterilized money, avoided crowds of people, and "look[ed] with hysterical eyes at anyone who cough[ed] around them." The author of the editorial anticipates that, in spite of everything, the growing apprehension toward the illness "will conclude, fortunately, in a joke."[28]

By the end of the third week of October, 250 people per day were dying in Barcelona; in Chile, barracks were ordered to be built to accommodate the growing number of patients; in Brazil, doctors continued to die, and the government resolved that a quarantine hospital be opened in Isla Grande under the leadership of Dr. Emilio Gomes. While Chile reported a daily influx in hospitals of 60 to 70 patients afflicted with the flu (resulting in 9 deaths per day), Argentine authorities decided to suspend classes in high schools and other teaching schools without any reliable statistics. Even more amazingly, the decision was carried out at the very same time in which the governmental authorities were fully engaged in publicizing that the illness was completely benign, and that it should therefore not concern the population. Despite the supposed lack of reason for concern, on October 21 *La Vanguardia* was forced to reduce its number of pages due to the growing impact of the virus among its employees, especially those who worked in the expedition and linotype sections.[29] *La Prensa* reported on October 22 that the Department of Hygiene had resolved to suspend classes for ten days in the teaching schools and national high schools located in Buenos Aires and its suburbs. After enumerating the different measures being taken to contain the contagion and improve the sanitary conditions of the city, such as the inspection of boats in the port and the cleanup of stream water, the author of the editorial concludes by saying, "as anyone can see, there does not exist any reason for alarm." Later on, the informative column reported the growing number of consultations taking place in the central medical center of the Municipal Health Service. The author explains that, during the course of a day, "a true caravan of patients were seen conferring, alarmed, about the seriousness of their illness. Doctors and practitioners had to answer 255 house calls and, like in earlier times, see four or five sick people in each house." *La Prensa* also reported the growing number of cases of the flu among doctors, elementary and middle school students, municipal employees, post office workers, and police officers as an indicator of the extent to which the different strata of the public sector found themselves affected. It highlighted with admiration the fact that "there was a doctor who, afflicted by the illness, completed his mission of attending to the sick while he was ingesting 'caches' of quinine."[30]

While the daily chronicles of the newspapers and magazines evince a narrative trajectory that oscillated between placating alarmism on the one hand and accurately portraying the impact of the illness on daily life on the other hand, a middle-ground approach began to surface in the final days of October. A series of observations in different publications would momentarily abandon the false dilemma that continued to place the press between the mission of bringing peace to the public and the obligation to report the sanitary scenario with accuracy. In an attempt to resolve the growing tension between the proposed need to avoid alarm and the ethical impera- tive of informing the public about the actual impact of the flu in the coun- try, *El Hogar* published an article in its October 25 issue titled "Proceeding without Coordination," in which the author points out that "the unexpected and extraordinary development of the prevailing epidemic brought with it the entourage of alarms inevitable in such cases." The author notes that, far from the alarm being the problem, the greatest difficulty was "that things are done in reverse of what would seem natural and logical, which, in truth, does not surprise us much, as we are accustomed to seeing ordinary problems of public interest be resolved in the least appropriate way."[31] In effect, *El Hogar* condemned the closing of education establishments, which complied with hygiene regulations and which carried forward a fundamen- tal mission in society, while "clubs without proper ventilation or sufficient cleanliness, frequented day and night by crowds of careless and heteroge- neous people" continued to operate despite the fact that they performed no socially relevant function.[32] For its part, *La Prensa* published a current affairs column on October 24 titled "Facing the Epidemic," in which the author maintains that "the relatively serious nature of some cases of the flu—very few, fortunately—in the last forty-eight hours cannot be cause for alarm." More than focusing on the theme of alarm in the present moment, how- ever, *La Prensa* stepped up its efforts to communicate the necessity of also considering possible future contingencies. Thus, the columnist argues that, although there had been no fatalities up to that point, one could not rule out that possibility. "Keeping this in mind," *La Prensa* indicated, "the fact that there is one victim to mourn should not frighten the population."[33]

Instead of dwelling on the subject of alarm, like countless editorials had done up to that point, "Facing the Epidemic" sets out to demonstrate that the Yrigoyen administration had spent its time and energy trying to gauge the hypothetical tenor of an excessive public reaction in the face of a pos- sible epidemic rather than evaluating the escalation of the epidemic itself. As *La Prensa* had pointed out, "our public health authorities, probably understanding that their fundamental job was to prevent alarm, have dis- played unparalleled zeal for taking away all importance given to the invad- ing condition, for which they considered it appropriate not to take any of the customary steps that are recommendable under circumstances such as those occurring in the municipality of the city."[34] Indeed, the relevant state agencies seem to have sidestepped their primary objective, targeting the consequences of the flu rather than the disease itself. In this manner, an alarm as contagious as the illness that causes it took the center stage. *La Prensa* then highlighted the two primary methods adopted by the govern- ment to eradicate alarm: denying the importance of the illness and avoiding taking substantive measures for fear of alarming the public. In sum, it was an elusively conceived alarm and not the flu that appears to have regulated the actions of Argentina's public health authorities, thereby divesting the society of the necessary mechanisms for ascertaining the extent of the spread of the influenza and for quelling sensible fears by reasonably containing the disease. Consequently, the absence of practical measures contributed to the increased incidence and virulence of the flu and, accordingly, the deepening of the alarm that authorities had sought to mitigate.

The possibility of a future fatality from the disease, to which *La Prensa* had alluded, came to fruition the following day when *La Nación* reported the first death from the flu. In an article titled "Where Do We Stand? Sanitary Contradictions," the newspaper critiqued the relationship between alarm and the sanitary measures taken by the government.[35] Although *El Hogar* was condemning the backwardness of inept politicians and *La Prensa* was expressing its indignation over the measures not taken for the sole purpose of preventing alarm, when the public health authorities finally decided to close the public places referenced by *El Hogar*, the move did not generate approval but, rather, the opposite. In fact, *La Nación* emphasized the contradictions within this alarmism, denouncing the fact that public health authorities "have refused, in the beginning and in recent days, to recognize the importance or seriousness of the prevailing disease, attempting, without a doubt, to communicate to the population a confidence opposed by definition to all futile alarmism." While *La Prensa* was condemning the government for intending solely to prevent alarm rather than evaluate conclusively the impact of the illness, as if both endeavors were mutually exclusive, *La Nación* attacked the harsh and abrupt character of the extreme set of measures that followed the country's first flu death. "There is, then," *La Nación* noted, "a contradiction in the method, which presumes certain confusion with respect to the real state of things." At the same time that government communiqués were transmitting optimism, the visible actions of various state departments began to insinuate the opposite. *La Nación* thus concluded that the most serious concern of all was "that one does not know what is wanted or what should be avoided."[36] In other words, the government's change in behavior was not necessarily accompanied by a change in rhetoric. As a result, this failure to communicate facts diligently left the press in the dark and forced multiple actors to come up with possible justifications for this communication crisis.

Damned If You Do, Damned If You Don't

While the Yrigoyen administration abruptly changed course between October 24 and 25, the articles published by *La Prensa* and *La Nación* during the respective moments of excessive inaction and excessive action converged in their critique of the fact that the level of alarm (or, more appropriately, the construction thereof) had risen on the administrative authority's barometer, displacing almost completely the underlying epidemiological reasons for such alarm. Nevertheless, La Prensa seemed to feel obligated to enter the same extra-epidemiological terrain that it attributed to the governmental management of public health measures. In fact, the author of the October 24 article "Facing the Epidemic" concludes that "it is necessary to recognize that the public health authorities have omitted a series of measures that, apart from their preventative effectiveness, are recommended for the reassuring persuasiveness that they exercise over the spirit of the masses."[37] In other words, even though La Prensa considered it absurd not to take preventative measures to avoid causing alarm, it also sought to persuade the political cadres of the administration that taking measures could be useful not only for sanitary prevention but also for political reasons such as quelling fear. From a position of overt opposition, La Nación condemned the sudden launch of excessive sanitary measures precisely because such behavior was incompatible with a government that claimed that there were no reasons for alarm. But even though the critiques launched by La Prensa and La Nación validated, to an extent, the government's strategy of subordinating practical measures to an undependable "alarm-ometer" of sorts, both newspapers coincided in recommending that resolute action be taken by the government, provided that such action was strictly tied to the concrete advance of the flu in the country. In the words of the editor of La Nación, "the fear of causing alarm is a puerile fear. A people, a great people, is not a group of nervous women and fearful children. Alarm does not necessarily have to be panic; the most natural is that it be precaution and foresight."[38]

On October 26 La Prensa echoed La Nación in a current affairs editorial titled "An Emergency Measure." The author conducts a brief report on the contradictory measures carried out by public health authorities. At one extreme was the initial optimism aimed at avoiding any possibility for alarm and the "parsimony in adopting defense measures that in such circumstances as these are of elemental prudence." At the other extreme was "the shock of alarm that will produce severe measures in the city, adopted or to be adopted rapidly by the same departments that until yesterday expressed the most satisfied optimism" in response to those who were recommending precautionary measures. In this way, La Prensa retraced its steps to place alarm as its central theme of discussion. If before October 24 it was unwise to do nothing only for the sake of avoiding panic, one day later it was equally wrong to do too much. According to La Prensa, this last approach, in effect, carried enough weight to generate concerns in the fragile minds of a public that was defenseless in the face of the vicissitudes of the flu. A public that, needless to say, the author of "Where Do We Stand?" did not consent to comparing with "a group of nervous women and fearful children." Thus, the municipal measures that prohibited the operation of theaters, bars, cafés, cabarets, and other public recreation centers after eleven o'clock at night, would, according to the analysis of the author of "An Emergency Measure," generate with its inconvenient and capricious nature precisely the alarm that the government had wanted to avoid by doing nothing at the beginning of October. "As the facts on which the restrictive regulations that are beginning to be put in place are based are not mentioned," maintains *La Prensa*, "the popular imagination tries to clear up the mystery, imagining that the notable change in strategy displayed, for example, by the recent decree by the Municipal Council, is caused by the serious development of the epidemic that has been proclaimed and believed to be harmless."[39]

The unforgiving logic of *La Prensa* implies that the government had failed both before, when it did nothing, and after, when it finally did act. The author concludes that the government should have begun to take measures beforehand and, furthermore, that it should have done so in a more methodical, gradual, and reasoned way, "to put out of people's minds the easily susceptible, fearful thoughts in relation to the sanitary state of the city." According to *La Prensa*, although there was no reason to fear the seriousness of the epidemic, "the unexpected nature of resolutions like the one mentioned can be the cause, unfortunately, of people suddenly losing their tranquility, which the authorities responsible for the care of public health had instilled in them, and the unleashing of worrying conjectures about what will occur in the metropolis." In the end, the sharp opposition of *La Prensa* to any type of measures taken by the government found an outlet in a proposal aimed at avoiding extremes and, primarily, at studying the empirical evidence in strictly epidemiological terms: "To avoid two dangerous extremes, irrational carelessness and unwarranted panic, it would be advisable that an officially authorized statement declare categorically and in precise terms what the true course of the epidemic in the city is."[40]

Following its policy of providing as little information as possible, the government did not respond with statistics but rather with measures of every tenor and caliber, including the disinfection of streets, movie theaters, churches, and streetcars; the inspection of ships, vacant land, trash dumps, and tenement housing; and the early closure of the academic year in educational establishments. The government also suspended the Day of the Dead festivities in the cemeteries, established a quarantine hospital on Marín García Island, closed down Buenos Aires nightlife, and launched an aggressive campaign to eradicate flies. The press, for its part, responded by insistently urging the government to focus on prevention and information. In this regard, *La Nación* indicated that "if there is uncertainty above, there cannot be security below, and if the people do not have a clear sense of the danger they are in, the vigorous and harsh prophylactic measures and sanitation of the environment will not be as effective as they could be."[41]

La Prensa emphasized preventative measures to "at the same time combat the illness and strengthen morale, which acts as a valuable collaborator with any prophylactic or healing regimen, [utilizing] all the methods that individual and collective hygiene advise in emergencies of this nature."[42] For its part, on October 29 *La Vanguardia* published a column titled "The Dirty and Neglected City," in which it recommended a series of measures to prevent infection, including "avoiding the overcrowding of people in enclosed bars, which produces a foul air eminently harmful for public health. It is, then, of good prophylaxis to avoid crowds in view of the danger of the epidemic."[43] In the March 1919 issue of the *Revista del Instituto Bacteriológico* of the National Department of Hygiene, finally, doctors Rodolfo Kraus and L. Kantor published "Studies on the Influenza Epidemic (1918)," an article that concludes with the issue of prophylaxis on an opposite note: "Allow us to say a few words about etiological prophylaxis of influenza. Various researchers worked on active and passive immunization, especially Kolle and Delius, experimenting on animals. Their work and work by Slatineanu, Cantani, and Latepie showed that it was not feasible to find the experimental basis in animals for man's immunization against the flu."[44]

The Emergence of Prophylaxis

Whether prophylaxis was feasible or not, its presence became the center of gravity of a discourse previously focused on alarm.[45] For example, the author who signed with the initials A. L. S. in *La Vanguardia* designed an actual catalog of preventative measures in an insert from November 4, titled "The Health Defense II," which read, "I will detail a few hygienic solutions intended as antiseptic methods for the mouth and nose, indicating thus a means of prophylaxis of immediate usefulness, since no one is ignoring that the flu is contagious and enters the organism through the respiratory tract."[46] But if there is a moment in which prophylaxis takes over the discursive plot of the story of the flu, it is found in the publication of a provocative caricature in the November 2 issue of the magazine *Caras y Caretas* (see fig. 10.1). Under the heading of "Prophylaxis against the Flu" and positioned above the caption, "Precautions, yielding infallible results, that should be taken to avoid infection from the epidemic," the caricature in question depicts a pedestrian, presumably from Buenos Aires, equipped with an assortment of necessary devices for combating infection. From the pedestrian's straw hat hang blocks of camphor, naphthalene, quinine, and ground cinnamon.[47]

As the character marches on with a confident gait, his face is covered by a sort of precarious gas mask from which projects a conspicuous oxygen tube attached to a pinwheel. His gloved hands carry a thurible and a cane

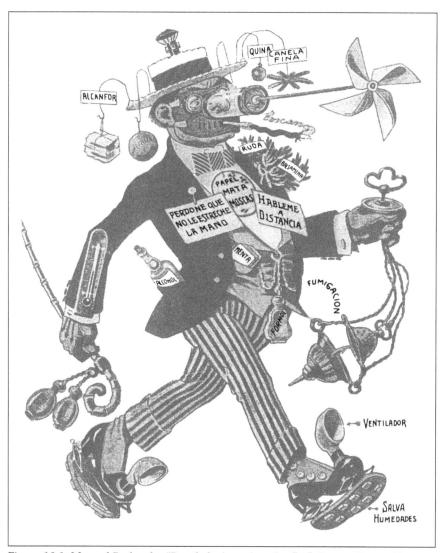

Figure 10.1. Manuel Redondo, "Prophylaxis against the flu," *Caras y Caretas*, November 2, 1918.

from which hang two grenade-shaped jars, one of them containing ammonia. Stuck on one of the sleeves of his jacket is a thermometer, while on his feet are shoes equipped with air holes and insulating soles called "humidity savers." His torso is also packed full of tools for fighting the flu. One of the pockets of his jacket contains a bottle of alcohol. One of the buttonholes of his lapel carries rue and balsam plants, and from the other hangs a sign with the caption, "forgive me if I don't shake your hand." Instead of a watch chain hanging from his vest is a bottle connected to a box of mints in his pocket. On the shirt we find flypaper and a sign that says "speak to me at a distance."

The multitude of gadgets carried by the pedestrian, and thus caricatured by *Caras y Caretas*, maintain a close relationship with what the periodical press had been reporting in regard to the methods that the Argentine public was adopting in response to the potential impact of the flu in their daily lives. For example, on October 18 *La Nación* had accused pharmacists of making a fortune from preaching the virtues of camphor, laxatives, and quinine. "But the most alarming in all of this is that many have embellished the prophylactic properties of alcohol, when this is, precisely, a factor that contributes to putting an individual in unfavorable conditions in every sense."[48] In an editorial from the following day, *La Nación* adopted a similar tone when it attributed the strong odor of camphor wafting through Buenos Aires to the misguided idea of a dishonest pharmacist who, having a surplus of camphor blocks, "found his salvation convincing some schoolteachers that the aromatic resin was the current panacea." The article explains how the news arrived to the sewers of the public health works, "home of a number of bums, and so yesterday the pedestrians on San Martín Street had the opportunity to admire a model of health showing off, as an accessory to his 'toilette' of rags, a straw hat with one of those aforementioned blocks [of camphor] hanging from the brim by a string."[49] Similarly, on October 31 *La Nación* published a report titled "Public Health in the Capital and in the Provinces: Development of the Flu; It Continues to Be Benign." The report contains different sections that describe the measures adopted to fight the epidemic, such as "The Extinction of Flies." In this section, the author details the municipal ordinances, aimed at the extermination of flies in the city of Buenos Aires, that have been in effect since 1913 without, by that point, having thoroughly accomplished their goal: "to disseminate the practice of the systematic destruction of the fly, the well-known universities in La Boca and Rosario have initiated a series of exhibitions of fly-catching devices and traps, intending additionally to distribute freely, to whomever asks, facsimiles of them and instructional pamphlets on the subject."[50] Meanwhile, in another section of the report, the author notes, "never as in these current circumstances has the benefit of recalling the old inscription of 'You are kindly requested not to shake hands' been so relevant."[51] Finally, in the first issue of "The Health Defense," published in *La Vanguardia* on November 2, the author A. L. S. echoed the warning when he affirms, "the practice of shaking hands should be put aside."[52]

The discursive nucleus of prophylaxis as the surreptitious replacement for the voice of alarm presents an etymological angle. Effectively, the word "prophylaxis" comes from the Greek term φύλαξις, the meaning of which ranges from the actions of observing to that of guarding and showing care. While the prefix indicates activity and the self-initiative of carrying out a task associated with the safekeeping and sheltering inherent in the term phylaxis, the term seems to take a detour, at first difficult to explain, when we discover its alternate meaning in the word "amulet." Referring to the etymological dictionary by Joan Corominas, we find that the term "phylacteria" comes from the same root that connotes "safeguard, preventative, amulet" and is defined as "a type of amulet, consisting in a piece of parchment with scriptural passages, that Jews were accusomed to wearing tied to the body." Furthermore, according to Corominas, "phylacterium" means "piece of parchment with verses from the Bible that the Pharisees and Medieval Jews carried as an amulet or as a religous attribute."[53] In his *Treasure of the Spanish Language* Sebastián de Covarrubias defines "phylacterium" as "precisely the trimming or the embellishment that is placed on the hems of clothing so that it keeps and conserves it, [and] without [which] it would unravel and split open easily." Nevertheless, the meaning is complicated when Covarrubias, as well as Corominas, recover the plural term "phylateria" that derives from the singular "phylacterium." On the one hand, Covarrubias defines it as a "throng of words that a deceitful speaker strings and spins in order to deceive us and persuade us of what he wants, because of the similarity of the many threads tangled together."[54] Corominas, on the other hand, rules out the hypothesis of the threads but thoroughly traces the use of the term phylateria in literary works: "it is evident that from the meaning of 'amulets or superstitious remedies,' 'inscriptions of magic words,' transformed into 'a barrage of words used by a trickster.'"[55]

The etymological derivations of prophylaxis color in the portrait of the pedestrian from *Caras y Caretas*, which is the nucleus around which orbit the public official with his slanted reports, the alarmed citizen, the doctor with his recommendations, the regular man in arms, and the sanitary-conscious subject who takes every precaution while interrogating a shared sense of hospitality toward a guest whose condition remains unknown.[56] In the words of the October 16 issue of *La Vanguardia*, "what is important for the public to know, and what has not yet been said, is how one should guard oneself against a plague that can become, we repeat, extremely harmful."[57] The caricature also visually portrays the saturation of the discourse resulting from the multiplicity of narratives surrounding the looming danger. It is a portrait laden with the double talk of conniving pharmacists, who strategically situated their advice on the border between science and superstition, thereby confining their gullible patients to fear and apprehension. Equipped with multiple phylacteria construed as indispensable but always insufficient to achieve immunity against the flu, Argentine citizens inhabit a social space flanked by weakness and illness. Citizens thus construed by epidemiological advice resort to covering their clothing with amulets to create more layers between them and the dangerous arena of social contact.[58]

Although the suppression of information at the beginning of October was intended to avoid alarm, it in fact ended up contributing to the prevailing narrative of the fear of fear. Moreover, even when the discursive focus shifted from fear to prophylaxis at the end of October, the employment of such radical measures did not accomplish the goal of dismantling the alarm but rather served to fuel the sensation of defenselessness. The historical evidence would come to corroborate, moreover, that the impact of the Spanish flu epidemic in Argentina, more than exposing sanitary weakness in the face of the flu, had revealed the unusually porous nature of the membranes regulating the narrative contours of alarmism in Argentine society at the beginning of the twentieth century.[59] With the worries over the flu having essentially passed by the middle of January 1919, Buenos Aires society would confront with similar clumsiness the dissemination of rumors regarding the possibility of a Soviet revolution commanded by Jews occurring in the nation. The incident resulted in the deployment of a truly overwhelming prophylaxis. The silencing of the press and the initial placation of alarm was followed by a colossal pogrom against the local Jewish community and the quelling of an imaginary Judeo-Soviet conspiracy. Like the flu, the conclusion of this affair was accompanied by cynical humorous comments regarding the supposed conspiracy and related panic.[60] The articulation of both incidents, to be sure, illustrate how prophylaxis without supporting information perpetuate a notion of social defense that is as pernicious as the most unwarranted alarm.

—Translated by Anne Garland Mahler

Notes

1. Mandatory references for the Spanish flu are Howard Phillips and David Killingray, eds., *The Spanish Influenza Pandemic of 1918–19: New Perspectives* (New York: Routledge, 2003), and its thorough bibliography. See also María-Isabel Porras-Gallo, *Un reto para la sociedad madrileña: La epidemia de gripe de 1918–19* (Madrid: Complutense / Comunidad Autónoma de Madrid, 1997). In the Argentine context, José W. Tobías obtained the prize Facultad de Ciencias Médicas with the submission of his doctoral thesis dealing with the flu, *La epidemia de grippe de 1918–19* (Buenos Aires: Las Ciencias, 1920).

2. The role of fear in Brazilian society is discussed in chapters 6 and 7 of this volume.

3. "Huésped peligroso," *El Hogar*, October 4, 1918.

4. On the Spanish experience, it is useful to consult chapters 5, 9, and 11 of this volume, as well as Ryan A. Davis, *The Spanish Flu: Narrative and Cultural Identity in Spain, 1918* (New York: Palgrave Macmillan, 2013); Beatriz Echeverri Dávila, *La gripe*

española: La pandemia de 1918–19 (Madrid: Centro de Investigaciones Sociológicas / Siglo XXI, 1993); Porras-Gallo, *Reto*; and María-Isabel Porras-Gallo, "Una ciudad en crisis: La epidemia de gripe de 1918–1919 en Madrid" (PhD diss., Universidad Complutense de Madrid, 1994). On the Brazilian case, see chapters 2, 6, and 7 of this volume, as well as the following books: Liane Maria Bertucci, *Influenza, a medicina enferma: Ciência e práticas de cura na época da gripe espanhola em São Paulo* (Campinas: Universidade Estadual de Campinas, 2004); Christiane Maria Cruz de Souza, *A gripe espanhola na Bahia: Saúde, política e medicina em tempos de epidemia* (Salvador: Editora da Universidade Federal da Bahia; Rio de Janeiro: Fundação Oswaldo Cruz, 2009); and Anny Jackeline Torres Silveira, *A influenza espanhola e a cidade planejada: Belo Horizonte, 1918* (Belo Horizonte: Argumentum, 2007).

5. "La 'grippe' en Río. Temores desvancidos," *La Nación*, October 12, 1918. "Brasil. Efectos de la epidemia," *La Nación*, October 16, 1918.

6. The Spanish government took a similar initiative, sending a commission to France when the second wave of the pandemic started. The commission comprised the physicians Gregorio Marañón, Gustavo Pittaluga, and Ruiz Falcó. María-Isabel Porras-Gallo, "Sueros y vacunas en la lucha contra la pandemia de gripe de 1918–1919 en España," *Asclepio* 60, no. 2 (2008): 261–88, 273.

7. "Brasil. La epidemia reinante," *La Nación*, October 17, 1918. On November 9, 1918, the magazine *Caras y Caretas* published a caricature titled "Current Contrasts," in which the page is divided in two. On the right side appears an emaciated man with empty pockets, accompanied by a scrawny black cat. On the left side appears a robust and well-dressed man, standing in front of a heavily armored box, smoking a Cuban cigar and accompanied by a healthy white cat. The captions below the pictures state, respectively, "I have the flu!" and "I have a pharmacy!" "Contrastes de actualidad," *Caras y Caretas*, November 9, 1918.

8. *La Vanguardia* was founded by Socialist leader Juan B. Justo in 1894 as the official press of the Argentine Socialist Party.

9. "Una nueva plaga: La 'grippe' radical," *La Vanguardia*, October 14, 1918. From the very beginning, the flu was referred to as "grippe" in most of the Argentine press. By the end of October most newspapers started to change it to "gripe," the term currently used in Argentina to refer to the flu.

10. "La defensa de la salud pública," *La Nación*, October 9, 1918.

11. "El fantasma del momento," *La Nación*, October 15, 1918. On the importance of Spain in the diffusion of the pandemic, see the introduction to this volume.

12. On this same topic, see also chapter 6 of this volume.

13. "Fantasma del momento."

14. Chapter 6 of this volume deals with similar reactions in Brazil.

15. "Alarmas peligrosas," *La Vanguardia*, October 16, 1918.

16. "La 'grippe' no debe alarmar: Su presentación benigna," *La Nación*, October 16, 1918.

17. "El bacilo de la influenza," *Caras y Caretas*, October 26, 1918.

18. "La grippe," *El Hogar*, October 25, 1918.

19. A trailblazing analysis of the cultural implications of the Spanish flu in Spain can be found in Davis, *Spanish Flu*. Chapter 4 provides unique insight on the cultural relevance of the Song of Forgetting and the figure of the Soldier of Naples with respect to the circulation of flu discourse.

20. As Silveira points out in chapter 6, this belief was shared in Belo Horizonte, Brazil.

21. "'Grippe' no debe alarmar."

22. "La defensa sanitaria," *La Nación*, October 16, 1918.

23. "Contagios," *El Hogar*, October 18, 1918.

24. In 1918 students of the University of Córdoba, at the time dominated by the Catholic Church, initiated a series of demonstrations that led to national recognition of the students' right to become an integral part of university government. The "Liminar Manifiesto," authored by the student Deodoro Roca detailed their demands for democratization within institutions of higher learning. These revolutionary reforms were soon legislated by the Argentine Congress during the administration of President Hipólito Yrigoyen, who viewed students' demands favorably. On the subject of the 1918 university reform, refer to Alberto Ciria and Horacio Sanguinetti, *La reforma universitaria: 1918–2006* (Santa Fe: Universidad Nacional del Litoral, 2006); Hugo Biagini, *La reforma universitaria: Antecedentes y consecuentes* (Buenos Aires: Leviatán, 2000); and María Candelari and Patricia Funes, *Escenas reformistas: La reforma universitaria, 1918–1930* (Buenos Aires: Universidad de Buenos Aires, 1997).

25. "Contagios."

26. "Uruguay: La epidemia de 'grippe,'" *La Nación*, October 18, 1918.

27. "La 'grippe' se acentúa su benignidad: Declaraciones oficiales," *La Nación*, October 18, 1918.

28. "El tema de la 'gripe': Víctimas y victimarios, la farmacopea popular, impresiones del momento," *La Nación*, October 19, 1918. Toward the end of October *El Hogar* would publish a commentary titled "Seriously," in which the author warned that those who had joked about the flu in Spain should now be taking the epidemic seriously. In this regard, the author urged Argentina to take caution against displaying similar attitudes. In November, nevertheless, the flu was one of the most depicted themes by the cartoonists of the Argentine graphic media. Moreover, the jokes did not limit themselves to the sphere of journalism. On November 3, for example, *La Vanguardia* published an insert titled "The Flu as a Joke," in which the author informed that "last night—Saturday night—thousands of young people on foot and in carriages filled within an hour the Corrientes Street thoroughfare, from Reconquista to Callao, and Mayo Avenue, from Perú to Entre Ríos, singing songs alluding to the flu and to the closing of the cafés and finishing with a chorus of a certain spicy flavor." "La gripe en broma," *La Vanguardia*, November 3, 1918.

29. "La epidemia de influenza se extiende en Buenos Aires," *La Vanguardia*, October 21, 1918.

30. "La epidemia de influencia: Clausura de los establecimientos de enseñanza," *La Prensa*, October 22, 1918.

31. "Procediendo sin concierto," *El Hogar*, October 25, 1918.

32. Once the local clubs and recreation centers were closed, *La Vanguardia* criticized that the same was not done with masses and funerals. Contemplating a funeral mass from afar, the author of "The Dirty and Neglected City" impugns this practice as contrary to the elemental rules of hygiene. "One can suppose that the air must have been foul in that environment where onlookers crowded together at the side of a dead person," the author notes, "whose death could be caused by a contagious

disease. Why that exception? It is unexplainable." "La ciudad sucia y descuidada," *La Vanguardia*, October 29, 1918.

33. "Frente a la epidemia," *La Prensa*, October 24, 1918.

34. Ibid.

35. "¿En qué quedamos? Contradicciones sanitarias," *La Nación*, October 25, 1918, 5. On October 26, the newspaper *La Vanguardia* reports the death of three infected people, two patients admitted to the Muñiz Hospital and an agent from the Central Police Department. "La epidemia de influenza. Tres casos fatales." *La Vanguardia*, October 26, 1918. Although it was at this moment when the official danger of fatality from the disease became clear, *La Vanguardia* had already reported a fatal case that occurred in the post office on October 15. "La Gripe. Nuevos casos en el correo. Un fallecimiento." *La Vanguardia*, October 15, 1918.

36. "¿En qué quedamos?"

37. "La defensa sanitaria," *La Prensa*, October 14, 1918.

38. "¿En qué quedamos?"

39. "Una medida de emergencia," *La Prensa*, October 26, 1918; "¿En qué quedamos?"

40. "Medida de emergencia." On November 1 *La Vanguardia* published a column titled "Public Health: The Government Takes Late and Poor Measures." The author denounces that, while the flu was spreading, the government was attributing the visibility of the epidemic to the invention of the opposing press. "But things took a serious turn," *La Vanguardia* adds, "alarm was widespread, and then the government dunces resolved to do something." "La salud pública: El gobierno toma medidas tarde y mal," *La Vanguardia*, November 1, 1918.

41. "¿En qué quedamos?"

42. "Frente a la epidemia."

43. "Ciudad sucia y descuidada."

44. Rodolfo Kraus and L. Kantor, "Estudios sobre la epidemia de influenza (1918)," *Revista del Instituto Bacteriológico* 2, no. 1 (1919): 69.

45. The importance of prophylaxis is also dealt with in chapters 2, 4, 5, 7, and 11 of this volume.

46. A. L. S, "La defensa de la salud II," *Vanguardia*, November 4, 1918.

47. "Profilaxis contra la gripe," *Caras y Caretas*, November 2, 1918. On November 9, 1918, the cover of the magazine *Caras y Caretas* depicted President Yrigoyen afflicted by the flu. The ills the president suffers are located on his face and represent current political problems. At the bottom of the picture a playful limerick encourages him to use cinnamon to fight this particular strand of flu. "¡Tomá canela!," *Caras y Caretas*, November 9, 1918.

48. "'Grippe' se acentúa su benignidad."

49. "Tema de la 'gripe.'"

50. "La extinción de las moscas" in "La salud pública en la Capital y en las provincias. Desarrollo de la Gripe. Continúa siendo benigna," *La Nación*, October 31, 1918.

51. "Se ruega no dar la mano," in "La salud pública en la Capital y en las provincias. Desarrollo de la Gripe. Continúa siendo benigna," *La Nación*, October 31, 1918.

52. A. L. S, "La defensa de la salud," *La Vanguardia*, November 2, 1918.

53. Joan Corominas, *Diccionario crítico etimológico castellano e hispánico* (Madrid: Gredos, 1980), 895–96.

54. Sebastián de Horozco Covarrubias, *Tesoro de la lengua castellana o española* (Barcelona: Horta, 1943), 546.

55. Corominas, *Diccionario crítico*, 896.

56. A sophisticated reading of the points of contact between hostility and hospitality can be found in the dialogue between Jacques Derrida and Anne Dufourmantelle in *Of Hospitality* (Stanford: Stanford University Press, 2000). In the Argentine context, see Diego Tatián, "Hostilidad/hospitalidad," *Pensamiento de los Confines* 11 (September 2002): 109–16.

57. "La gripe: Algunos datos útiles," *La Vanguardia*, October 16, 1918.

58. For a discussion of the cultural impact of the concept of contagion in the urban United States, see the chapter "Communicable Americanism" in Priscilla Wald, *Contagious: Culture, Carriers, and the Outbreak Narrative* (Durham, NC: Duke University Press, 2008), 114–56. Regarding the concept of immunity, see Robert Esposito, *Immunitas: Protección y negación de la vida* (Buenos Aires: Amorrortu, 2005); and Ed Cohen, "Emplotting Immunity: Inscribing Defense in the Bio-Medical Imagination," *Queen: A Journal of Rhetoric and Power* 4, no. 1 (2009), www.ars-rhetorica.net/Queen/Volume41/Articles/Cohen.html.

59. Otis's membrane model is a fitting point of departure for reflecting on the cultural importance of borders in literary, scientific, and political accounts of the nineteenth century. Laura Otis, *Membranes: Metaphors of Invasion in Nineteenth-Century Literature, Science, and Politics* (Baltimore: Johns Hopkins University Press, 1999).

60. Curiously, the incidents that occurred in Argentina in January 1919 were designated "La Semana Trágica," or the tragic week, a term also of Spanish origin. For a bibliographic look at La Semana Trágica, consult Allen Metz, "La Semana Trágica: An Annotated Bibliography," *Inter-American Review of Bibliography* 40, no. 1 (1990) 51–92. Regarding the pogrom that resulted from La Semana Trágica, see Emilio J. Corbiére, "¿Pogrom en Buenos Aires?," *Todo Es Historia* 378 (1999) 28–44.

Chapter Eleven

Epidemic Disease, Local Government, and Social Control

The Example of the City of Alicante, Spain

JOSEP BERNABEU-MESTRE AND
MERCEDES PASCUAL ARTIAGA

Throughout history, urban societies, the social structures that form them, and their capacity for reaction have been called into question as a result of periodic mortality crises caused by infectious diseases of epidemic proportions. In the contemporary age alone, the European Mediterranean area has suffered outbreaks of yellow fever and cholera in the nineteenth century and an epidemic of influenza in 1918–19.[1] Infectious processes of this kind usually cause intense and complex reactions due to the health-related, social, economic, political, and demographic consequences that they bring.[2] Terror, panic, instinctive selfishness, a moral explanation of the disease analyzed in terms of guilt and innocence, the call for measures to exclude or isolate those affected, and the search for scapegoats are just some of the collective reactions that have emerged in different periods of history whenever a society has been threatened by an epidemic.[3]

Society's attitudes to the sick and the value placed on health and illness have varied throughout history, but what has remained constant is the social isolation that victims of a disease have been subjected to, particularly during an epidemic.[4] The sudden and spectacular way in which epidemics tend to start, the way their incidence increases, the large number of deaths they cause, and the numbers of people affected underlie such significant social aggressiveness.[5]

But despite the fact that epidemic diseases do not tend to make any distinction between social groups or classes, their repercussions tend to be greater in sectors of society where poverty and a lack of resources make people far more vulnerable. Not only are victims isolated, but various health, social, and political control processes are usually implemented that affect the most socioeconomically disadvantaged members of the population, those who are often thought to be the cause of the disease or responsible for it spreading.[6] Given that the social class to which one belongs greatly impacts the differential risk of falling ill, it is feasible that this realization would therefore have influenced the development and implementation of instruments of control by ruling classes throughout history to benefit themselves and their interests.[7] In reality, many of these considerations may be valid for any episode of disease, but historical evidence shows that it is during an epidemic when the greatest mechanisms of control have arisen. It is then that they are brought to bear with the greatest impact on those suffering the consequences of the outbreak.

This chapter concentrates on the sociosanitary, cultural, and political control mechanisms that, as a result of epidemics such as the 1918 influenza, the municipal authorities of Alicante, Spain, adopted with regard to the most underprivileged members of society (in socioeconomic and hygienic-sanitary terms) and thus the most vulnerable.[8] Although the focus is mainly on events that occurred as a result of the influenza epidemic that affected the city in the autumn of 1918, a comparative analysis of the 1804 yellow fever epidemic and the cholera epidemics of the mid-nineteenth century show the continuity and similarity in the arguments upheld by the political and sanitary discourses that justified them, despite the changes that occurred in scientific and medical knowledge and the developments in hygiene and public health.[9] In addressing these questions, we have consulted documents from the Alicante Municipal Archive, including Actas del Ayuntamiento (Council Minutes), the Sección de Beneficencia y Sanidad (Charitable Works and Sanitation Section), the printed press during the 1918 influenza epidemic, and other sources such as the *Boletín Oficial de la Provincia de Alicante* (Alicante Province Official State Gazette).[10]

Epidemic, Hunger, and Misery in Alicante in 1918

In 1918 the city of Alicante had fifty-five thousand inhabitants living in eight urban districts (Casas Consistoriales, San Fernando, Hernán Cortés, Teatro, El Carmen, Santa María, San Antón, and the Ensanche, the latter two being the most heavily populated) and various rural areas. The municipal government was in the hands of right-wing liberals, but conservative minorities and left-wing and republican groups under the umbrella of the Alianza de las Izquierdas (Alliance of the Left) were also represented.[11]

When the influenza outbreak reached Alicante in 1918, it coincided with a serious socioeconomic crisis that had worsened in the last few months of 1917, with the greatest effects felt in districts such as San Antón and the Ensanche, where most of the working-class proletariat population (i.e., those with the fewest economic resources) lived. Alicante had experienced protests and strikes, particularly the national strike of August 1917, which was repressed by the armed forces with serious consequences for many working families, some of whom saw relatives imprisoned.[12] The commerce that had led to Alicante's status as a port city had been brought to a virtual standstill by the crisis affecting the national and regional economy, as well as by the difficulties that the war raging across Europe and the world meant for transportation, particularly shipping.[13] The lack of work, the freezing of wages, the shortage of primary foodstuffs, and price increases left the working classes in a state of helplessness. In the midst of a major social conflict, the problems of hunger, unemployment, and disease quickly became the habitual bedfellows of the proletariat.[14]

From a demographic-sanitary viewpoint, in 1918 the mortality rate in Alicante was fifteen percentage points above the average for nonepidemic years, and the number of deaths had doubled. Of 2,206 deaths, 664 were recorded in the month of October, at the height of the epidemic. As occurred elsewhere throughout the world, those most affected by the influenza outbreak were people between twenty and thirty-nine years of age; in other words, the most productive group in social and economic terms, which undoubtedly meant that the impact of the outbreak was that much greater. The epidemic was most virulent and caused the highest death rates in the districts of San Antón and the Ensanche, which, as stated previously, were home to large numbers of the working class.[15] These were people with the fewest socioeconomic resources, and both of these areas (particularly San Antón) had serious deficiencies in terms of hygiene and sanitation (table 11.1).[16]

The district of San Antón lay outside the city walls, and its development owed much to the tobacco factory that opened in 1801, which became the most important industrial establishment in Alicante.[17] It gave work to thousands of women, who gradually settled on the slopes of the Benacantil Mountain beneath the Santa Bárbara castle.[18] These workers settled in a disorganized fashion in areas that were increasingly unsuitable, building veritable slums that led to a sharp rise in densification, degradation, and social exclusion, particularly in the neighborhood of Las Provincias (see fig. 11.1).[19]

Documentary evidence exists from the early nineteenth century regarding the poor hygiene of the homes and urban areas of Las Provincias and other parts of the city, such as Santa Cruz and the upper part of La Villavieja. These conditions only worsened during epidemics, when the largest number of cases and the most dramatic situations were recorded.

Table 11.1. Mortality rates (per thousand inhabitants) in the urban areas of Alicante in October 1918

Districts	Males	Females	Population (inhabitants)
Casas Consistoriales	8.14	11.46	5,385
San Fernando	10.15	13.70	7,411
Hernán Cortés	10.26	8.09	3,855
Teatro	11.42	12.88	7,045
El Carmen	3.09	10.98	4,999
Santa María	6.46	6.90	5,996
San Antón	13.73	14.17	9,162
Ensanche	15.52	19.45	11,443
City Total	9.85	12.2	55,296

Source: Official Municipal Statistics, Boletín Oficial de la Provincia de Alicante, 1914–18.

In the yellow fever epidemic of 1804, even though the first cases appeared in the center of the city rather than the outlying or poorer areas (the unhygienic conditions of which meant that disease would spread on a periodic basis), the main objective for the authorities was to prevent the poor from catching the disease and spreading it, since they were the ones who lived in such unhealthy conditions:

> [We] hav[e] verified that the first people to have fallen ill live in the center of the city, immediately affecting adjacent houses. . . . The lack of improvement in the more wretched inhabitants, among whom epidemics tend to start, gives grounds to our suspicion, and we must make every effort to prevent the infection from reaching these people, whose scant resources, lack of clean clothes and appropriate sanitation, and who live with little or no ventilation and practically one on top of another, cause the outbreak to spread on a massive scale.[20]

Such considerations were expressed again as a result of the cholera epidemics of 1833 and 1834. Faced with the threat of a new outbreak, the Alicante authorities took measures to meet the needs of the poor should the disease take hold in the city. The wealthier members of society were called on to give voluntary donations "to come to the aid of public poverty."[21] The aim was for "the immense majority of this town, made up of poor people, not to be caught up in the double horror of hunger and infection at the same time." The municipal health authorities would be in charge of "researching and investigating causes of ill-health among the population and the town's

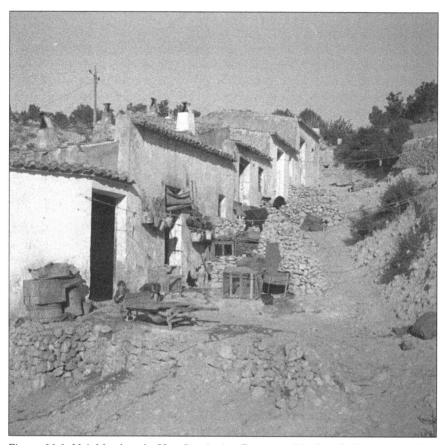

Figure 11.1. Neighborhood of Las Provincias. Francisco Sánchez Collection, Archivo Municipal de Alicante. Reproduced with permission from the Concejal Delegado de Cultura of Alicante.

neighborhoods, so as to reduce or contain the damage that Asian cholera may cause."[22] In 1849 a Permanent Commission on Health for the city was formed, consisting of a doctor, a pharmacist, and a municipal alderman, all of whom, after touring the city and surrounding areas, were to produce a report detailing all health and sanitation problems and provide proposals to correct or remove them. Among the sources of health problems that the commission detected was the former convent of Santo Domingo, on Calle Mayor next to the Puerta de Elche. The building was rented out to a large number of extremely poor families. The commission criticized the dirt, stench, and miserable conditions the inhabitants lived in, which were so bad that it felt there was nothing that could be done to make the building a healthier place to live, and it was feared that any disease originating there could affect the rest of the population. The Department of Health proposed evacuating the building.[23]

In a context of ongoing surveillance aimed at ensuring that the so-called partial causes of ill health were destroyed and the outbreak of cholera prevented, the authorities needed to control the least well-off social classes and prevent "poor families, young workers, water carriers, laborers, and so on from living piled up in small rooms." Visits were to be made to examine the degree of cleanliness in homes and to point out and classify those that, due to their poor state of upkeep, should be whitewashed, forcing the owners "to oversee this work, as it brings undeniable benefits."[24] As far as was possible, and while the epidemic raged, the local authorities were in charge of preventing families or individuals from living in large groups in narrow, poorly ventilated rooms by providing the needy (free of charge) with the necessary means to disinfect their premises, as long as they were in agreement.[25]

A similar situation occurred in 1853, when the threat of the proximity of the cholera outbreak in northern Europe triggered an interest in the Alicante authorities with regard to the hygienic conditions in which the population was living. The authorities insisted on the need to carry out preventive home visits with the purpose of inspecting both the dwellings and the lifestyle of the poor.[26] But whereas any preventive action during the possibility of an epidemic was limited to increased vigilance, when an epidemic did actually strike, the policy changed to one of strict control, even segregation. Various documents in Alicante's municipal archive evidence the control exerted over the hygienic conditions in some areas of the city as a result of the 1854 and 1855 outbreaks. In April and May 1855, the aldermen on the Health Commission were entrusted with conducting a visit to some of the city's neighborhoods due to the derelict state they were in, to propose measures that would remedy "the lack of policing and of health, both inside the homes and in the streets."[27] In July of the same year, a "good governance" edict ordered doctors to make weekly home visits in their corresponding districts, accompanied by local aldermen. Beggars and nonlocal vagrants were ordered to leave, and special attention was paid to the waste dumps in the Arrabal Roig area. A visit was also ordered to the San Antón neighborhood to locate all vagabonds there and expel them.[28] Many of these measures and attitudes that arose as a result of the yellow fever and cholera epidemics were repeated with the outbreak of influenza in 1918. Just as in the nineteenth century, the same neighborhoods and areas of the city were identified as sources of ill health and places besieged by poverty, misery, and malnutrition.

Following the control and disappearance of the cholera epidemics, certain critical voices, such as the hygienist doctors, continued to denounce the lack of hygiene and sanitation in the most disadvantaged neighborhoods of the city.[29] In 1910 the republican doctor and Alicante city councilor,

Antonio Rico, presented various motions and called for the areas of Las Provincias, Santa Cruz, and the upper part of La Villavieja to be knocked down or at least declared as areas for surveillance. Despite such calls, no action had been taken by 1918, according to Lorenzo Carbonell, also a city councilor and a spokesman for the Alianza de las Izquierdas. Not until the 1918 outbreak of influenza, in the face of "the shame and danger to the city of the hovels known as Bonetes [*sic*] and many others of the same type that exist on the slopes of the Castle," were urgent calls made for the city council to "take the necessary measures to ensure they [these hovels] disappear."[30]

In May 1918, with serious threats of an epidemic, further complaints were made to the mayor regarding the deficient housing conditions of the working class, with instructions to avoid or correct such deficiencies that could have an effect on the general health of the neighborhood: "Allow me to appeal to your zeal so that, with all authority and interest, you inspect said houses and inform me of their state, proposing all measures or provisions that should be taken."[31]

The Fight against the Influenza Epidemic

Once the epidemic had been declared in September 1918, the measures applied by the local authorities to control the spread of the disease included disinfecting all manner of places, premises, objects, and even people.[32] On one hand, these measures were based on contemporary medical theories regarding the origin and method of contagion. But they also illustrated the importance of physical conditions and social surroundings to disease processes, something emphasized in the nineteenth-century miasmatic theories of disease, which were applied to some of the initiatives for tackling the yellow fever epidemic and the subsequent outbreaks of cholera.[33]

Many of the measures taken to control the infection involved instances of rigidly structured administrative and political control, such as that carried out by the so-called disinfection brigades, which entered private homes where cases of influenza had occurred.[34] As with the epidemics of the nineteenth century, the aim was to ensure that hygiene rules were followed in the private, as much as in the public, sphere.[35]

In the case of the 1918 outbreak of influenza, the municipal authorities of Alicante adopted clearly intimidating strategies, with severe economic sanctions for anyone not meeting the established standards of hygiene. The media even called for a health dictatorship to ensure that all rules were followed to the letter.[36] In reality, the control measures enacted by the municipal authorities enjoyed wide support, as the notion that the epidemic was a public health problem that affected everyone gained strength. In such a context, the media repeatedly called on everyone to comply with all sanitary regulations (particularly those relating to hygiene), stressing the need for involvement from all social classes, implying that if one part of the population did not follow the scientific precepts laid down, the efforts of the rest of the city could be rendered useless.[37]

As part of this concern to ensure the collaboration of all sectors of society in the fight against the epidemic, several people condemned the major inequalities that existed with regard to the disease. Some in the media criticized (or drew attention to) the fact that most of those affected were people who lived in crowded, unhealthy, poorly ventilated homes in narrow streets outside the city, whereas few cases were recorded in the center of the city.[38] Las Provincias was the main focus point of the influenza outbreak and the area that suffered most as a consequence of the epidemic, due to the number of people living in unsanitary hovels without the slightest notion of hygiene. In some instances the media went further and called on the wealthier classes in the city to help the needy by providing them with food, finding suitable shelter for the sick, and, above all, "evacuating all living beings from the caves and hovels in Las Provincias and El Castillo, where fellow beings live in their own filth and with no medical assistance of any kind."[39] As we have seen, the focus of attention was directed once again at those sectors of the population with the fewest resources. Those who were considered high-risk groups and who were perceived as a clear danger to society as a whole because of this were subjected to serious sanitary and administrative means of control.

The political discourse concerning the outbreak was heard loudest precisely when the epidemic reached its most alarming stages. On October 14, 1918, a special city council session was held with the sole purpose of analyzing the city's desperate sanitary conditions. As the highest level of authority in the city, it described what it considered to be the "true state of sanitation in Alicante" as being "of [the] most alarming proportions, with mortality reaching five times its usual levels. With the greatest number of fatalities occurring in homes with the lowest levels of hygiene and which are not fit for habitation, namely, on the hills around the Santa Bárbara castle." The mayor of the city also reminded those in attendance at the session that hundreds of families were suffering the effects of both influenza and poverty and stressed the need to ensure the collaboration of all citizens "to reestablish public health and mitigate the cruelties of misery." And, true to these arguments, one of the most important agreements reached was "to proceed to clean up the whole of the area known as Las Provincias, and the upper part of the Carmen and Raval Roig neighborhoods."[40]

This decision was carried out with unusual speed. In a session held on November 8, 1918, the city council reported that the evacuation and demolition of all the aforementioned areas had begun on October 18, four days after the special session during which the resolution had been passed. It also stipulated that the occupants of the homes had been given a period of forty-eight hours to leave their premises. More than eighty homes were destroyed in just two days with apparently no opposition or resistance. The buildings demolished were both those deemed by the architects to be in a state of ruin and those that, although not in ruins, failed to meet the technicians' standards of hygiene and suitability for habitation.

Various measures were taken with regard to the population affected by this evacuation. Some families were relocated to different areas of the city, while those who had emigrated from other parts of Spain were forced to return to their places of origin (Murcia, Cartagena, Lorca, Albacete, Cádiz, etc.), for which the council paid their travel expenses. Other families were put up at the Santa Bárbara castle, which had been adapted for this purpose following an agreement with the Ministry of War.[41] The measures summarized here were supported by most of the political groups represented on the city council; only members of the Alianza de las Izquierdas were critical. Although they did not oppose the measures adopted, they regretted that it took an epidemic of this nature for the authorities to realize the dangers posed by some areas of the city, clearly referring to the pockets of poverty and ill health found in Las Provincias and the other neighborhoods considered to be sources of infection.[42]

The more conservative sectors of Alicante society widely applauded the measures taken. The newspaper *El Correo*, mouthpiece of the *mauristas* (a right-wing political group with representatives on the city council), wrote of the evacuation of Las Provincias using expressions such as "neighborhoods where the battle for sanitation will be waged." The daily newspaper *El Tiempo*, official voice of the *dinásticos* (another right-wing group), stated that tearing down Las Provincias could be the first step toward eradicating the epidemic.[43] In an article published on November 3 with the headline "The Misery of the Upper Neighborhoods," the same newspaper played down the virulence of the epidemic, as it was surprised by the fact that the death toll among the more needy members of the population was not as great as had been expected:

> Despite the victims of the epidemic, it could not be denied that the outbreak had been so acute and of such virulence. If it had reached them, the death toll among people from the upper neighborhoods, in those narrow streets and filthy homes, where human beings lived piled on top of one another, without resources, food or the most rudimentary conditions of hygiene would have been horrendous. The houses are veritable warrens, inhabited by poor and wretched people, and must necessarily be breeding grounds for any plague. It is a duty of humanity to remove from these homes those sick people living there, because it is God's will, and transfer them to hospitals.[44]

Two days later, *El Tiempo* again dealt with the issue in an article titled "So Much Could Have Been Done: The Credit Operation," which criticized the fact that not all possible measures had been implemented:

> Days have passed, and the epidemic has gained ground in humble homes lack-
> ing in hygiene and resources; the cleanup of el Carmen and el Arrabal Roig,
> the main sources of the influenza infection, has not been verified.... The
> poor families that live in filthy homes, unable to care for their loved ones, lack-
> ing even the basics with which to feed themselves, are still in their disgusting
> holes, piled up with the sick, the young ones starving, vehicles for propagation
> and innocent victims of these terrible ills.[45]

As well as illustrating the wide social support for the measures described,
these testimonies also made a point of stating that the people responsible for
the epidemic and the way it spread were the citizens who suffered its effects
the most, without providing any critical consideration of the factors and causes
behind these pockets of poverty and marginalization.[46] In fact, five years after
the epidemic, in a report dated October 16, 1923, the medical department
of the city council presented extensive details on the sanitary situation of the
southern district that should have been used to conduct an inquiry into the
evacuation, demolition, and destruction of caves and the cleanup of homes
in the buildings known as Venta del Tío Vicente el de las Rejas and Venta del
Sordo. Instead, it mentioned the well-known Garrut caves on the Calle Sevilla
and others in La Montañeta and San Fernando castle.[47]

This report, prepared by Dr. Pascual Pérez, dean of the Cuerpo Municipal
de Beneficencia y Sanidad (Municipal Department of Charitable Works),
referred to a memorandum written as a result of the 1918 influenza epidemic that recommended these areas be destroyed because they were permanent sources of infection that their inhabitants, as vectors, spread to the
rest of the city. As well as expressing feelings of humanity, shame, and honor,
the report spoke of how these people lived "like a troglodyte or some ver-
min in its den." It went on to say that nothing had changed and that the
original considerations still applied. In other words, the authors of the 1923
report would have endorsed every one of the conclusions reached by the
1918 report.

The diagnosis of the situation, exemplified in the case of the Venta del
Tío Vicente el de las Rejas building, shows the extreme conditions of ill
health and marginalization that surrounded these sectors of the population.
Moreover, it helps explain the excessive death toll that occurred during the
epidemic and the discourse that led to the controlling measures proposed
and carried out, albeit only partially. The building in question was described
as a yard or courtyard, formed by a group of "tiny rooms" that were home to
an anthill ("without such a euphemism, a vulgarity would be required") of
human beings being eaten away at by carrion:

> It is shameful, it is embarrassing, it turns our cheeks red to consider that a fam-
> ily lives in each one of these hovels, where men and women, elders and minors,
> all sleep together in the most denigrating promiscuity. They eat their meals on

their beds, because there is no space for a table, and there they perform their bodily functions, because there is just a single and highly repugnant lavatory, which is for the sole use of the building's owner, with all the other inhabitants "tout a l'egout," or rather, just outside. . . . In the angle formed by the two sections of the corridor, there is a well that is said to be dry, and it seemed an ideal place for microbes to germinate and mosquito larvae to develop. . . . And so, what remedy can a hygienist suggest? Just one—the red pencil; to proceed like the Army when one of its "Docker" buildings is invaded by pestilential disease, which is to burn it and reduce the rotten heap, home to multiple diseases, to ashes. . . . But as one must not commit the inhumanity of leaving the families that live there without any shelter, until somewhere suitable is found to put them up, it is right to proceed with an intense process of disinfecting all walls, floors, and household items, without forgetting the smallest details and with thorough auditing to ensure continued cleanliness.[48]

What this testimony shows is that, rather than being an "intolerable social problem," as other health problems had become, these slums came to be considered the cause that explained the disease phenomenon and therefore inevitably subject to control or auditing.[49] To explain this attitude of the municipal authorities, it is important to remember how long it took the Valencia region and Spain in general to modernize, in terms of sanitation, and the repeated negligence in resolving a situation that, as successive epidemics had shown, became a problem for the whole of society and one that worsened the conditions and accentuated the inequalities and exclusion of the most disadvantaged sectors of society.[50]

A Few Final Considerations

The epidemic outbreak of influenza in 1918 exacerbated the existing social and economic difficulties that the city of Alicante was experiencing at the time. Hunger, unemployment, and the progressive deterioration of hygiene and sanitary conditions, which most strongly affected the poorest classes, were all added to the problems of the influenza outbreak. As had occurred in the yellow fever and cholera epidemics that affected the city in the nineteenth century, the fact that it was specifically the most socioeconomically disadvantaged members of society who were most affected by the epidemic led to a causal link being established between the outbreak and the conditions of poverty, misery, and ill health in which a high number of families lived. Their homes were considered sources of infection and the very origin of the disease, and the inhabitants, vehicles of propagation and contagion. All these circumstances allowed the municipal authorities, with the support not just of most of the political groups represented on the city council but also of public opinion (as represented by the media), to implement a complex process of social, administrative, and sanitary control of these sectors of the population, the most extreme example of which occurred in the neighborhood of Las Provincias.

The evacuation and demolition of homes in the area; segregation, with most families accommodated in the Santa Bárbara castle; and expulsion, attenuated by the expression "facilitating the return to their places of origin," were the three main measures that allowed the local powers that be, using the disease as a tool, to exercise strict social control over the most underprivileged sectors of the population, in economic, social, cultural, and political terms. Historical experiences such as those discussed here help us to reevaluate current strategies for dealing with epidemic processes and thereby strengthen the health objectives with which society has expected to enter the twenty-first century.[51]

Acknowledgments

We would like to thank the Alicante Municipal Archive for their collaboration and help with the graphical materials and the management of documents. This work was produced as part of the following research projects: "The Conditioning Historical-Health Factors in the Spanish Nutritional Transition (1874–1975)," HAR2009-13504-C02, Spanish Ministry of Science and Innovation; and Prometeo/2009/122, Group Alicante of Studies Advanced in History of the Health and Medicine, Generalitat Valenciana.

Notes

1. For the case of Spain, see José Luís Bertrán Moya, *Historia de las epidemias en España y sus colonias (1348–1919)* (Madrid: Esfera de los Libros, 2006).

2. Howard Phillips and David Killingray, introduction to *The Spanish Influenza Pandemic of 1918–1919*, ed. Howard Phillips and David Killingray (New York: Routledge, 2003), 12–15.

3. François Lebrun, preface to *Peurs et terreurs face* à *la contagion: Choléra, tuberculose, syphilis, XIXe–XXe siècles*, ed. Jean-Pierre Bardet, Patrice Bourdelais, Pierre Guillaume, François Lebrun, and Claude Quetel (Paris: Fayard, 1988), 7–12.

4. Chapters 4 and 9 also discuss this attitude during the Spanish flu.

5. Henry Sigerist, *Civilización y enfermedad* (Mexico City: Biblioteca de la Salud, 1987), 89. See also Charles Rosenberg, *Explaining Epidemics and Other Studies in History of Medicine* (Cambridge: Cambridge Univesity Press, 1992).

6. Sigerist, *Civilización y enfermedad*, 106–7.

7. María Angeles Durán, *Desigualdad social y enfermedad* (Madrid: Tecnos, 1983), 23–24.

8. In chapter 9 of this volume, Davis sees sanitary measures like those studied in this chapter as central to the creation of what he terms "sanitary Spain." In chapter

8, León-Sanz deals with how nongovernmental organizations treated workers from Pamplona, Spain.

9. Mercedes Pascual Artiaga, *Fam, malaltia i mort: La ciutat d'Alacant i la febre groga de 1804* (Simat de Valldigna: Xara, 2000). Patrice Bourdelais, ed., *Les hygiénistes: Enjeux, modèles et pratiques, XVIIIe–XXe siècles* (Paris: Belin, 2001).

10. The newspapers that were published in Alicante in 1918 and used in the analysis were as follows: *El Día*, a liberal newspaper that acted as the mouthpiece for the political majority that backed the municipal government; *La Unión Democrática*, the mouthpiece for the Partido Republicano Progresista (Progressive Republican Party); *El Luchador: Diario Republicano de Alicante*, the mouthpiece for the minority Alianza de las Izquierdas (Alliance of the Left); *El Correo*, the mouthpiece of the *mauristas*, one of the right-wing conservative groups involved in Alicante politics; *El Heraldo de Alicante*, considered the mouthpiece for the radicals; and *El Tiempo*, the mouthpiece for the *dinásticos*, another right-wing conservative group that sat on the city council. Other newspapers were also consulted that did not have such a well-defined political affiliation, such as *El Diario de Alicante*, *La Correspondencia de Alicante*, and what was known as the *Periódico para Todos*. For the press in Alicante, see Francisco Moreno Sáez ed., *La prensa en la ciudad de Alicante durante la dictadura de Primo de Rivera (1923–31)* (Alicante: Instituto de Cultura Juan Gil-Albert, 1995).

11. Salvador Forner and Mariano García, *Cuneros y caciques* (Alicante: Patronato Municipal del Quinto Centenario de la Ciudad de Alicante, 1990), 209–15.

12. Regarding the protests and strikes of 1917, see Francisco Moreno Sáez, *Las luchas sociales en la provincia de Alicante (1890–1931)* (Alicante: Unión General de Trabajadores, 1988), 296–97. To deal with the situation and the criticisms coming from all political sectors and to help the people most in need, in 1918 the municipal government set up a Prosubsistence Board. *Libro de actas del ayuntamiento constitucional de Alicante*, session of January 19, Archivo Municipal de Alicante (hereafter AMA). Measures of this kind, such as what was known as the *sopa de pobres* (soup for the poor), had been applied throughout the nineteenth century, when economic crises worsened the precarious living conditions of the most disadvantaged. See Pascual Artiaga, "El reto de la alimentación en una ciudad mediterránea: Alicante en el siglo XIX; Nota de investigación," in *Medicina rural i cultura popular al País Valencià*, ed. Joaquím Guillem Llobat and Frasquet Gabriel (Gandía: CEIC Alfons El Vell, 2009); and Edict by the mayor Tomás España on the large number of beggars filling the streets and subscription to pay for the cheap soup and ration of bread for the poor, October 1850, Alicante, *Beneficencia*, leg 2/29, AMA.

13. For more details on the critical situation of Spain, see the introduction to this volume.

14. Miguel Angel Alzamora Rodríguez, "1918: Carestía y enfermedad en la ciudad de Alicante," in *Les respostes socials davant la malaltia i la mort*, ed. Josep Bernabeu-Mestre, Josep Xavier Esplugues, Mercedes Pascual Artiaga, and Vicent Terol Reig (Valencia: Denes, 2008).

15. The Ensanche consisted of newly created neighborhoods built in the late nineteenth century, when cities were no longer big enough to accommodate the immigrant population that flocked to them, attracted by the process of industrialization.

16. On the demographic-sanitary impact of the epidemic of flu of 1918–19 in the city of Alicante, see Josep Bernabeu-Mestre, ed., in collaboration with Andreu

Nolasco Bonmatí, Marisa Bardisa Escuder, Vicente Bartual Méndez, José María Gutiérrez Rubio, Luis López Penabad, and José Miguel Mataix Piñero, *La ciutat davant el contagi: Alacant i la Grip de 1918–19* (Valencia: Conselleria de Sanitat i Consum, Generalitat Valenciana, 1991), 37–64.

17. Caridad Chapuli Valdés, *La fábrica de tabacos de Alicante* (Alicante: Caja de Ahorros del Mediterráneo, 1989); Teresa Lanceta Aragonés, *Mujeres e industria tabaquera en Alicante* (Alicante: Abisal, 2013).

18. Regarding the harsh living and working conditions that tobacco workers of Alicante had to endure, see the contemporary medical topography testimony of Evaristo Manero Mollá, published in 1883. Bernabeu-Mestre, María Eugenia Galiana Sánchez, Ana Paula Cid Santos, and Josep Xavier Esplugues, "Overexploitation, Malnutrition and Stigma in a Women's Illness: Chlorosis in Contemporary Spanish Medicine, 1877–1936," in *Gender and Well-being in Europe: Historical and Contemporary Perspectives*, ed. Bernard Harris, Lina Gálvez, and Elena Machado (Hampshire: Ashgate, 2009), 160–61.

19. Joan Calduch Cervera and Santiago Varela Botella, *Guía de arquitectura de Alacant* (Alicante: Comisión de Publicaciones del CSIC, 1979), 91–93.

20. Board of Health, Doctor's report, September 13, 1804, Alicante, leg. 1/ 6 bis., *Sanidad*, AMA.

21. Board of Health, "Precautions Taken in Alicante Due to the Proximity of the Cholera Outbreak," suppl., *Boletín Oficial de la Provincia de Alicante* (hereafter *BOPA*), July 27, 1834.

22. Board of Health, *BOPA*, July 27, 1834.

23. Board of Health, *Sanidad*, April 1849, leg. 2/1, AMA; *BOPA*, no. 16, February 5, 1849.

24. *BOPA*, no. 59, May 16, 1849.

25. Real Orden, March 30, 1849, instructions given by the Board of Health, *BOPA*, no. 45, April 13, 1849.

26. *BOPA*, no. 112, September 19, 1853.

27. Board of Health, *Sanidad*, April 26, 1855, Alicante, leg. 2/105, AMA.

28. Junta Municipal, decree of the good government, *Sanidad*, July 23, 1855, leg. 2/ 91, AMA.

29. Antonio Oliver Jaén, "Les propostes higienistes de José Guardiola Picó per a la ciutat d'Alacant," in *Higiene i salubritat en els municipis valencians (1813–1939)*, ed. Josep Bernabeu-Mestre Josep, Elena Robles, and Josep Xavier Esplugues (Benissa: Seminari d'Estudis sobre la Ciencia / Institut d'Estudis Comarcals de la Marina Alta, 1997).

30. Lorenzo Carbonell, *Libro de Actas del Ayuntamiento*, October 14, 1918, AMA.

31. Board of Health, *Sanidad*, May 21, 1918, Alicante, leg. 27/42, AMA.

32. Measures that had been applied since the spring of 1918 and resolutions passed to prevent the spread of the epidemic recorded in other towns, *Sanidad*, leg 27/54, AMA.

33. María José Baguena Cervellera, "La microbiología," in *Las ciencias médicas básicas en la Valencia del siglo XIX*, ed. José María López Piñero (Valencia: Alfons El Magnànim / IVEI / Institut d'Estudis Juan Gil-Albert, 1988), 199–262.

34. These same measures were used in other parts of Spain, as shown in chapters 5, 8, and 9 of this volume.

35. Social control measures such as those represented by the disinfection brigades and commissioners had already reached an important degree of institutionalization as a result of the cholera epidemics of the nineteenth century. Patrice Bourdelais, "Le chólera: Presentation," in *Peurs et terreurs face a la contagion*, ed. Jean-Pierre Bardet (Paris: Fayard 1988), 17–41.

36. This is how the newspaper *La Región* put it in a news item from October 14, 1918. This attitude of exercising power dictatorially in epidemic crisis situations was something that had repeatedly occurred since the plague epidemics of medieval times. David S. Reher, "Les ciutats i les crisis a l'Espanya moderna," *Estudis d'Història Agrària* 5 (1984): 112. Davis deals extensively with this topic in chapter 9 of this volume.

37. This was how it was stated, for example, by the newspaper *El Tiempo*, mouthpiece for the *dinásticos*, in an editorial from October 8, 1918.

38. Editorial in *Diario de Alicante*, October 4 and 23, 1918; editorial in *Periódico para Todos*, October 15, 1918.

39. Editorial in *La Región*, October 12, 1918.

40. Antonio Bono Luque (mayor of the city of Alicante), *Libro de actas del ayuntamiento*, extraordinary session of October 14, 1918, AMA.

41. The matter of evacuating the cave dwellings that existed on the hills of the castle and the call to adapt the premises of the castle itself as a home had already been dealt with in the meeting of the Provincial Board of Health on October 10 and was discussed again on October 20. *Libro de actas de la junta*, sig. 169, AMA, 201–7.

42. Editorial in *El Luchador*, October 28, 1918.

43. Editorial in *El Correo*, October 28, 1918; editorial in *El Tiempo*, October 30, 1918.

44. "The Misery of the Upper Neighborhoods," *El Tiempo*, November 3, 1918. On this topic in the Portuguese context, see chapter 4 of this volume.

45. "So Much Could Have Been Done: The Credit Operation," *El Tiempo*, November 5, 1918.

46. See Paul Farmer, *AIDS and Accusation: Haiti and the Geography of Blame* (Berkeley: University of California Press, 1983); Farmer, *Infections and Inequalities: The Modern Plagues* (Berkeley: University of California Press, 1999).

47. Ayuntamiento Constitucional de Alicante, secretaría, Negociado de Sanidad, dossier relating to the evacuation, demolition, and destruction of caves and the cleanup of homes in the buildings known as the "Venta del Tío Vicente el de las Rejas" and "Venta del Sordo," *Sanidad*, 1923–25, leg. 36/79, AMA.

48. Ibid.

49. Josep Luis Barona, *Salud, enfermedad y muerte: La sociedad valenciana entre 1833 y 1939* (Valencia: Alfons el Magnànim, 2002).

50. Josep Lluís Barona, Josep Bernabeu-Mestre, and Enrique Perdiguero, "Health Problems and Public Policies in Rural Spain, 1854–1936," in *Health and Medicine in Rural Europe (1850–1945)*, ed. Josep Lluís Barona and Steven Cherry (Valencia: Seminari d'Estudis sobre la Ciencia / Universitat de València, 2005), 63–82. As noted in the introduction to this volume, this process of transforming and modernizing was taking place across all of Spain.

51. Paul Farmer, "Social Inequalities and Emerging Infectious Diseases," *Emerging Infectious Disease* 2, no. 4 (1996): 259–69.

Chapter Twelve

The Gendered Dimensions of Epidemic Disease

Influenza in Montreal, Canada, 1918–20

Magda Fahrni

In recent years, a number of social historians of medicine have begun to apply the insights of gender history to their studies of health and illness. This chapter builds on such work by examining the influenza pandemic of 1918–20 through a gendered lens, revealing the ways in which the epidemic reaffirmed (and, very occasionally, altered) the roles and responsibilities assigned to men and women respectively in Montreal, Canada's early twentieth-century metropolis.

On the surface, the Montreal epidemic might appear to have been gender-neutral. Historians of other places have pointed out that, globally, more men than women died of influenza during the 1918–20 pandemic and suggest that this disparity was caused by the larger numbers of men present in the public sphere—as paid workers and as active members of the armed forces during the Great War—and thus at greater risk than women of exposure to the virus.[1] In Montreal, by contrast, men and women died in roughly equal numbers during these epidemics—perhaps because, in a metropolis such as Montreal, built in part on so-called light industry, unmarried women participated in paid labor in large numbers and were thus also at risk of contracting the virus.[2] Montreal women were also exposed to the virus because, as we shall see, they were the primary caregivers during the epidemic—although this was surely the case elsewhere as well. Nonetheless, despite mortality rates that differed little by sex, this epidemic, like others, had gendered dimensions and implications. The management of the epidemic drew on, and benefited from, well-established gendered roles and divisions of labor in Montreal. Moreover, the campaigns waged against influenza in 1918–20 both valorized and ultimately reinforced the gendered nature of such roles and responsibilities. This chapter begins by interrogating the gendered dimensions of caregiving during the epidemic. It then examines the obituaries of doctors, priests, and nuns felled by influenza and highlights the gendered qualities attributed to these caregivers who lost their lives during the epidemic. Finally, it explores some of the public health solutions proposed in the immediate wake of the epidemic and underlines the ways in which the suggestions of female middle-class reformers drew on women's particular experiences of the epidemic and differed slightly from those of medical, municipal, and religious authorities.

Inspired by the work of such social historians of medicine as Nancy Tomes, Nancy K. Bristow, Judith Leavitt, Naomi Rogers, and Esyllt Jones, this chapter draws on a wide variety of primary sources, including the records of the municipal, provincial, and federal governments; the papers of voluntary associations such as the Montreal Soldiers' Wives' League and the Fédération Nationale Saint-Jean-Baptiste (Saint John the Baptist National Federation); the archives of Montreal's Catholic archbishop and of the Sœurs Grises (Gray Nuns) of Montreal; and local and provincial medical and public health publications.[3]

Gendered Responses to Influenza

In October the Spanish Influenza took hold of Regalia [Montreal], so that no one could think of anything else. The influenza took hold—with a strangling sort of hold that squeezed the life out of the city. Regalia was not worse than other cities, of course: it was not so bad as some. But it was bad enough. The colds—the coughing and sneezing of September—turned by microscopic degrees into the influenza of October and then the plague went round invisibly, like a thief in the night, and laid its microbe on its victim; and if it laid it on *hard*—that victim died.[4]

In the space of six months, pandemic influenza killed 50,000 Canadians— roughly the same number as died in World War I. Of this total, 14,000 deaths took place in the province of Quebec. In Montreal in particular, between September 1918 and January 1919, almost 20,000 people fell ill with influenza and more than 3,600 died.[5] A second wave of influenza descended on the city in the winter of 1920. Less severe than the fall 1918 wave, it nonetheless affected 4,336 Montrealers between January and April and took the lives of 431 of them.[6]

In Montreal, as elsewhere in Canada, the global menace that was the influenza pandemic of 1918–20 met with largely local responses. No real countrywide public health infrastructure existed in Canada at this time—the federal Department of Health was not established until 1919, in part as a belated response to the epidemic.[7] The pandemic was thus lived to a considerable degree as a local event, even though the residents of these localities knew that they were linked to localities elsewhere and that the "virus" employed regular means of communication and transportation (ships, trains, mail lines), as they watched the epidemic approaching in newspaper headlines and in letters from friends and relatives elsewhere in Canada or in nearby New England.[8]

Montreal was at this time the metropolis of Canada; its medical and municipal authorities were attuned to public health developments in other North American and European cities.[9] Yet a study of the 1918–20 epidemics also reminds us of Montreal's idiosyncrasies—its particular linguistic and religious configuration, for instance, as a city housing French-speaking Catholics, English-speaking Protestants and Catholics, and a small but significant Jewish community. Montreal was also a transportation hub: a port city and a railway center, it was a receiving city for both rural migrants from the Quebec countryside and immigrants from overseas, as well as a way station for Canadians heading to the United States and for residents of the United States heading north. It was a commercial center and a key manufacturing city, with a well-established financial elite and an important industrial workforce. As in other industrial cities, Montreal's manufacturing districts were densely populated, its working-class neighborhoods characterized by crowded and sometimes dilapidated housing.[10] The large proportion of the population that was Catholic is important to this story. Not only did religious communities, male but especially female, provide much of the unpaid labor force during the epidemic—as nurses, home visitors, and stretcher-bearers—but the large number of Catholic institutional buildings (boarding schools, orphanages, hospitals, asylums) housing hundreds of people may have had implications for the rapid spread of influenza in the city and in the province more broadly.[11] Among the first cases of influenza in Quebec, for instance, were the young boys boarding at the Collège du Sacré-Cœur in Victoriaville. Finally, during the Great War, Montreal was a mobilized city, despite significant opposition in some quarters to military participation and particularly to conscription. This too may well have shaped the spread of the disease: among the first cases of influenza in the Montreal region were soldiers in the barracks at Saint-Jean-sur-Richelieu, not far from the city limits.[12]

Municipal authorities such as the Department of Health; the Board of Health (reconvened at the onset of the flu outbreak); and the Administrative Commission, an official body of short duration, established by the province in 1918 to better manage the municipality's finances, were on the frontlines of the war against influenza as demonstrated in the following poster:

CITÉ DE MONTRÉAL
SERVICE DE SANTÉ

EN GARDE
CONTRE LA GRIPPE ESPAGNOLE

Évitez les excès de toute sorte.
Toussez dans un mouchoir ou à l'abri de la main.
Ne parlez pas directement dans la figure des gens.
Gargarisez-vous trois ou quatre fois par jour avec la solution suivante qui
coûte très peu: eau bouillie, une pine; sel, deux cuillérées à thé; permanga-
nate de potasse, une demi-cuillérée à thé.
Ne vous servez ni du verre, ni de la pipe d'un autre.

SI VOUS ÊTES MALADE

Gardez la chambre.
Appelez le médecin.
Et continuez à faire tout ce qui est dit ci-dessus.[13]

They were directed, to some degree, by the Conseil d'Hygiène de la
Province de Québec (Public Health Council of the Province of Quebec),
the provincial body that established emergency regulations and attempted
to ensure that these were respected by the different municipalities. The
council also appears to have kept abreast of what scientific research was conducted during the epidemic.

To a certain degree, these state departments, particularly those at the municipal level, attempted to coordinate the work of physicians during the epidemic.
Medical doctors fought influenza in long-established local hospitals, including those originally founded to deal with contagious disease. They also worked
in the makeshift hospitals set up during the epidemic by the municipality: in
the Meurling Refuge, for instance, in orphanages and in the Catholic and
Protestant schools temporarily emptied of their regular clientele. Finally, doctors visited the ill in their homes—a site of many, perhaps most, of the ill—for,
as Montreal novelist J. G. Sime noted about the fall 1918 wave of the epidemic,
"it was impossible to move any of the sufferers into hospitals: the hospitals in
Regalia [Montreal] filled up, during the wave of the influenza, as if by magic,
and soon there was room for no fresh case."[14] Yet Montreal, like other North
American localities, confronted an urgent shortage of physicians during the epidemic. This shortage was due in part to the fact that doctors had volunteered or
been assigned to Canada's military infrastructure during the war.[15]

The role of nurses in combating influenza was thus almost certainly as
important as that of doctors: given that there existed in 1918–20 no known
preventative measures nor a surefire cure for influenza, basic components

of healthy living—bed rest, fresh air, sunshine—played just as important a role in the management of influenza as "modern" twentieth-century science and medicine. The importance of nurses was widely acknowledged during the epidemic. Two key organizations of lay nurses were active in Montreal during this medical crisis. The first was the Victorian Order of Nurses, a primarily English-speaking association of professional visiting nurses who, in the space of only five weeks, ministered to over 5,500 Montrealers—Catholic, Protestant, and Jewish—stricken with influenza.[16] The second was the French-speaking Gardes-Malades de Ville-Marie, similarly constituted of certified lay nurses. The contributions—indeed, the sacrifices—made by these lay visiting nurses were lauded with great enthusiasm by the daily press.[17] Yet lay nurses, like doctors, were in short supply during the epidemic: one bourgeois Montreal woman described them as "*affreusement rares*" (horribly rare).[18]

The majority of women with experience in nursing in Montreal, however, were the members of female religious communities such as the Sœurs Grises (Gray Nuns) and the Sœurs de la Providence (God's Nuns). During the epidemic, nuns ministered to patients—primarily, but not exclusively, Catholic—in the hospitals run by their own religious communities, in the city's emergency hospitals, and in the homes of the ill. Again, Montrealers were quick to acknowledge the selfless devotion of nursing sisters: Archbishop Paul Bruchési, for example, called attention to the "admirable conduct" of male and especially female religious communities during the epidemic.[19] Meanwhile, a number of Montrealers wrote to the editor of *Le Devoir*—a newspaper that catered to the city's French-speaking intelligentsia—to point out the devotion of various male and female religious communities: the Sœurs de la Providence, the Frères des Écoles Chrétiennes (Brothers of Christian Schools), the Sœurs Franciscaines (Franciscan Nuns), and the Missionnaires de l'Immaculée-Conception (Missionaries of the Immaculate Conception), all of whom, since the epidemic had begun, could be found at the bedsides of the poor and the ill.[20]

Alongside doctors and lay and religious nurses, a large number of volunteers—civic-minded or reform-minded citizens, Montrealers struck by the pathos and neediness of their neighbors—worked tirelessly to alleviate the worst effects of the epidemic. Many of these volunteers were women; some of them were activist women already engaged, in normal times, in various associations and causes. Idola Saint-Jean, for instance—a feminist, a university instructor, and a well-known social and political activist—ran an Emergency Bureau in downtown Montreal for influenza victims and their families. Her team of female volunteers dispatched doctors and nurses to those in need and provided these families with clothing and food.[21] Voluntary influenza work was aided by the fact that a large number of Montreal women were already mobilized by the Great War effort. Journalist Madeleine Huguenin

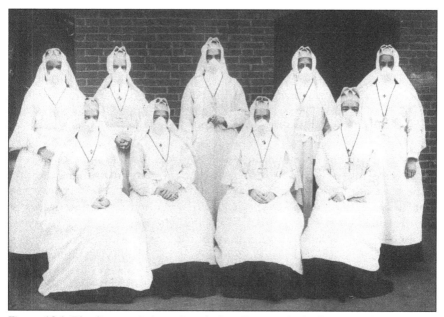

Figure 12.1. The Sœurs missionnaires du Bon-Pasteur de Québec providing care to victims of influenza in 1918. Image no. PH-D-22, 4-03, Archives des Soeurs du Bon-Pasteur de Québec (ABPQ). Reproduced with permission from the ABPQ.

put the efforts of the Dames de la Croix-Rouge Canadienne-Française (Ladies of the French-Canadian Red Cross) at the service of influenza victims; Helen Reid of the Canadian Patriotic Fund recruited nurses to care for the ill in the city's Protestant community; and the ladies of the Montreal Soldiers' Wives' League brought bed linens, clothing, food, and fuel to members of soldiers' families stricken with influenza.[22]

Not all influenza volunteers were women. "Flying squads" of policemen and firemen provided families in need with food and fuel, prepared meals, and lit stoves.[23] Likewise, male members of the clergy, particularly the Catholic clergy, were to be found at the bedside of the ill and the dying, administering the last rites but also acting as stretcher-bearers. Some of the work carried out by these men might well have been considered feminine in the early twentieth century; one might ask whether male members of the clergy, in particular, were a third gendered category, that of feminized men. Yet we might also see these male volunteers—the policemen and firemen in particular—as standing in for absent or ill husbands and sons. And as we shall see, the obituaries of priests felled by influenza for the most part described these members of the clergy in terms rather similar to those used to describe physicians struck down during the epidemic.

The efforts of doctors, lay nurses, nuns, religious brothers and priests, and volunteers of both sexes were thus essential to the battle against influenza. Yet it was the female family members of those stricken with influenza, particularly mothers, who found themselves on the veritable frontlines of this war.[24] As *La Bonne Parole*, the newspaper published by the Fédération Nationale Saint-Jean-Baptiste, the principal association of Catholic women in Montreal, noted, "The epidemic that has swooped down upon our country, and that has brought grief and death to so many families, requires every woman to redouble her zeal at home and to concentrate all her attention upon her domestic duties."[25] Many of these women, of course, were recipients of the aid furnished by other, mobilized, women, and one trope present in the sources is that of the "grateful mother," an archetype that historian Ellen Ross has shown was popular among visiting nurses in London during the same period.[26] One French-Catholic influenza victim, for instance, reportedly told the press that the visits of nuns were like the "good Lord who enters into our home."[27] An English-Protestant mother, for her part, wrote to thank the Montreal Soldiers' Wives' League for the food that it had sent her and asked for further provisions for the following week. Grateful though this mother no doubt was, she was clearly also resourceful and not above asking for help that she had good reason to think would be forthcoming.[28]

The fact that we have few records of the words of influenza victims reflects the unequal power relations between the women who participated in influenza relief work and the women who benefited from, and sometimes actively sought, their help.[29] Home visits were a long-established practice by the early twentieth century, in Montreal as elsewhere, and they inevitably involved a moralizing dimension; although, as historian Michelle Perrot remarks, "moralizing does not preclude compassion."[30] During the influenza epidemic, unequal social relations were compounded by the physical and emotional fragility of the ill and the dying.[31] Yet I would suggest that during a medical crisis such as this one, the moralizing dimension was perhaps less present than in normal times, particularly since cases of influenza were so numerous and widespread. Although the poorer districts of the city appear to have been hardest hit by the epidemic, the poor were not the only Montrealers to contract influenza.[32]

Not all Montreal women benefited from the extensive influenza relief campaign. It appears that single women boarding in rooming houses were particularly liable to be forgotten by home visitors—or perhaps particularly unlikely to seek out help.[33] Moreover, neighbors could not always be counted on to lend a hand. One family of Russian immigrants, for instance, in which the father and three children were ill, appealed in vain to their neighbors for assistance: the latter refused to help for fear of contracting the disease.[34] While in this case, neighbors' reluctance may have been exacerbated by xenophobia, several examples suggest that French-Canadian and English-Canadian Montrealers also had little contact with their neighbors during the epidemic.[35]

The influenza labor force was thus divided between professional workers (doctors, nurses) and volunteers, and between laypersons and members of the clergy. These distinctions did not fall neatly along gender lines, but they were gendered nonetheless. Women—religious nursing sisters, lay nurses with professional training, social reformers long concerned with public health in Montreal, and civic-minded volunteers motivated to act by the extent of the misery that they saw around them during the epidemic—made up a very large proportion of the influenza labor force. This was seen as fitting—indeed, as only natural—for care of the ill and the weak had long been viewed as women's domain. That it was seen to be natural did not mean that it went unremarked: on November 4, 1918, roughly five weeks after the first appearance of epidemic influenza in Montreal, a journalist writing for *La Patrie* (a daily newspaper aimed at the French-speaking popular classes), for instance, commented admiringly that "the part that women have played in the battle against the influenza epidemic will probably never be entirely known. Every day, we discover new examples of [their] devotion."[36] This appreciation for women's devoted efforts during Montreal's flu epidemic appears to contrast with what historian Lorraine O'Donnell has found for Toronto's 1937 polio epidemic, during which, she argues, women's caregiving—both the paid labor of nurses and the unpaid work of mothers—received little recognition. According to O'Donnell, time-intensive and labor-intensive "ways of caring tended to fall to the lot of mothers and nurses; there was a gender dimension to the distribution of prestige and power in the medical care given during the epidemic, and women received little of either."[37] The public appreciation of women's caregiving expressed during Montreal's flu epidemic, however, largely neglected the daily and exhausting efforts of ordinary mothers and tended to focus on the more public devotion of nurses, nuns, and Ladies Bountiful. For a sense of the more private work of mothers and wives, we need to turn to more private kinds of records. In her diary, for instance, Lady Lacoste (Marie-Louise Globensky) recounted the travails of her daughter Jeanne, whose seven children were ill with influenza in October 1918: "*Leur grippe est légère mais tout de meme il faut donner beaucoup de soins, c'est une tâche fatigante pour la mère*" (Their flu isn't serious, but it still requires a lot of care; it's a tiring task for the mother), commented Lacoste on October 15. The next day, writing of the heavy work involved in disinfecting sick children's bedrooms, Lacoste noted, "*Pauvre Jeanne a les bras pleins*" (Poor Jeanne has her arms full).[38]

Gender and Discourses of Heroism

Canadian historian Esyllt Jones has analyzed the discourse of what she calls "feminine heroism" during the influenza epidemic in Winnipeg.[39] We might add to Jones's astute analysis the fact that there also existed a discourse of "masculine heroism" during the epidemic. Yet these two discourses were not identical. An examination of the obituaries of doctors, priests, and nursing sisters published during and shortly after the epidemic reveals the gendered qualities attributed to these medical professionals and spiritual advisers.[40] This observation echoes, to some degree, what Nancy K. Bristow has discovered for the American context. Although Bristow claims that much of the praise lavished by citizens on doctors and nurses during the epidemic was "gender-neutral, heralding heroic qualities shared by doctors and nurses alike," she notes that "while both men and women were heroes, in many accounts the nature of their heroism, as described by their contemporaries, proved gender-specific."[41]

The obituaries of Montreal doctors, priests, and nuns who died after contracting influenza "*au chevet des malades*" (at the bedside of the ill) portrayed all of these caregivers and spiritual advisers, male and female, as heroic, and as "*victimes du devoir*" (victims of duty) and "*victimes de leur dévouement*" (victims of their devotion).[42] More intimate sources used the same language: Lady Lacoste (Marie-Louise Globensky), for instance, wrote in her diary of the death from influenza of Dr. Jules Frémont, the brother of her son-in-law. Noting that Frémont had contracted the flu while treating four sick members of a poor family, Lacoste eulogized, "*Il succombe en vaillant combattant, victime de son devoir*" (He succumbs as a valiant combatant, a victim of duty) and, elsewhere in her diary, reiterated her opinion that Frémont was a "*victime de son dévouement.*"[43] But it is nonetheless possible to discern gendered differences in these descriptions. Doctors felled by the epidemic were lauded for their devotion but also for their skill, expertise, intellectual curiosity, good judgment, hard work, energy, and vigor. Their studies and career paths were described in detail. They were hailed as members of a fraternity of medical professionals, as men who had excelled in their studies and their chosen profession and, often, as men who had worked hard but also played hard: doctors who met death during the epidemic were described, variously, as a "big eater and big smoker" or as a "lively companion" and lauded for their sense of (masculine) camaraderie.[44] Descriptions of their energy and vigor were all the more common given that these doctors, like other victims of the epidemic, were often felled in the prime of their life, in their thirties or early forties. The abbé Élie-J. Auclair, editor of Montreal's *La Semaine Religieuse*, insisted on the youth of the victims, lamenting the fact that "young priest-professors, with the future ahead of them," and doctors, "also young, and already very well-known," were struck down "in the prime of their youth, full of strength, in the prime of their life."[45] Dr. Joseph Gauvreau, writing in *L'Union Médicale du Canada*, likewise noted, "Among our doctors who have died on the job, during this flu epidemic, what is striking is the vigor they all shared, the uniformity of their age, the appearance of their barely matured youth."[46]

Priests, too, were among the influenza victims. As Franco-American Ellen Drouin, writing to her daughter in Montreal during the influenza epidemic, noted, "They have lost a good many priest and Brothers in Canada."[47] Perhaps surprisingly, differences between descriptions of deceased physicians and those of deceased priests were, all things considered, minimal. Priests were praised for their devotion and their ability as well, and their studies and career paths were also described in detail. The obituary of the abbé Joseph-Antoine Messier, for instance, noted that he died after two months of devotion at the bedside of influenza victims and insisted on his "lively and penetrating intelligence."[48] The abbé Bruno-Adrien Joubert, who died in December 1918 of the flu, was described by the abbé Élie-J Auclair as someone who was young and who "loved life, enjoyed his ministry and gave himself to it without stinting."[49] Father Wilfrid Valiquette was described as "*tendre et dévoué*" (tender and devoted)—qualities perhaps more feminine than those generally used to describe doctors.[50]

On rare occasions, the obituaries of nuns resembled those of priests or even doctors, in that the emphasis was placed on the vocation—indeed, on the career path. The obituary of a Gray Nun identified simply as "*la sœur Rodier*," for instance, stressed her artistic and musical talents.[51] In general, however, descriptions of nursing sisters who died in the line of duty during the epidemic emphasized their caregiving, eminently feminine qualities. Nuns were said to be victims of their charity as well as of their devotion.[52] The daily press pointed out their bravery and good works, lauding "*l'admirable dévouement des religieuses*" (the admirable devotion of the nuns) and their "*zèle incomparable*" (incomparable zeal) and remarking that the admirable actions of nuns were not rare; rather, Montrealers had long been accustomed to nuns' acts of heroism.[53] Religious communities sometimes adopted the rhetoric of heroism themselves. The annalist of the Gray Nuns, for instance, insisted on the heroic devotion of the nuns in her community, on the "*heureuses héroïnes*" (happy heroines).[54] She compared these nuns to "*d'intrépides soldats, qui tressaillent en entendant résonner le clairon, [et] répondent à l'appel*" (fearless soldiers, who thrill with joy upon hearing the sound of the bugle and respond to the call).[55] Evidently, this rhetoric of heroism carried particular weight in the context of the Great War—a context in which devotion, duty, self-sacrifice, and death were glorified as patriotic.[56] The numerous influenza deaths that occurred among nuns were seen as deaths on a feminine battlefield, on the home front rather than in Europe. The Gray Nuns annalist described two nuns, ill with influenza, who were "laid out calmly upon their beds of pain, like the soldier who rests after a day of battle."[57]

One might argue that in comparing nuns to soldiers, observers were masculinizing them—a phenomenon parallel, perhaps, to the feminization of male clergy who attended to the ill at their bedside. The heroism of these nursing sisters did resemble that of soldiers, in that it appeared to consist of bravery, sacrifice, and even physical strength. Yet in other ways it was a typically "feminine" heroism, in that it was perfectly compatible with the maternal role attributed to women, even those who were not themselves biological mothers. The kinds of deeds and gestures lauded and legitimated by this rhetoric of heroism were not, in fact, that different from the expectations made of women in ordinary times at the dawn of the twentieth century.

Nancy K. Bristow, in her interesting analysis of the gendered expectations surrounding the work of doctors and nurses respectively during the influenza epidemic in the United States, notes that the epidemic could be seen as a defeat for physicians. Their failure to either prevent or cure influenza was a devastating blow to their self-confidence and, more generally, to the masculine authority associated with medical science. American nurses, on the other hand, tended to reflect positively on their experiences during the epidemic, during which they "found in their work confirmation as women and as nurses." Unlike (male) doctors, of whom one expected mastery—indeed, victory—over the microbe, (female) nurses were expected "to demonstrate qualities of selflessness and compassion as they nurtured and cared for, rather than cured, their patients."[58] Bristow's analysis raises interesting questions for the Montreal case. Although, as we have seen, the obituaries of doctors, priests, and nuns alike lauded the devotion of these caregivers to the ill and the dying, it is quite clear that the professional devotion of physicians, so highly praised, was not particularly effective, in the sense that many of their patients died nonetheless. The fact that medical men were largely powerless to treat or cure victims of influenza must surely have been a blow to their sense of masculine expertise and mastery over disease.

Women Propose Solutions in the Wake of the Epidemic

The two waves of influenza experienced by Montrealers in 1918 and 1920 provided the opportunity for public reflection on the health of the population, and some of these reflections were explicitly gendered. In particular, among the myriad suggestions made during and immediately after the epidemic were proposals that built on women's specific experiences of the epidemic and the knowledge that they had acquired during this medical crisis. This local, concrete knowledge is perhaps what historian Maureen Flanagan meant when she alluded to "a women's vision of the city"—a vision that was not innate but, rather, conceived in and nourished by what reform-minded women experienced and witnessed during the epidemic.[59]

We know of one apparently ordinary woman who, in the throes of the influenza epidemic, wrote to city hall to criticize Montreal's everyday insalubrities and to call for greater intervention on the part of the Board of Health. She was an exception: almost all of the other letters written to municipal authorities about the epidemic that I have found appear to have been written by men. She was an exception also in that she wrote anonymously, signing her letter simply "Hygiène Générale." This was one of only two anonymous letters concerning the epidemic that I have found in the municipal archives. The pronouns used by "Hygiène Générale" suggest that she was a woman, as do the author's lengthy discussions of candy shops, butchers' stalls, and grocery stores.[60] This anonymous, no doubt "ordinary" woman thus drew on her feminine experience and knowledge of the city to make public health recommendations for the future.

Most of the Montreal women in contact with municipal authorities during and immediately after the epidemic, however, were organized, bourgeois women, active in social and urban reform long before the arrival of influenza. Women such as Idola Saint-Jean, responsible for the French-language section of the Uptown Emergency Health Bureau, and her Anglophone counterpart Anna S. Lyman, responsible for the English-language section of the same emergency bureau, relayed to municipal authorities and to the local press accounts of what they and their assistants had witnessed during the epidemic: dire poverty, dilapidated housing, barely or shabbily furnished homes, and several members of the same family ill, bedridden, and without assistance of any kind.[61] Many of these problems, of course, predated the epidemic.[62] But the home visits conducted during the epidemic and the attention accorded public health matters by medical and municipal authorities, as well as by the press, brought such long-standing matters to the forefront of public attention. Small wonder, then, that the solutions advocated by reform-minded women in the wake of the epidemic appeared remarkably familiar: laundered clothing, cleaner and better housing, the razing of slums, and the eradication of seedy back alleys.[63] It seems to have been difficult for these activist women to separate the strictly medical aspects of the influenza experience from the larger question of poor living conditions. Such a blurring of the two problems was no doubt exacerbated by the fact that strictly medical solutions to the influenza epidemic were in visibly short supply.

Gender on the Influenza Battlefield

A gendered analysis of Montreal's experience of the 1918–20 influenza pandemic enables us to understand who cared for the ill and in what capacity;

how this caregiving was received, perceived, and acknowledged; and what kinds of lessons were drawn from this medical crisis. Given the relative helplessness of medical professionals facing the influenza virus and the lack of solutions provided by modern science, basic measures of care—fresh air and sunlight but also rest, nourishment, and clean and decent clothing and bedding—were essential. During the epidemic, as prior to the epidemic, such basic measures of care were often provided by women: the women of families afflicted by the flu, to begin with, but also volunteers, lay nurses, and Catholic nuns. To some degree, then, influenza relief efforts put to use and even valorized local and intimate knowledge, acquired on the ground through years of housewifery, mothering, and other forms of care gendered feminine rather than modern scientific and medical innovations. Likewise, the solutions advocated by reform-minded women in the wake of the epidemic were relatively basic proposals for improving housing and living conditions. While this local knowledge or experience was not exclusively feminine, much of it was in effect transmitted and put into practice by women. A gendered analysis also helps us to understand the place of men in the campaign against influenza, along with discourses of masculine heroism that had little to do with the Great War that constituted the backdrop to the epidemic. Sharing the terrain with female nurses, nuns, and volunteers were doctors, priests, even firemen and policemen. Always lauded for their devotion and their loyalty, and sometimes for their vigor, both intellectual and physical, these were the male (and almost always masculine) heroes on the influenza battlefield.

Notes

An earlier version of this chapter was published, in French, as "'Elles sont partout . . .': Les femmes et la ville en temps d'épidémie, Montréal, 1918–1920," *Revue d'Histoire de l'Amérique Française* 58, no. 1 (2004): 67–85. My thanks to the *Revue d'Histoire de l'Amérique Française* for giving me permission to republish this piece here. I would also like to thank my very competent research assistant, Valérie Poirier, as well as Sophie Doucet, who pointed me to Lady Lacoste's diary. Final thanks go to the Université du Québec à Montréal's PAFARC and to the Fonds Québécois de la Recherche Sur la Société et la Culture for the generous funding they provided in the form of two important research grants.

1. Andrew Noymer and Michel Garenne, "Long-Term Effects of the 1918 'Spanish' Influenza Epidemic on Sex Differentials of Mortality in the USA: Exploratory Findings from Historical Data," in *The Spanish Influenza Pandemic of 1918–19: New Perspectives*, ed. Howard Phillips and David Killingray (New York: Routledge, 2003), 202–17; Peter Tuckel, Sharon Sasler, Richard Maisel, and Andrew Leykam, "The Diffusion of the Influenza Pandemic of 1918 in Hartford, Connecticut," *Social Science History* 30, no. 2 (2006): 170–71.

2. Francis Dubois, Jean-Pierre Thouez, and Denis Goulet, "A Geographical Analysis of the Spread of Spanish Influenza in Quebec, 1918–1920," in *Epidemic*

Encounters: Influenza, Society, and Culture in Canada, 1918–20, ed. Magda Fahrni and Esyllt Jones (Vancouver: University of British Columbia Press, 2012), 145–46.

3. Nancy Tomes, *The Gospel of Germs: Men, Women, and the Microbe in American Life* (Cambridge, MA: Harvard University Press, 1998); Nancy K. Bristow, "'You Can't Do Anything for Influenza': Doctors, Nurses and the Power of Gender during the Influenza Pandemic in the United States," in Phillips and Killingray, *Spanish Influenza Pandemic*, 58–70; Judith Walzer Leavitt, *Typhoid Mary: Captive to the Public's Health* (Boston: Beacon, 1996); Naomi Rogers, "Germs with Legs: Flies, Disease, and the New Public Health," *Bulletin of the History of Medicine* 63 (1989): 599–617; Esyllt W. Jones, *Influenza 1918: Disease, Death, and Struggle in Winnipeg* (Toronto: University of Toronto Press, 2007).

4. J. G. Sime, *Our Little Life: A Novel of To-Day* (New York: Stokes, 1921), 345; italics in the original.

5. Between September 23, 1918, and January 27, 1919, there were 19,399 cases of influenza and 3,639 deaths related to influenza reported in Montreal. Séraphin Boucher, director, Department of Health, to Charles A. Hodgetts, MD, medical adviser, Commission of Conservation, February 12, 1919, Ottawa, VM1, S3, D5241, Conseil de Ville, Archives de la Ville de Montréal (hereafter AVM), 1, 2. Elsewhere, the municipal government reduced its estimate of the total number of cases to 19,299. The 3,639 deaths thus constituted 18.85 percent of those taken ill with the disease. Cité de Montréal, "L'épidémie d'influenza," *Bulletin d'Hygiène* 5, nos. 1–6 (1919): 2.

6. Doctor Séraphin Boucher, *Rapport du Service de Santé de la Cité de Montréal 1920* (Montréal: Pigeon, 1921), 23.

7. Janice P. Dickin McGinnis, "The Impact of Epidemic Influenza: Canada, 1918–1919," *Historical Papers* 12, no. 1 (1977): 120–40.

8. Although a few physicians attributed the epidemic to a "virus," the workings of the influenza virus were not fully understood until the 1930s. Most contemporary observers spoke of the influenza "bacillus." According to the *Canadian Municipal Journal*, "In very few cases were the local public health departments prepared though there was plenty of notice given, for before it reached Canada the Spanish 'flu' had almost travelled the world." *Canadian Municipal Journal* 14, no. 11 (November 1918): 362. In chapter 2 of this volume, Bertucci deals extensively with the problem of identifying the specific agent of the flu pandemic and the debates among physicians in Brazil.

9. On "inter-city cooperation in matters of disease control" in an earlier period, see John B. Osborne, "Preparing for the Pandemic: City Boards of Health and the Arrival of Cholera in Montreal, New York, and Philadelphia in 1832," *Urban History Review / Revue d'Histoire Urbaine* 36, no. 2 (2008): 29–42.

10. Terry Copp, *The Anatomy of Poverty: The Condition of the Working Class in Montreal, 1897–1929* (Toronto: McClelland and Stewart, 1974); Bettina Bradbury, *Working Families: Age, Gender, and Daily Survival in Industrializing Montreal* (Toronto: McClelland and Stewart, 1993). On these same conditions in Alicante, Spain, see chapter 11 of this volume.

11. Sobral, Lima, and Silveira e Sousa (chapter 4) and Cruz de Souza (chapter 7) show similar reactions in, respectively, Portugal and Brazil.

12. As noted by Porras-Gallo in chapter 5 of this volume, the first cases of influenza were also soldiers in Spain.

13. Poster, fonds VM 1, S3, D5241-01, Archives de la Ville de Montréal (AVM). Reproduced with permission from the AVM.

14. Sime, *Our Little Life*, 348.

15. Elzéar Pelletier to Monsieur J. S. Croteau, Conseil Local d'Hygiène, Lake Weedon, P. O. St. Gérard, October 23, 1918, contenant 15, registre 84; Elzéar Pelletier to Monsieur A. G. Godbout, Risborough and Marion Marlow, P. O. St. Ludger, October 29, 1918, contenant 16, registre 88; E.-M. G. Savard, Inspecteur en Chef, contenant 16, registre 88; Circulaire à MM, Inspecteurs Régionaux, February 11, 1920, all in Fonds du Conseil d'Hygiène de la Province de Québec, E88, Archives Nationales du Québec à Québec. See also "Doctors Are Victims," *Montreal Herald and Daily Telegraph*, October 10, 1918; and "L'épidémie de grippe espagnole," *La Patrie*, October 1, 1918. On shortages of doctors and nurses in other Canadian locales during the influenza epidemic, see Jones, *Influenza 1918*, 67; Bristow, "You Can't Do Anything," 58.

16. Minute book, Board of Management, February 1919–January 1923, VON for Canada, Local Association of Greater Montreal; Minutes, Twenty-First Annual General Meeting of the Local Association of Greater Montreal, March 14, 1919, VON for Canada, both in Archives of the Victorian Order of Nurses, Montreal.

17. "La lutte contre le mal fait naître de beaux dévouements," *La Patrie*, October 17, 1918.

18. Journal de Lady Lacoste (Marie-Louise Globensky), October 19, 1918, P155, S8, SS2, D1, Fonds Famille Landry, Archives Nationales du Québec à Montréal (hereafter ANQM). See also entry for October 17, 1918.

19. "Lettre de Mgr L'Archevêque de Montréal aux communautés religieuses de son diocèse sur leur conduite admirable durant l'épidémie, 23 décembre 1918," *La Semaine Religieuse de Montréal*, 72, no. 27 (1918): 418–22.

20. "Les Sœurs de la Providence," *Le Devoir*, October 18, 1918; "Hommage au dévouement," *Le Devoir*, October 30, 1918; "Hommage," *Le Devoir*, November 4, 1918; "Une page sur l'épidémie," *Le Devoir*, November 12, 1918.

21. "L'épidémie et la part des dames," *La Patrie*, October 30, 1918.

22. "La situation reste la même," *La Patrie*, October 17, 1918; Montreal Soldiers' Wives' League, *Annual Report of the Montreal Soldiers' Wives' League, 1918*, vol. 2, file 30, MG 28 I 311, National Archives of Canada. The Red Cross was also a key institution during the pandemic in Portugal and Brazil, as noted by Nunes (chapter 3), Bertucci (chapter 2), and Cruz de Souza (chapter 7).

23. "Le Bureau d'urgence," *Le Devoir*, October 21, 1918, 1; "Pour enrayer le fléau plus efficacement," *Le Devoir*, October 21, 1918, 3; "Lutte sans relâche," *La Patrie*, October 21, 1918, 3.

24. This was all the more the case since municipal and medical authorities advised against visits from extended family members during the epidemic. "More Stringent Rules to Curb 'Flu Epidemic," *Montreal Daily Star*, October 10, 1918; "Extreme Cases Are Reported by Host of Workers," *Montreal Daily Star*, October 21, 1918.

25. "L'épidémie qui s'est abattue sur notre pays, et qui sème la désolation et la mort dans tant de familles, oblige chaque femme à redoubler de zèle au foyer et à concentrer toute son attention sur ses devoirs domestiques." "Chronique des Œuvres," *La Bonne Parole*, October 1918, 3.

26. Ellen Ross, *Love and Toil: Motherhood in Outcast London, 1870–1918* (New York: Oxford University Press, 1993), 174; Jessica M. Robbins, "Class Struggles in the Tubercular World: Nurses, Patients, and Physicians, 1903–1915," *Bulletin of the History of Medicine*, 71, no. 3 (1997): 427. Dr. Séraphin Boucher, director of the city's Department of Health, noted in 1921 about visiting nurses: "On me rapporte qu'en général, les mères de famille écoutent volontiers l'enseignement qui leur est donné" (It was reported to me that, in general, mothers of families listen willingly to the education given them"). Dr. Séraphin Boucher, *Bulletin Sanitaire* 21, no. 4 (1921): 1. See also *Bulletin Sanitaire*, 3e trimestre de 1919, 19.

27. "Bon Dieu qui pénètre chez nous." "La lutte contre le mal fait naître de beaux dévouements," *La Patrie*, October 17, 1918, 10.

28. Montreal Soldiers' Wives' League, "Report of the Hon. Corresponding Secretary and of the Office Work," in *Annual Report*.

29. On the scarcity of firsthand accounts of influenza victims, see chapter 13, where Belling deals with the case of Katherine Anne Porter.

30. "La moralisation n'exclut pas la compassion." Michelle Perrot, *Les femmes ou les silences de l'histoire* (Paris: Flammarion, 1998), 230.

31. On the "unequal power relations" between middle-class women and poor flu victims, see Jones, "Contact across a Diseased Boundary: Urban Space and Social Interaction during Winnipeg's Influenza Epidemic, 1918–1919," *Journal of the Canadian Historical Association*, n.s., 13 (2002): 137. See also Robbins, "Class Struggles," 423.

32. "Pour les orphelins," *Le Devoir*, October 22, 1918; "Moins de nouveaux cas," *La Patrie*, October 19, 1918; Journal de Lady Lacoste (Marie-Louise Globensky), entries from September 27–November 10, 1918, P155, S8, SS2, D1, ANQM. Bernabeu-Mestre and Pascual Artiaga also point out in chapter 11 that the poorest districts of the city of Alicante, Spain, were hardest hit by the epidemic. As noted by Sobral, Lima, and Silveira e Sousa in chapter 4, the Portuguese experience was similar to the Canadian one.

33. "Many Answered Urgent Appeal to Help Nurses," *Montreal Daily Star*, October 10, 1918; "Everyone Helps to Fight Disease," *Montreal Daily Star*, October 23, 1918.

34. "Le nombre des cas nouveaux diminue sensiblement," *Le Devoir*, October 18, 1918. Both chapters 6 and 7 of this volume treat the effects of the fear of becoming ill in Brazil.

35. "La lutte contre le fléau se poursuit et le dévouement ne fait pas défaut," *La Presse*, October 16, 1918; "Extreme Cases Are Reported"; "Relief Bodies Report General Improvement Now," *Montreal Daily Star*, October 31, 1918. The *Star's* example of a woman killed by influenza after having cared for a neighbor suggests not only that some neighbors were more generous than others but also that the others had good reason to be wary. "Bad Housing is Portion of Poor," *Montreal Daily Star*, November 2, 1918. Counterexamples, however, are provided in J. G. Sime's novel *Our Little Life*, set in Montreal during the epidemic and published in 1921. In the novel some Montreal women nurse their neighbors during the epidemic apparently without a second thought. See pages 347–48, 371, 374, and 388. Also see chapters 3 and 9 of the present volume for other examples of the increased prevalence of national identity and the role of national borders during the pandemic.

36. "La part que les femmes ont prise dans la lutte contre l'épidémie d'influenza ne sera probablement jamais entièrement connue. Chaque jour, on découvre encore de nouveaux dévouements." "L'admirable dévouement des femmes," *La Patrie*, November 4, 1918.

37. Lorraine O'Donnell, "A 'Dread Disease': The 1937 Polio Epidemic in Toronto" (major research paper, York University, 1989), 52.

38. Journal de Lady Lacoste (Marie-Louise Globensky), October 15 and 16, 1918, P155, S8, SS2, D1, ANQM.

39. Jones, "Diseased Boundary."

40. Sime, *Our Little Life*, 348.

41. Bristow, "You Can't Do Anything," 65.

42. L.-J.-A. Derome, *Le Canada Ecclésiastique: Almanach annuaire du clergé canadien; Pour l'année 1919* (Montreal: Librairie Beauchemin, 1919), 14–15, 18–19; "L'épidémie d'influenza: Dix religieuses ont succombé," *La Patrie*, November 19, 1918, 5.

43. Journal de Lady Lacoste (Marie-Louise Globensky), October 12 and 21, 1918, P155, S8, SS2, D1, ANQM.

44. "Gros mangeur et grand fumeur"; "Un gai compagnon." See the obituaries of doctors published in *L'Union médicale du Canada* 47, no. 11 (1918): 526–34.

45. "Jeunes prêtres-professeurs, pleins d'avenir"; "Jeunes aussi, et de haute notoriété déjà"; "En pleine jeunesse, en pleine force, en pleine vie." Élie-J. Auclair, "Le dimanche, 13 octobre 1918," *La Semaine Religieuse* 72, no. 17 (1918): 259–60.

46. "Chez nos médecins morts au poste, durant cette épidémie de grippe, ce qui frappe c'est la vigueur commune, l'uniformité de l'âge, la physionomie de leur jeunesse à peine mûrie." Joseph Gauvreau, "Bulletin: La leçon de nos morts," *L'Union Médicale du Canada* 47, no. 11 (1918): 523.

47. Ellen Drouin to Alma Drouin, September 30, 1918, Alma Drouin Collection. Private Collection, West Lafayette, Indiana.

48. "Intelligence vive et pénétrante." Les Cloches de Saint Boniface, "M. L'Abbé J.-A. Messier: Aumônier de l'Hôpital de Saint-Boniface," *La Semaine Religieuse* 73, no. 7 (1919): 104.

49. "Aimait la vie, se plaisait à son actif ministère et s'y dépensait sans compter." L'Abbé Elie-J. Anclair, "L'Abbé Adrien Joubert," *La Semaine Religieuse* 73, no. 1 (1919): 10–15. On the "zeal" of religious brothers and priests, see, for example, L'Abbé Elie-J. Anclair, "L'Abbé Henri Charlebois," *La Semaine Religieuse* 72, no. 26 (1918): 412–13.

50. "Le Père Wilfrid Valiquette," *La Semaine Religieuse de Montréal* 72, no. 24 (1918): 376–80.

51. "Chez les Sœurs Grises de la rue Guy," *La Semaine Religieuse de Montréal* 72, no. 21 (1918): 331–34.

52. "Mort d'une religieuse," *La Patrie*, November 16, 1918.

53. "L'admirable dévouement des religieuses," *La Patrie*, October 28, 1918.

54. Annales des Sœurs de la Charité (Sœurs Grises) de l'Hôpital Général de Montréal destinées aux maisons de l'Institut, October 16 and 17, 1918, vol. 15, 1917–18, Archives des Sœurs Grises de Montréal.

55. "L'Influenza ou Grippe Espagnole, en 1918," Dossier: Épidémies, Grippe Espagnole, 1918, 1920, Archives des Sœurs Grises de Montréal.

56. Philippe Ariès, *Essais sur l'histoire de la mort en Occident* (Paris: Seuil, 1975), 61. On the masculine heroism promoted in Canada before and during the Great War, see Mark Moss, *Manliness and Militarism: Educating Young Boys in Ontario for War* (Toronto: Oxford University Press, 2001); and Paul Maroney, "'The Great Adventure': The Context and Ideology of Recruiting in Ontario, 1914–17," *Canadian Historical Review*, 77, no. 1 (1996): 95–96.

57. "Étendues tranquillement sur leur lit de douleur, comme le soldat qui se repose après la journée du combat," November 18, 1918, Annales des Sœurs de la Charité (Sœurs Grises) de l'Hôpital Général de Montréal, vol. 15, 1917–18, Archives des Sœurs Grises de Montréal.

58. Bristow, "'You Can't Do Anything," 58, 69.

59. Maureen Flanagan, *Seeing with Their Hearts: Chicago Women and the Vision of the Good City, 1871–1933* (Princeton: Princeton University Press, 2002), 5.

60. "Hygiène Générale" à Messieurs les membres du Bureau d'Hygiène, October 14, 1918, Montréal, VM 1, S 3, D 5241-02, Fonds du Conseil de Ville, AVM.

61. "L'admirable dévouement des religieuses," 8; "Les taudis," *Le Devoir*, April 22, 1919, 1.

62. Copp, *Anatomy of Poverty*.

63. Procès-verbal, Bureau de Santé, October 24, 1918, Montréal, VM 21, S 2, D 12, AVM; Idola Saint-Jean à Monsieur le Président et aux Membres du Bureau de Santé, November 16, 1918, VM1, S3, D5241-02, Fonds du Conseil de Ville, AVM; Anna S. Lyman, Report of the Uptown Emergency Health Bureau, English Section, November 18, 1918, VM1, S3, D5241, Fonds du Conseil de Ville, AVM, 4.

Chapter Thirteen

Remembering and Reconstructing

Fictions of the 1918–19 Influenza Pandemic

CATHERINE BELLING

Anguish verged on overwhelming the very medium that carried it, perhaps causing the air to bleed black ash or gray dust.

—Myla Goldberg, *Wickett's Remedy*

A single death is a tragedy; a million deaths is a statistic.

—Attributed to Josef Stalin

Narrative is the medium that must carry and communicate the burden of
past suffering. In Myla Goldberg's historical novel, a Boston family learns in
the fall of 1918 that the eldest son has died of influenza in the army. Lydia,
his sister, is walking home from the hospital—where she has just learned
of her little nephew's death from the flu—when from the street she hears
the terrible sound of her family's grieving. She knows it is being replicated
throughout the city and imagines that the air itself must be damaged by the
weight of so much pain. She imagines the air bleeding ash, or dust, the fall-
out not of a single damaged body but of a kind of holocaust.[1]

A profound cultural and ethical implication of major epidemics is the
loss of access to personal narratives. When the collective replaces the individual as protagonist, and the health of the public takes precedence over
that of the individual, the resulting reductionism elides the particular and
the subjective. As Stalin is said to have observed (and the irony of this attri-
bution is apt), there is a paradox in the multiplication of personal catastrophe throughout a society, where the moral and emotional significance of
an event is in inverse proportion to its extent or its incidence. The human
imagination can inhabit the meaning of a single human calamity; multiply it
across an entire population and the mind is overwhelmed. A million deaths,
let alone the fifty or a hundred million caused by the pandemic, cannot be

recounted as a meaningful story; they can only be counted, reduced to statistics, and trusted to speak for themselves—and they can speak only by reducing the particulars of suffering to intangible abstractions.[2]

It makes sense that individual, embodied, deeply subjective representations of the pandemic, and particularly of the disease's felt effects on the lived bodies of the infected, would be missing, overshadowed by the enormity of global social disruption. The excess of this compounded suffering verges on the absurd; the hyperbolic writing it demands is an affront to writerly decorum. Either one must tell a small fraction of the story, by implication diminishing the whole, or one must attempt to take it all on and find that language itself cannot carry the burden. Historians revert to statistics, while literary writers may be inclined to find a different story to tell. There is a dearth of literary representations (fictional or autobiographical) of the 1918–19 pandemic by those who were there, especially compared to the wealth of literature that emerged from World War I.[3]

In this chapter I examine some of the few literary representations of the Spanish flu pandemic to have been published in English, showing that fiction can go some way to enhancing our ability to imagine the pandemic as the sum of multiple richly felt and suffered experiences by particular individuals. At the same time, however, the accounts that exist, one based on the author's own illness in 1918 and others extrapolating from historical records, reveal a second challenge to imagining what the pandemic was like: it seems that the experience of suffering from the flu was, in part because of the mental effects of the virus, oddly resistant to being remembered and described. Not only did the statistical enormity of the pandemic challenge the medium of narrative, but so too did the nature of the influenza itself.

My expectation when I began work on this chapter was to find that fiction about the pandemic might work as an antidote to the odd collective amnesia that, throughout the twentieth century, characterized our apprehension of it. What I have found instead is that the fiction tends to replicate, albeit in microcosm, the pandemic's resistance to subjective articulation by those who lived through it.

My discussion begins by showing how this resistance is captured in two distinctly different texts, the historical play *1918*, written in the 1980s by the American dramatist Horton Foote, and a fictional history of a futuristic avian flu pandemic, set in 2012, by Canadian journalist Craig DiLouie. Their generic differences highlight what they share: a sense of the incommunicability of the individual's experience of being infected with influenza during a pandemic and a strategic effort by the author to overcome this challenge. I then discuss the only literary account of the 1918 pandemic by a writer who actually contracted the disease herself: *Pale Horse, Pale Rider*, by the American journalist and novelist Katherine Anne Porter. This author's use of modernist stream of consciousness to convey the effects of the disease points both to the difficulty of recounting the experience in conventional, nonliterary discourse and to her influence on the last two books I examine, both of which were published in 2006, at the height of current public discussion of an anticipated avian flu pandemic. These novels are by two contemporary American writers of literary fiction: Thomas Mullen's *The Last Town on Earth* and Myla Goldberg's *Wickett's Remedy* are the result of deliberate efforts by their authors, working in a period of renewed interest in the pandemic, to restore individuals' experience of the flu to public discourse, albeit in the form of fiction. These accounts explicitly incorporate the pandemic's challenge to memory, the threat its statistical immensity poses to the telling of stories. In its inadequate struggle to contain and express the experience of the influenza, the discourse of literary fiction carries traces, the ash and dust if not the vivid blood, of a trauma that is now almost impossible to apprehend even while, increasingly, we anticipate and try to imagine a recurrence.

The Thin White Line and *1918*

Accounts of infection with pandemic flu have a revealing characteristic in common: they describe the recovery from the illness starting with a moment of "waking up," as if from a nightmarish sleep. Patients recall the most serious period only with difficulty, as an experience all but lost to the subject's autobiographical account of being ill. This febrile loss of contact with reality may well be a contributing factor (along with the high fatality rate, of course) to the shortage of direct accounts of infection with the disease.

I begin my discussion with two very different literary works about pandemic influenza that have in common the trope of awakening from a period somehow lost to the flu. The first, Craig DiLouie's 2008 novel, *The Thin White Line: A History of the 2012 Avian Flu Pandemic in Canada*, presents imaginary first-person accounts by recovered patients in a speculative fiction about a future pandemic; the second, Horton Foote's play *1918*, uses the form of the drama itself to delineate a character's experience of the flu as an incommunicable lacuna. This derealization at the level of the individual patient is a probable contributor, by limiting the number of detailed firsthand accounts of being sick that were available, to a similar lacuna in cultural recollection of the pandemic, a sleep from which we arguably began to awake in the 1990s.

In *The Thin White Line*, a man describes catching the flu. Walking home from work, he collapses in the street and spends "the next two weeks unconscious"; when he wakes up, he cannot "believe the state of the world" and recalls that he "felt like Rip Van Winkle, sleeping through history and waking up in a strange world I barely knew anymore." "Time lost all meaning," observes another flu patient; "This torture went on for what felt like years. It's what Hell must be like."[4]

Although the novel deals ostensibly with an avian flu (H5N1) pandemic in the twenty-first century, the 2012 disease and its effects are modeled explicitly on the 1918–19 pandemic (an H1N1 virus like the current swine flu that appeared in 2009). An early description of its clinical characteristics has a footnote (the notes are evidently external to the fictional document): "All symptoms for infection with the Avian Flu strain of the H5N1 virus are based on accounts of the Spanish Flu of 1918–1919, and not the symptoms of the few cases of humans contracting bird flu over the past few years."[5]

Although DiLouie does not document the sources informing his novel's first-person patient accounts, those he does provide are, like those in historical fictions of the 1918 disease, characterized by the distortion of time, loss of contact with external reality, and an inability to recall the acute period of illness, resulting in a sense of "sleeping" (or, nightmarishly, dreaming) "through history." Just as recovery seemed to be an awakening from sleep so, the phenomenological effects of febrile delirium, possibly in combination with the effects of this particular influenza virus on the brain, may have played a part in the pandemic's resistance to narration. One fictional character, to which we shall return, describes his illness as a struggle to "protect his mind from his body."[6]

This sense of a mind under siege is also evident in Horton Foote's play *1918*, set in small-town Texas. (The play was written in the early 1980s.) Foote, born in 1916, modeled the male protagonist, Horace Robedaux, on his own father. Horace comes home sick and tells his wife, Elizabeth, "I ache all over. I have heard so much about the symptoms of the flu that I don't know whether I'm getting it or I'm imagining it." The delirium that quickly follows is unambiguous. "I feel dizzy. Everything looks so peculiar," he says, and by the time the doctor arrives, he is having auditory hallucinations, asking, "Can you hear them?"[7] Horace collapses in his wife's arms, and his loss of consciousness marks the end of the play's first act. Act 2 opens ten days later, when he wakes up, lucid for the first time since becoming ill.

The illness itself takes place between the two acts, a literal intermission or lacuna in the story of the play. The second act begins with Hector waking up in bed, asking, "Where am I?" He wonders whether he had the flu, and his wife answers, "Yes. Don't you remember?" She asks him this question three times in the scene, since his memory has been distorted: "I kept dreaming that you told me the baby was dead. . . . It was the fever. I know I must have had a very high temperature. I dreamed all kinds of crazy things." It was not a dream, though, and the baby has died, and now his wife has to break the news again: "It wasn't a dream, Horace. She died a week ago. . . . I told you at the time. Don't you remember any of it?"[8] Horace has returned from the flu to a terribly changed world, but for the audience, as for Horace, the experience of illness itself cannot be retrieved.

This gap is of course partly due to the limitations of realist drama, which necessarily represents only what can be externalized through behavior or recounted in dialogue. The bedridden and delirious do not make effective dramatic protagonists, not least because their experience is inherently surreal, demanding a different kind of language, a more flexible medium, than realist theater can provide.

The first-person narration of illness experience (fictional or not) has been called an "extreme test case" for narratology, since illness threatens and disrupts embodied experience, the "disintegrating body" a threat to "the very possibility of narration."[9] The diseased body, perhaps especially in acute response to overwhelming viral infection, does not have much time for the mind that watches its inward events and tries to record them. The bodily events of pandemic influenza could be horrific. The symptoms that Foote tactfully conceals along with Horace's experience of the flu have been documented elsewhere, though until fairly recently were largely elided by the disease's seemingly innocuous name and its more familiar seasonal incarnations. Margaret Humphreys points out that panic responses tend to be proportionate neither to the lethality or likelihood of an infection but to the "putridity" of its physical symptoms. As a counterexample to diseases like smallpox and cholera, which induce panic, she lists the benignly "pitiful respiratory distress of Spanish influenza." In his history of the pandemic, John Barry repeatedly reminds us that this was "only influenza"—but as he lists its ghastly impact on bodies, his refrain quickly becomes ironic.[10]

First-person patient accounts of the flu do not go into much physical detail, probably because the delirious mind was not experiencing bodily sensations in a way that was easy to describe literally. External observers, however, describe symptoms far exceeding the "pitiful respiratory distress" noted by Humphreys. A doctor in *The Thin White Line* calls this influenza "Ebola of the lungs." A character in Dennis Lehane's novel *The Given Day* describes sailors taken from an infected ship in Boston harbor in this fashion: with "pinched skulls and caved-in cheeks, their sweat-drenched hair and vomit-encrusted lips, they'd looked dead already. Three of the five bore a blue tint to their flesh, mouths peeled back, eyes wide and glaring." A physician in Thomas Mullen's novel *The Last Town on Earth* gets a letter from a friend, a doctor at Fort Devens, the military cantonment outside Boston. Dated September 20, 1918, the letter is clearly modeled on an actual one written on September 29 by a Fort Devens doctor who signed it "Roy." The letter was found decades later by a Scottish doctor, Norman Grist, and published in the *British Medical Journal*. According to Mullen's fictional version, the "symptoms rivaled the breadth of the epidemic in their horror. Even if only a few people had suffered this disease, it still would have been a terror to be scarcely believed." These symptoms include bleeding from the nose, ears, and eyes; sodden blood-filled lungs; and the characteristic cyanosis that

Roy and his fictional counterpart both note with a particular kind of horror as threatening even the racial identity of the patient. Although Mullen does not quote the letter directly, his description closely approximates Roy's actual document: "Victims became cyanotic, starved of oxygen—parts or all of their bodies turned blue, sometimes such a dark hue that the corpses of white men were indistinguishable from those of coloreds."[11] Roy wrote, "Two hours after admission they have the Mahogany spots over the cheek bones, and a few hours later you can begin to see the Cyanosis extending from their ears and spreading all over the face, until it is hard to distinguish the coloured men from the white. It is only a matter of a few hours then until death comes."[12]

The visible external effects of the disease would have been only a minor aspect of the patients' illness experience. It was more difficult to ascertain how the flu felt than how it looked. A vivid description of the disease's clinical effects that hints at the patients' experience comes in *The Last Town on Earth* when Doc Banes finds a body:

> The blankets cover[ed] only the feet, as if Leonard had tried to kick them off in his final throes of agony. On the wall beside him was blood that had been coughed there or perhaps wiped by his fingers, which were also a dark red. There was blood on the pillow and blood on the sheets, and his entire jaw looked as if he had dipped it in reddish black ink. His eyes were white and opened wide, so wide Doc wondered if his eyelids had somehow been sucked into the space behind them. There was blood on the small table beside the bed, blood on the corner of a framed photograph . . . , an old portrait of a stern father and expressionless mother and three young sons in suit coats and shorts, blood on its lower left-hand corner and blood in the center, where he must have brushed against it one last time.[13]

This violent scene is visible to the doctor and to the reader, through his eyes, but it also lets us infer a glimpse of Leonard's experience: what his horrible, unclosed eyes saw last was the portrait, presumably of his family, his blood marking a dying effort to maintain contact with a reality outside himself.

Patients who survived the Spanish flu were changed by it. The memories of influenza, it seems, are surreal, and to write them is seemingly to write nonsense or dreams or poetry. Perhaps this meant that even those who might vividly describe injuries to the body (like those caused by the war) would have found themselves incapable of representing to others the experience of having the flu. Only the most articulate, and those unafraid of writing outside the conventions of the real, might find language for it.

In her essay "On Being Ill" Virginia Woolf describes the effects of disease, in particular the flu, on perception and experience. She quotes an imaginary "invalid" saying, "I am in bed with influenza," and then asks, "but what does that convey of the great experience: how the world has changed its shape" because of the disease? In 1926, when Woolf published the essay, the world certainly had changed, but her focus here is not on how disease changes the world but rather on how it changes the mind's grasp of the world. The subjective experience of being ill affects both perception and the ability to describe it. The medium mutates under the influence of disease. Although Woolf did not write about the 1918 pandemic explicitly, perhaps because her focus was so intently on the individual and private, influenza recurs throughout her public and private life and writing. Not only did her mother die of the disease, but Woolf herself was repeatedly bedridden by it. The distortion it imposed on her view of reality was both liberating and debilitating for her work, providing insight and despair: "What wastes and deserts of the soul a slight attack of influenza brings to light."[14] It was likely the freedom of modernist prose as Woolf developed it, though—where narration tracks subjective, internal reality—that made possible the one first-hand literary account we do have of a patient's experience of pandemic flu, the novella *Pale Horse, Pale Rider* by Katherine Anne Porter.

Pale Horse, Pale Rider

Katherine Anne Porter was twenty-eight years old in 1918, working as a newspaper reporter in Denver, when she contracted influenza. She was sick enough that her obituary had been set in type and her father had planned her funeral.[15] Twenty years later she published *Pale Horse, Pale Rider*, a novella in which her clearly autobiographical protagonist, Miranda, almost dies of the flu. We can surmise that Porter based her account of Miranda's illness on her memory of having the flu, rather than imagining it whole cloth or deducing it from the accounts of others.

At the center of *Pale Horse, Pale Rider*, narrated in the third person, but entirely from Miranda's point of view, is a sustained account of her illness, tracing the disease's assault on consciousness, memory, and the medium of language itself. As soon as Miranda falls ill, her (and our) hold on external reality becomes tenuous, a process of trying to restore missing events: "I think I have been asleep all day. Oh, I do remember. There was a doctor here."[16]

As the illness takes hold, delirious monologues construct Miranda's perceptions. While dreamlike (or nightmarish), they are also recognizably embedded in the corporeal experience of fever and infection. Temperature swings are realized by an imagination liberated from the limits of rationality: "I wish I were in the cold mountains . . . and all about her rose the measured ranges of the Rockies . . . chilling her to the bone with their sharp breath. Oh, no, I must have warmth—and her memory turned and roved after another place." She sees a sailing ship in a jungle, "moored near by, with a gangplank weathered to blackness touching the foot of her bed." Bed and jungle coexist, and Miranda is able to leave her sick body: "Without surprise, watching from her pillow, she saw herself run swiftly down this gangplank to the slanting deck, and standing there, she leaned on the rail and waved gaily to herself in bed, and the slender ship spread its wings and sailed away into the jungle."[17] This surreal escape from the sickbed might suggest why the bedridden body itself would be so hard for the patient to describe.

When the landlady, Miss Hobbe, discovers Miranda has the flu and tries to throw her out of the building, and Adam, the young soldier who loves her, fights for her to stay, Miranda is both present and elsewhere: "The air trembled with the shattering scream and the hoarse bellow of voices all crying together. . . . There was her door half open, Adam standing with his hand on the knob, and Miss Hobbe with her face all out of shape with terror was crying shrilly, 'I tell you, they must come for her *now*, or I'll put her on the sidewalk. . . . I tell you, this is a plague, a plague, my God, and I've got a houseful of people to think about!'"[18] It is apparently true that Porter's landlady tried to evict her for fear of contagion. Is Miranda's version Porter's exact memory recorded as fiction, or did she learn of the event later and incorporate it into her reimagining? Even while in pain, and vomiting, Miranda feels "hilarious and lightheaded" and, as the fever progresses, her sense of temporal orientation is increasingly distorted: "There were no longer any multiple planes of living, no tough filaments of memory and hope pulling taut backwards and forwards holding her upright between them. There was only this one moment and it was a dream of time."[19] The past tense reminds us, though, that the narrator is not in the midst of delirium but is describing it in retrospect from a more rational vantage point. Even this most vivid account is, necessarily, mediated.

An ambulance takes Miranda to the hospital, and the narrative breaks off, a space on the page marking the interim in which she has simply "floated into darkness." Later she awakens briefly in the hospital but is unable to communicate. She says to a doctor, "I'm not unconscious . . . , I know what I want to say," but "to her horror she heard herself babbling nonsense, knowing it was nonsense though she could not hear what she was saying."[20]

Porter articulates the division between delirious self and detached self even as the dissociation moves beyond the imagined corporeality of the self watched in its real bed: "Her mind, split in two, acknowledged and denied what she saw in one instant, for across an abyss of complaining darkness her reasoning coherent self watched the strange frenzy of the other coldly."[21] She cannot judge the reality or meaning of what her sick self knows. Porter marks this struggle as an effort to represent, to hold onto language: "Oblivion, thought Miranda, her mind feeling among her memories of words she had been taught to describe the unseen, the unknowable, is a whirlpool of gray water turning upon itself for all eternity." As she approaches this oblivion, language itself fails: "Death is death, said Miranda, and for the dead it has no attributes. Silenced she sank easily through deeps under deeps of darkness until she lay like a stone at the farthest bottom of life, knowing herself to be blind, deaf, speechless, no longer aware of the members of her own body, entirely withdrawn from all human concerns, yet alive with a peculiar lucidity and coherence."[22] She is not dead—she is lucid, but it is an animal lucidity, a "will to live," not a human, linguistic, being. It is only when she begins to recover that Miranda can remember her diseased and inarticulate body with words: "Pain returned, a terrible compelling pain running through her veins like heavy fire, the stench of corruption filled her nostrils, the sweetish sickening smell of rotting flesh and pus; she opened her eyes and saw pale light through a coarse white cloth over her face, knew that the smell of death was in her own body."[23] Only in describing and recognizing her damaged body as her own does Miranda reinhabit it and, unwillingly, return to the troubled eloquence of being once more fully human rather than motivated purely by that inarticulate animal will to live.

As one who, remarkably, has survived, Miranda is an occasion for celebration by those who have cared for her, yet she does not share their sense of victory: "She struggled to cry out . . . but heard only incoherent sounds of animal suffering. She saw doctor and nurse glance at each other . . . their eyes alive with knowledgeable pride. They looked briefly at their handiwork and hurried away." Her body has become "a curious monster, no place to live in," and her return to the living is unwanted, not least because she learns that Adam has died of the flu. (Porter's own body was permanently marked by the disease: when she recovered, all her black hair had fallen out, and what grew back was completely white.) Miranda envies Adam and is mystified by "the whole human conviction and custom of society, [that had] conspired to pull her inseparable rack of bones and wasted flesh to its feet, to put in order her disordered mind, and to set her once more safely in the road that would lead her again to death."[24]

It is surely risky to speculate about the actual neurological effects of the influenza virus on patients' minds and hence on their memories and their stories, but I will venture to suggest an improbable connection. There certainly is evidence that the 1918 virus could affect the brain; as Barry puts it, "the virus's impact on the mind was . . . real."[25] Febrile delirium in general is associated with disturbances in the formation of long-term memory, but this may have been something more. A famous study of one hundred patients admitted to the Boston Psychopathic Hospital in 1919 who had the influenza during the pandemic and were later diagnosed as psychotic found a significant connection between influenza infection and subsequent development of schizophrenia, and Barry lists a range of psychiatric sequelae noted at the time by the New York City Department of Health, including "mental depression" and "protracted prostration [which] led to hysteria, melancholia, and insanity with suicidal intent."[26] The return to health after influenza may well have been like awakening to a new and sinisterly different world, apprehended with a mind oddly divided.

The last words of Porter's story point convincingly to the silence of those who went through the disease and recovered: "No more war, no more plague, only the dazed silence that follows the ceasing of the heavy guns; noiseless houses with the shades drawn, empty streets, the dead cold light of tomorrow. Now there would be time for everything."[27] This time, for most, should not be used for recollecting the plague that had left such damage behind. Porter herself was a rare exception, *Pale Horse, Pale Rider* a possibly unique narration that allows us, now, to try and follow a 1918 influenza patient to the core of that experience. Except, of course, that by Porter's own account her experiencing mind was hardly more present in the diseased body, or in the external reality of the pandemic, than we can be now. Fortunately, we have her story and the imaginative identification it provokes to help us reconstitute both her experience and its paradoxical and threatening intangibility.

I complete this chapter by considering two novels about the pandemic published in 2006. Each struggles in a different way with the problem of recounting the experience of particular patients infected by the flu in the context of its overwhelmingly multiplied incidence. Both authors state explicitly their intention to try and remedy our historical amnesia.

Thomas Mullen's *The Last Town on Earth* describes the efforts of the inhabitants of Commonwealth, a small town in the Pacific Northwest, to keep the influenza out of the town through strict, self-imposed isolation. It fails, and quarantining the outside world proves to be profoundly harmful. Myla Goldberg's novel, *Wickett's Remedy*, recounts the experiences of a Boston woman, Lydia Wickett, whose husband, and many in her family, die in the pandemic. She becomes a nurse and assists in studies of the flu pathogen by attempting to infect convicts who had volunteered for the experiments. Plot particulars of both novels are based on the historical record; Commonwealth resembles the town of Gunnison, Colorado, which succeeded in protecting itself from the flu by complete isolation, and the experiments in Goldberg's novel are based on those carried out by the US Public Health Service on Gallups Island in Boston Harbor. These recorded events provide contexts and plot for the accounts, establishing the pathological social matrices in which patients' private experiences of the disease find voice.

Both Goldberg and Mullen have articulated their intentions in various interviews. In the Random House edition's "Reader's Guide," Mullen has stated, "Not only would [this novel] fill a gap in the literary canon but it would also help retrieve some of the fading memories."[28] Similarly, in an interview, Goldberg claims that the pandemic has been "effaced" and tells how, in writing her novel, she "wanted to address how we forget things, how we replace facts with interpretation; . . . the frailty of memory, both individual and collective."[29]

The Last Town on Earth

In Mullen's novel the character whose experience of the flu is most vividly conveyed is sixteen-year-old Philip Worthy, a young man involved in the shooting of a soldier who attempts to breach the town's cordon sanitaire. Because of his contact with this soldier and another who arrives soon after, Philip is put in quarantine in case he is infected. Although he *is* ill, Doc Banes misses this fact, and on his first night home Philip experiences what seems to be an ominous mental prodrome of the influenza:

> Something kept him from rising. It certainly wasn't the pleasantness of his dreams; indeed, he'd suffered from nightmares. . . . [He] stayed in bed because the outside world seemed so much less welcoming than he'd expected. . . . It felt like he'd walked into some altered rendition of his life, painted by a malevolent artist intent on revising Philip's most halcyon memories. As if not the flu but some other plague had descended upon the town while Philip was away, robbing everything of its warmth and casting a sinister hue on every familiar sight.

As in Porter's account, the virus itself seems to distort perception. Once ill, Philip retreats into delirium, too, in this case a "hellish train ride" to which he keeps returning, in "an overcrowded car so hot from the press of bodies that he felt the sweat pool . . . in his armpits and groin. . . . He was standing in the car . . . , but when he opened his eyes he saw he was actually lying down in his bed. He closed his eyes again and things made more sense: his legs ached and his foot throbbed because he was in this dark train car, his toes occasionally stepped upon."[30] As Mullen shows with Philip's character, the mind looks for stories, or invents them, to make sense of inexplicable sensations or to fill the gaps when the brain cannot perceive reality directly. For Philip, the fever dream makes "more sense" than reality can.

Philip does experience odd moments of lucidity, but even these are experienced in the context of the hellish train ride, as if it has become his new reality, the site of a battle between psyche and soma:

> How long had he been on that train? Days. . . . Time was a chimera dancing before him to distract him from the only thing that mattered: getting healthy. . . . His body dared not consider health—it took all its strength to fight on and stay alive while in this siege. Just as the town had been under siege from all sides. Now the same scenario was playing itself out, but this time the flu-infected world was his body and the safe haven of Commonwealth was his

mind. He needed to protect his mind from his body. If his mind could stay healthy, if he could properly quarantine it, then maybe his body would give up this gruesome battle. He thought about that, then realized it made no sense. He was already losing his mind—his brain had already fallen victim to his body. The flu had broken the quarantine.[31]

Mullen makes the body-mind division explicit. Philip becomes a microcosm of the town of Commonwealth, his body inhabited by his mind as the town is by its people. He comes to realize, though, that the body and its infectibility (and its vulnerability to temptation—the disease has in fact been brought into Commonwealth by men sneaking to the next town to visit the brothel) cannot be contained by the will of the mind.

When Philip finally recovers, and when he gets up for the first time, ten days later, both he and the world appear changed: "He seemed to be remembering how to talk, his tongue awkward, his body stumbling"; the "world looked different," for "ten days . . . had passed with no reliable record except disturbing dreams, conversations he wasn't sure were real or imagined."[32] Like Horace and Miranda, Philip has no reliable record of the time of his illness. And, just as in Foote and Porter's accounts, Philip learns on recovering that Elsie, the girl he has fallen in love with, has died of the flu. At least in the fictions it has produced, the disease has at its center a dangerous inattention, a kind of irresponsibility that is potentially lethal for those one loves. The problem with pandemics is that the individual patient is never the only patient, never the center of attention in a story about one special illness, never the only one who needs to be cared for and to be heard.

Mullen says that readers of his novel "have told me that its subject reminded them of a great-aunt or a great-grandfather who lost a spouse or parents or children to the epidemic. I have been struck by the fact that their stories always end with some variation of the line: 'but she never talked about it.' There seemed to be a wall of silence surrounding survivors' memories of the 1918 flu, which, after the passing of many generations, is quickly leading to the very erasure of those memories."[33] Myla Goldberg's novel, the least realist account of the pandemic, and thus the most free to pay explicit attention to its own methods of representation, incorporates Mullen's concern explicitly. Why *did* they "never talk about it?"

Wickett's Remedy

While her novel does not include any single account of the flu from the perspective of a patient, Goldberg thematizes the problem of conveying that experience, directly confronting the struggle to remember and tell that we are coming to associate with the pandemic. Unlike Mullen, Goldberg focuses insistently on her medium, narrative. For instance, where both authors describe pulmonary congestion as a creature inhabiting the lungs, Goldberg links this entity to language itself. Mullen's Philip feels "something inside his chest, something large and waxy and heavy, something that had attached itself to his rib cage and woven its fibers into his muscles and ligaments," but Goldberg's narrator shows how a patient is given a horrible new voice by the disease even as it also renders her (the patient but not the narrator) inarticulate: "thick, labored speech rose in intensity to become the voice of sickness itself. It was as if a large, phantom hand was squeezing her chest from inside to expel the cobwebby air that powered her words."[34]

Goldberg tries to channel the many-tongued voice of the pandemic, using a multivocal text to convey a multiplicity of perspectives on the pandemic (at least in Boston) and its sequelae. To this end, each chapter ends with documents—letters, newspaper cuttings, snippets of conversation. Most significant, though, is Goldberg's use of a parallel counternarrative, or metanarrative, told in the collective second-person plural voice of "The Dead." The novel's central narration is repeatedly interrupted, and illuminated, by a text printed literally in its margins. If the medium of univocal narration is overwhelmed by the multiplicity and the feverish forgetfulness of the pandemic, then Goldberg creates in her writing a different kind of medium, quite literally the clairvoyant medium who can transmit the voices of the dead, of those able to recount knowledge never accessible to the living. The Dead do not know everything; as they say, "*Our collective knowledge is surpassed only by Our collective amnesia, which encompasses millions of moments lived and subsequently forgotten.*"[35] But from their chorus emerge corrective contradictions that make it impossible for the reader to forget the noisy heteroglossia of pandemics, where so many different voices are competing with equal urgency to be heard.

I will show how this works in just one scene. The central narrative is told from Lydia's perspective. She enters the sickroom where her brother, Malachy; his wife, Alice; and their children are all in bed: "the air was dense with the smells of fever sweat, phlegm, and unwashed sheets and seemed, by its very thickness, responsible for the prostration of its inhabitants. Whether sickness alone or a combination of poor health and poor light contributed to the family's complexions, their skin reminded Lydia of potato broth, save for Brian's lips—which were tinged blue." Lydia notices that Alice is in an awkward position and imagines that her "original intention in lying on her side had been to watch over her children, but fever had reduced her gaze to a glazed stare." The mother is too sick even to see her own children, and when Alice's own mother tries to comfort her, she does not recognize her, calling her "Devil." Lydia notices in Alice the same dissociation of mind and body captured by Porter and by Mullen: Alice accidentally hits her head against the bed frame but does not seem to notice. Lydia observes that "if it had hurt, Alice's face betrayed nothing. Sickness had turned her into a spectator of her own body."[36] (Unless, of course, she does feel pain, but sickness has rendered her body incapable of conveying what she feels. Frighteningly, the effect on an observer would be the same.)

A similar problem arises for Lydia when she remembers that her brother mentioned the flu in a letter but "she had not recalled that remark until she was told he was dead." She feels this inattention as guilt, an "indictment" "too tenuous to survive exposure to the air, but incontrovertible within the confine of her body."[37] This corporeal knowledge is both absolute and inexpressible. Perhaps this is why so many who remembered the flu would not talk about it.

Alice dies and Goldberg's medium offers us Alice's posthumous recollection of being ill. Paradoxically, though, if unsurprisingly, we learn little more than Lydia can tell. In the margin, the Dead tell us that "*Alice remembers only feeling awfully tired and deciding to lie down.*" Amnesia affects the dead too, and the flu still eludes us despite Goldberg's efforts to address its opacity. Alice's mother does not recall things clearly either. Lydia describes Alice's body as grotesque: her "mouth was frozen in a grimace, her eyebrows raised in astonishment. She looked neither asleep, nor at peace." The Dead tell us what Alice's mother recalls: "*Jennie Feeney is certain her daughter looked beautiful.*" They also tell us, though, that "*Jennie Feeney remembers blessed little of that terrible day.*"[38] Our trust in Lydia's own perception is also threatened, despite Goldberg's use of a supposedly dispassionate third-person narrator. Rather than giving us the whole story, the many voices of the text simply draw our attention to how little they can tell.

This is perhaps most true in the case of six-year-old Brian's postmortem memory. He spends his last night in the hospital, and Lydia is told that a nurse had been with him when he died. What Brian remembers is "*a lady with bird wings on either side of her head. He thought she was an angel, but once he could not breathe anymore he realized she was nothing at all.*"[39] Rather than consolidating memory, death renders it obsolete. The Dead can tell their stories, add their versions, but Goldberg refuses us a trustworthy voice. The unnarratable cannot be remembered.

In *The Forgotten Pandemic* Alfred Crosby asks (and tries to tell): "what happened, not to statistics, but to people and families and communities?" "The answer isn't easy to give," he says, "because it consists of thousands of separate stories. Shall we therefore examine the stories of a dozen or so individuals? That would be like judging an elephant by examining a dozen cells."[40] Crosby decides to tell the stories of the cities, because there is more data about them than about how the pandemic unfolded in rural areas. He cannot claim to tell the whole story. But then who can?

Two reviews of Myla Goldberg's novel articulate the challenge of writing a pandemic in microcosm. For one reviewer, the vivid account of a part is enough to convey the whole: the book is "about the great influenza pandemic of 1918—or at least, about one poignant and beautifully observed corner of it, in which nevertheless the whole meaning of that fatal episode is captured."[41] Another reviewer finds Goldberg too inclusive: "While her thoroughly researched attempt to capture the broad sweep of an epidemic is admirable, it reminds us, nevertheless, that part of fiction's task is to select: to single out, from a mass of events and individuals, the representative few who will engage our emotions and come to stand for all the others."[42] Goldberg's intent was not to capture "the whole meaning," to recall or reconstruct, but rather to ask *how* we recall and reconstruct, how even those who were there cannot remember exactly or retell without distortion—and how the meaning of events lies less in what happened than in how they are reinvented, retold, in stories later on.

Our medium, the telling, is inherent in the sense we make of reality. Maia Saj Schmidt points out that the "the techniques of fiction [are valuable] in the narrativization of so-called facts, because despite the impossibility of accessing truth, it is perhaps possible to get ever closer to truth by exploring the subtleties and ambiguities of its representation."[43] Goldberg explores the problem of representation in her novel and through this exploration moves closer to the difficult truth about the Spanish flu. Much of it is already out of our reach, and probably always was, even during the pandemic itself.

Notes

Parts of chapter 13 appeared in a slightly different form in Catherine Belling, "Overwhelming the Medium: Fiction and the Trauma of Pandemic Influenza in 1918," *Literature and Medicine* 28.1 (2009): 55–81.

1. I use the word "holocaust" in its generic sense and am not trying to equate the pandemic with the Holocaust. There are of course a great many differences too obvious to note. Comparisons, though, concerning witnessing and remembering mass suffering, might be of value, for in both cases the trauma extends beyond the individual or family and yet cannot be felt or conveyed on this scale, but only one story, one teller, at a time. Shoshana Felman writes about Claude Lanzmann's film *Shoah*: "What is testified to is limit-experiences whose overwhelming impact constantly puts to the test the limits of the witnesses and of the witnessing, at the same time that it constantly unsettles and puts into question the very limits of reality." "In an Era of Testimony: Claude Lanzmann's *Shoah*," *Yale French Studies* 79 (1991): 40. One might suggest that global pandemic, albeit in a different way, also puts history to the test.

2. On the severity and main characteristics of the pandemic, see the introduction to this volume.

3. See, for example, John M. Barry, *The Great Influenza: The Epic Story of the Deadliest Plague in History* (New York: Viking, 2004), 393–94. Looking only at works in English, the World War I literary canon includes the writing of poets such as Rupert Brooke, Wilfred Owen, and Siegfried Sassoon and of novelists like Ernest

Hemingway, John Dos Passos, and Robert Graves, to name only a few. It is beyond the scope of this chapter to compare the two bodies of writing, but two factors are likely to have led to the comparative absence of flu literature: the overshadowing effect of the war, which was qualitatively different from previous experience (where epidemics were a fairly familiar experience, albeit never on the same global scale), and the longer period over which the war would have been experienced by an individual, producing more complex plot lines than the rapid descent into incoherence that characterized the flu.

4. Craig DiLouie, *The Thin White Line: A History of the 2012 Avian Flu Pandemic in Canada* (Calgary: Future Shock Books, 2008), 64, 65.

5. Ibid., 195n4. Similarly, an illustration for the section describing the isolation in Canada of the H5N1 virus has the caption "The 2012–13 Avian Flu virus as seen in a negative-stained transmission electron micrograph collected from a canine kidney cell culture 18 hours after infection"; the caption, in turn, has a footnote disclosing that the picture, a "public domain image captured from the Centers for Disease Control website," "actually shows the 1918 Spanish Flu virus as recreated" by a CDC microbiologist. DiLouie, *Thin White Line*, 56, 199n15. DiLouie does not say why he relies on the Spanish flu rather than recorded accounts of avian flu to construct his imaginary pandemic.

6. Thomas Mullen, *The Last Town on Earth* (New York: Random House, 2006), 334.

7. Horton Foote, *1918* in *Courtship, Valentine's Day, 1918: Three Plays from the Orphans Home Cycle* (New York: Grove, 1994), 138, 140, 143.

8. Ibid., 149.

9. Shlomith Rimmon-Kenan, "What Can Narrative Theory Learn from Illness Narratives?," *Literature and Medicine* 25 no. 2 (2006.): 245.

10. Margaret Humphreys, "No Safe Place: Disease and Panic in American History," *American Literary History* 14, no. 4 (2002): 849; Barry, *Great Influenza*, 231, 232, 236, 241.

11. DiLouie, *Thin White Line*, 45; Dennis Lehane, *The Given Day* (New York: Morrow, 2008), 71; Mullen, *Last Town on Earth*, 129.

12. In his first description of the influenza's symptoms, John M. Barry also notes this odd race confusion, as observed by Paul Lewis among sailors: "some showed just a tinge of blue around their lips or fingertips, but a few looked so dark one could not easily tell if they were Caucasian or Negro. They looked almost black." Barry, *Great Influenza*, 2. Barry doesn't give a source for this detail. It is probably the same letter, from which he quotes directly on page 187.

13. Mullen, *Last Town on Earth*, 218.

14. Virginia Woolf, "On Being Ill," in *The Moment and Other Essays* (New York: Harcourt Brace, 1947), 12, 9.

15. For details, see Darlene Harbour Unrue, *Katherine Anne Porter: The Life of an Artist* (Jackson: University Press of Mississippi, 2005), 63.

16. Katherine Anne Porter, *Pale Horse, Pale Rider* (New York: Modern Library, 1939), 229.

17. Ibid., 231, 232.

18. Ibid.; ellipsis in the original.

19. Ibid., 234, 241.

20. Ibid., 242, 245.

21. Ibid., 251. Rita Charon gives a vivid clinical account of the interactions between an ill subject and a body that "is and is not the self" in *Narrative Medicine: Honoring the Stories of Illness* (New York: Oxford University Press, 2006), 90.

22. Porter, *Pale Horse, Pale Rider*, 251, 252. In a longer version of this chapter, I would be able to show how Porter's writing is, in passages like this, clearly influenced by the modernist prose of Woolf, most notably the account of illness in her first novel, *The Voyage Out.*

23. Porter, *Pale Horse, Pale Rider*, 255.

24. Ibid., 247, 259–60.

25. Barry, *Great Influenza*, 381.

26. For the link between influenza infection and schizophrenia, see Karl A. Menninger, "Psychoses Associated with Influenza," *Journal of the American Medical Association* 72 (1919): 238. The citations about psychiatric sequelae come from Barry, *Great Influenza*, 238.

27. Porter, *Pale Horse, Pale Rider*, 264.

28. Mullen, *Last Town*, 400.

29. Simon Houpt, "Triumph of the Nerd," review of *Wickett's Remedy*, by Myla Goldberg, *Globe and Mail* (Toronto, Canada), September 24, 2005.

30. Mullen, *Last Town on Earth*, 219, 332.

31. Ibid., 334.

32. Ibid., 354, 355.

33. Ibid., 399.

34. Ibid., 332–33; Myla Goldberg, *Wickett's Remedy* (New York: Anchor Books, 2006), 133.

35. Goldberg, *Wickett's Remedy*, 178; italics in the original.

36. Ibid., 129–32.

37. Ibid., 166.

38. Ibid., 133, 145, 146.

39. Ibid., 161.

40. Alfred W. Crosby, *America's Forgotten Pandemic: The Influenza of 1918*, 2nd ed. (Cambridge: Cambridge University Press, 2003), 66.

41. A. C. Grayling, "An Inspirational Novel of Influenza, Love, Life, and Death," review of *Wickett's Remedy*, by Myla Goldberg, *Lancet* 366, no. 9503 (2005–6): 2077.

42. Andrea Barrett, "Flu Season," review of *Wickett's Remedy*, by Myla Goldberg, *New York Times*, September 18, 2005.

43. Maia Saj Schmidt, "Literary Testimonies of Illness and the Reshaping of Social Memory," *Auto/biography Studies* 13 (1998): 75.

Selected Bibliography

This selected bibliography shows only the most relevant books and articles about the Spanish influenza pandemic and the history of epidemic diseases cited in the chapters in this volume.

Abrão, Janete Silveira. *Banalização da morte na cidade calada: A hespanhola em Porto Alegre, 1918*. Porto Alegre: EDIPUCRS, 1998.

Bardet, Jean Pierre, Patrice Bourdelais, Pierre Guillaume, François Lebrun, and Claude Quétel, eds. *Peurs et terreurs face à la contagion: Choléra, tuberculose, syphilis, XIXe–XXe siècles*. Paris: Fayard, 1998.

Barry, John M. *The Great Influenza: The Epic Story of the Deadliest Plague in History*. New York: Viking, 2004.

Bashford, Alison. *Imperial Hygiene: A Critical History of Colonialism, Nationalism and Public Health*. New York: Palgrave, 2004.

Bernabeu-Mestre, Josep, ed., in collaboration with Andreu Nolasco Bonmatí, Marisa Bardisa Escuder, Vicente Bartual Méndez, José María Gutiérrez Rubio, Luis López Penabad, and José Miguel Mataix Piñero. *La ciutat davant el contagi: Alacant i la grip de 1918–19*. Valencia: Conselleria de Sanitat i Consum, Generalitat Valenciana, 1991.

Bertolli Filho, Claudío. *A gripe espanhola em São Paulo, 1918: Epidemia e sociedade*. São Paulo: Paz e Terra, 2003.

Bertrán Moya, José Luís. *Historia de las epidemias en España y sus colonias (1348–1919)*. Madrid: La Esfera de los Libros, 2006.

Bertucci, Liane Maria. *Influenza, a medicina enferma: Ciência e práticas de cura na época da gripe espanhola em São Paulo*. Campinas: Universidade Estadual de Campinas, 2004.

Beveridge, William I. *Influenza: The Last Great Plague; An Unfinished Story of Discovery*. New York: Prodist, 1977.

Bourdelais, Patrice. *Epidemics Laid Low: A History of What Happened in Rich Countries*. Translated by Bart K. Holland. Baltimore: Johns Hopkins University Press, 2006.

———, ed. *Les hygiénistes: Enjeux, modèles et pratiques, XVIIIe–XXe siècles*. Paris: Belin, 2001.

Byerly, Carol R. *Fever of War: The Influenza Epidemic in the U.S. Army during World War I*. New York: New York University Press, 2005.

Cooter, Roger. "Of War and Epidemics: Unnatural Couplings, Problematic Conceptions." *Social History of Medicine* 16, no. 2 (2003): 283–302.

Crosby, Alfred W. *America's Forgotten Pandemic: The Influenza of 1918*. 2nd ed. Cambridge: Cambridge University Press, 2003.

Davis, Ryan A. *The Spanish Flu: Narrative and Cultural Identity in Spain, 1918*. New York: Palgrave Macmillan, 2013.

Echeverri Dávila, Beatriz. *La gripe española: La pandemia de 1918–19*. Madrid: Centro de Investigaciones Sociológicas / Siglo XXI, 1993.

Evans, Richard J. *Death in Hamburg: Society and Politics in the Cholera Years, 1830–1910*. London: Penguin Books, 1987.

Farmer, Paul. *Infections and Inequalities: The Modern Plagues*. Berkeley: University of California Press, 2001.

Fee, Elizabeth, and Daniel M. Fox, eds. *AIDS: The Burdens of History*. Berkeley: University of California Press, 1988.

Frada, João José Cúcio. *A gripe pneumónica em Portugal continental, 1918: Estudo socio-económico e epidemiológico com particular análise do concelho de Leiria*. Lisbon: Sete Caminhos, 2005.

Garrett, Laurie. *The Coming Plague: Newly Emerging Diseases in a World Out of Balance*. New York: Penguin, 1995.

Girão, Paulo Jorge Marques. *A pneumónica no Algarve*. Lisbon: Caleidoscópio, 2003.

Golden, Janet, ed. *Framing Disease: Studies in Cultural History*. New Brunswick, NJ: Rutgers University Press, 1992.

Honigsbaum, Mark. *Living with Enza: The Forgotten Story of Britain and the Great Flu Pandemic of 1918*. London: Macmillan, 2009.

Johnson, Niall. *Britain and the 1918–19 Influenza Pandemic: A Dark Epilogue*. London: Routledge, 2006.

Johnson, Niall, and Juergen Mueller. "Updating the Accounts: Global Mortality of the 1918–1920 'Spanish' Influenza Pandemic." *Bulletin of the History of Medicine* 76, 1 (2002): 105–15. doi:10.1353/bhm.2002.0022.

Johnson, Steven. *The Ghost Map: The History of London's Most Terrifying Epidemic and How It Changed Science, Cities and the Modern World*. New York: Riverhead, 2006.

Jones, Esyllt W. *Influenza 1918: Disease, Death, and Struggle in Winnipeg*. Toronto: University of Toronto Press, 2007.

Knobler, Stacey, Alison Mack, Adel Mahmoud, and Stanley M. Lemon, eds. *The Threat of Pandemic Influenza: Are We Ready? Workshop Summary*. Washington, DC: National Academies Press, 2004.

Kolata, Gina. *Flu: The Story of the Great Influenza Pandemic of 1918 and the Search for the Virus That Caused It*. New York: Farrar, 1999.

Lederberg, Joshua. "Infectious Disease as an Evolutionary Paradigm." *Emerging Infectious Diseases* 3 (1997): 417–23.

Lupton, Deborah. *Medicine as Culture: Illness, Disease and the Body in Western Societies*. London: Sage, 2003.

Markel, Howard. *When Germs Travel: Six Major Epidemics That Have Invaded America*. New York: Pantheon, 2004.

Martínez, Manuel. *València al límit: La ciutat de València davant l'epidèmia de grip de 1918*. Simat de la Valldigna: Edicions La Xara, 1999.

Morens, David M., and Anthony S. Fauci. "The 1918 Influenza Pandemic: Insights for the 21st-Century." *Journal of Infectious Diseases* 195 (2010): 1018–28. doi:10.1086/511989.

Oldstone, Michael B. A. *Viruses, Plagues and History*. Oxford: Oxford University Press, 2000.

Pandemic Influenza Storybook. Centers for Disease Control. US Department of Health and Human Services, 2008. www.flu.gov/pandemic/history/storybook/index. html.

Phillips, Howard, and David Killingray, eds. *The Spanish Influenza Pandemic of 1918–1919: New Perspectives.* London: Routledge, 2003.

Porras-Gallo, María-Isabel. "The Place of Serums and Antibiotics in the Influenza Pandemics of 1918–1919 and 1957–1958 Respectively." In *Circulation of Antibiotics: Journeys of Drug Standards, 1930–1970,* edited by Ana Romero, Christoph Gradmann, and María Santesmases, 141–60. Madrid: European Science Foundation. ESF Networking Program DRUGS. Preprint no. 1. 2010. http://drughistory.eu/downloads/Madrid_Preprint.pdf.

———. *Un reto para la sociedad madrileña: La epidemia de gripe de 1918–19.* Madrid: Complutense / Comunidad Autónoma de Madrid, 1997.

Porter, Dorothy. *Health, Civilization and the State: A History of Public Health from Ancient to Modern Times.* Abingdon: Routledge, 1999.

Porter, Roy. *The Greatest Benefit of Mankind.* London: Fontana, 1999.

———. *The Cambridge Illustrated History of Medicine.* Cambridge: Cambridge University Press, 2001.

Quinn, Tom. *Flu: A Social History of Influenza.* London: New Holland, 2008.

Ranger, Terence, and Paul Slack, eds. *Epidemics and Ideas: Essays on the Historical Perception of Pestilence.* Cambridge: Cambridge University Press, 1992.

Rosen, George. *A History of Public Health.* Expanded ed. Baltimore: Johns Hopkins University Press, 1993.

Rosenberg, Charles E. *Explaining Epidemics and Other Studies in the History of Medicine.* Cambridge: Cambridge University Press, 1992.

Sigerist, Henry. *Civilización y enfermedad.* Mexico City: Biblioteca de la Salud, 1987.

Silveira, Anny Jackeline Torres. *A influenza espanhola e a cidade planejada: Belo Horizonte, 1918.* Belo Horizonte: Argumentum, 2007.

Slack, Paul. *The Impact of Plague in Tudor and Stuart England.* 1983. Reprint, Oxford: Oxford University Press, 2005.

Smolinski, Mark S., Margaret A. Hamburg, and Joshua Lederberg. *Microbial Threats to Health: Emergence, Detection and Response.* Washington, DC: National Academies Press, 2003.

Sobral, José Manuel, Maria Luísa Lima, Paulo Silveira e Sousa, and Paula Castro, eds. *A Pandemia Esquecida: Olhares comparados sobre a pneumónica, 1918–1919.* Lisbon: Imprensa de Ciências Sociais, 2009.

Souza, Christiane Maria Cruz de. *A gripe espanhola na Bahia: Saúde, política e medicina em tempos de epidemia.* Salvador/Rio de Janeiro: Editora da Universidade Federal da Bahia / Fundação Oswaldo Cruz, 2009.

Taubenberger, Jeffery K., and David M. Morens. "1918 Influenza: The Mother of All Pandemics." *Emerging Infectious Diseases* 12, no. 1 (2006): 15–22. doi:10.3201/eid1201.050979.

Tognotti, Eugenia. "Scientific Triumphalism and Learning from the Facts: Bacteriology and the 'Spanish Flu' Challenge of 1918." *Social History of Medicine* 16, no. 1 (2003): 97–110. doi:10.1093/shm/16.1.97.

Tomes, Nancy. *The Gospel of Germs: Men, Women, and the Microbe in American Life.* Cambridge, MA: Harvard University Press, 1998.

Van Hartesveldt, Fred R., ed. *The 1918–1919 Pandemic of Influenza: The Urban Impact in the Western World.* New York: Mellen, 1993.

World Health Organization. *Handbook for Journalists: Influenza Pandemic.* Geneva: World Health Organization, 2005. www.who.int/csr/don/Handbook_influenza_pandemic_dec05.pdf.

Contributors

CATHERINE BELLING is an associate professor of medical humanities and bioethics at Northwestern University's Feinberg School of Medicine. Her research concerns contemporary fears of health care, and relationships between anxiety, narration, and interpretation in fiction, medicine, and bioethics. Her book *A Condition of Doubt: On the Meanings of Hypochondria* (Oxford: Oxford University Press, 2012), won the 2013 Kendrick Book Prize (Society for Literature, Science, and the Arts), and her essay, "Narrative Oncogenesis: The Problem of Telling when Cancer Begins," *Narrative* 18, no. 2 (2010): 229–47, won the 2010 Schachterle Prize. She has served on the Board of Directors of the American Society for Bioethics and Humanities and is the executive editor of the journal *Literature and Medicine* (published by Johns Hopkins University Press).

JOSEP BERNABEU-MESTRE is a professor of the history of science at the University of Alicante in Spain. His principal field of research is the history of public health (public health and nutrition, mother and child health care, and historical epidemiology in contemporary Spain). Most prominent among his latest publications are *Nutrición, salud y sociedad: España y Europa en los siglos XIX y XX* (in collaboration with Josep Lluís Barona) (Valencia: Seminari d'Estudis sobre la Ciència / PUV, 2011) and "La prévention et la protection sociale dans la lutte contre la mortinatalité et la mortalité néo-natale précoce: Réflexions à partir de l'expérience espagnole, 1924–1936," *Annales de Démographie Historique* 1 (2012): 181–204.

LIANE MARIA BERTUCCI earned her PhD in history from State University of Campinas, Brazil, and did postdoctoral research at the University of São Paulo. She is currently a professor of the history of education at Federal University of Paraná in Curitiba, Brazil. Her fields of research include the history of health and work as related to education, health science, healing practices, and public health. Her publications include *Influenza, a medicina enferma* (Campinas: Universidade Estadual de Campinas, 2004); "Entre doutores e para os leigos: Fragmentos do discurso médico na influenza de 1918," *História, Ciências, Saúde: Manguinhos* 12, no. 1 (2005): 143–57; "Bacilo versus vírus: Olhares de médicos brasileiros sobre a gripe de 1918," in *A pandemia esquecida: Lisboa*, ed. José Manuel Sobral, Maria Luísa Lima, Paula

Castro, and Paulo Silveira e Sousa (Lisbon: Imprensa de Ciências Sociais, 2009); and "Os paulistanos e as faces do medo durante a gripe espanhola," in *As doenças e os medos sociais*, ed. Y. N. Monteiro and M. L. T. Carneiro (São Paulo: Fap-Unifesp, 2013).

RYAN A. DAVIS received his PhD from Emory University and is currently an assistant professor in the Department of Languages, Literatures, and Cultures at Illinois State University. His research on modern Spain focuses on the intersection between literary and medical discourses, "fringe" discourses (e.g., hypnotism), and the creative fiction of physicians. He is the author of *The Spanish Flu: Narrative and Cultural Identity in Spain, 1918* (New York: Palgrave Macmillan, 2013). His published work has also appeared in the *Journal of Spanish Cultural Studies*, *Revista de Estudios Hispánicos*, *Decimonónica*, and *Ometeca*.

ESTEBAN DOMINGO is a professor of research with the Spanish Research Council (CSIC), Centro de Biología Molecular "Severo Ochoa" (CBMSO) at the Universidad Autónoma de Madrid in Spain. He received his PhD in biochemistry from the University of Barcelona in 1969. He has more than thirty years of experience working as a professor of virology in Spain, the United States, and France and has spent more than seven years working in international laboratories, with experience in sequencing influenza virus genes. He serves on the editorial board of several journals of virology. He is editor or coeditor of *Origin and Evolution of Viruses* (London: Elsevier Academic Press, 2008); *Quasispecies: Concepts and Implications for Virology* (New York: Springer, 2006); and *Foot and Mouth Disease: Current Perspectives* (Boca Raton: CRC, 2004).

MAGDA FAHRNI is an associate professor in the Department of History at the Université du Québec à Montréal. She is the author of *Household Politics: Montreal Families and Postwar Reconstruction* (Toronto: University of Toronto Press, 2005); the coauthor of *Canadian Women: A History*, 3rd ed. (Toronto: Nelson Education, 2011); and the coeditor of *Epidemic Encounters: Influenza, Society, and Culture in Canada, 1918–20* (Vancouver: University of British Columbia Press, 2012) and of *Creating Postwar Canada: Community, Diversity, and Dissent, 1945–1975* (Vancouver: University of British Columbia Press, 2008). She is currently writing a sociocultural history of accidents in the context of industrial modernity.

HERNÁN FELDMAN obtained his law degree from the Facultad de Derecho y Ciencias Sociales de la Universidad de Buenos Aires and received his doctoral degree in Latin American Literature from Indiana University. He is currently an assistant professor at Emory University, where he teaches courses on Río de la Plata literature and culture. Professor Feldman's main interests are intellectual history, political philosophy, critical legal studies, and film. In 2011 he published his book, *Una patria amurallada: Políticas de contención en la Argentina aluvial (1870–1904)* with Prometeo Libros. Professor Feldman has also published essays in journals such as *Revista Iberoamericana, Journal of Latin American Cultural Studies, Revista Canadiense de Estudios Hispánicos, Estudios Interdisciplinarios de Latinoamérica y el Caribe, Hispamérica,* and *Latin American Literary Review.*

PILAR LEÓN-SANZ is an associate professor of the history of medicine and medical ethics at the University of Navarra. She also has been a research fellow at the Wellcome T. C. for the history of medicine at University College London (2002, 2010), a visiting scholar at Harvard University (2011), and a member of the Steering Committee Phoenix European Thematic Network on Health and Social Policy (2006–9). She is currently a member of the project "Emotional Culture and Identity" (Institute for Culture and Society, UN). Her research interests include topics related to medicine in eighteenth-century Spain, especially music therapy, and the practices of health care professionals during the nineteenth and twentieth centuries. Her publications include "Medical Assistance Provided by la Conciliación, a Pamplona Mutual Assistance Association (1902–84)," in *Welfare and Old Age in Europe and North America: The Development of Social Insurance,* ed. Bernard Harris (London: Pickering & Chatto, 2012), 137–66; "El carácter terapéutico de la relación médico-paciente," in *Emociones y estilos de vida: Radiografía de nuestro tiempo* (Madrid: Biblioteca nueva, 2013), 101–30; "Evolution of the Concept of Emotion in Medicine: A Music-Therapy Approach," in *The Emotions and Cultural Analysis* (Burlington: Asghate, 2012); *Health Institutions at the Origin of the Welfare Systems in Europe* (Pamplona: Eunsa, 2010); *La Tarantola Spagnola: Empirismo e tradizione nel XVIII secolo* (Lecce: Besa, 2008); *Vicente Ferrer Gorraiz Beaumont y Montesa (1718–1792), un polemista navarro de la ilustración,* with Dolores Barettino (Pamplona: Gobierno de Navarra, 2007); *La implantación de los derechos del paciente* (Pamplona: Eunsa, 2004).

MARIA LUÍSA LIMA is a professor of social psychology at ISCTE-Institute University of Lisbon in Portugal. She has published in various edited collections and academic journals, including the *Journal of Applied Social Psychology, British Journal of Health Psychology, Risk Analysis,* and *Journal of Environmental Psychology.* She was the president of the Portuguese Psychological Association and the representative of psychology at the Social Sciences Research Council of FCT (National Research Funding Agency). She is also a coeditor of *A Pandemia Esquecida: Olhares comparados sobre a pneumónica, 1918–1919* (Lisbon: Imprensa de Ciências Sociais, 2009).

MARIA DE FÁTIMA NUNES is a professor of history and a research unit director at the Centro de Estudos de História e Filosofia da Ciência (Scientific and Technological Foundation) at the Universidade de Évora in Portugal. She teaches courses on history, history of culture, and history of science (from the eighteenth to the twenty-first century), with emphasis on scientific and musicology subjects, including the first, second, and third Bologna cycles. She supervises PhD students in history and the history and philosophy of science, with specialization in museology, as well as master students, including master mundus and PhD mundus. Her main works include *Imprensa periodica cientifica, 1772–1851: Leituras de "sciencia agrícola"* (Lisbon: Estar, 2002); *Ideia cientifica de Europa: Metrologia, memoria e ciência em Evora, Lisboa* (Casal de Cambra, Portugal: Caleidoscópio, 2004); *Imagens da ciência em Portugal, sec. XVIII–XX* (Lisbon: Caleidoscópio, 2005); and, with A. Fitas and M. Rodrigues, *Filosofia e história da ciência em Portugal no século XX* (Casal de Cambra: Caleidoscópio, 2008); Augusto Fitas, J. P. Princípe, Maria Fátima Nunes, and Martha Cecilia Bustamante, coords., *A Atividade da Junta de Educação Nacional* (Lisbon: Caleidoscópio / CEHFCi, 2012); J. M. Brandão and Maria Fátima Nunes, eds., *Ciência, Crise e Mudança* (Livro de Resumos: ENHCT, 2012) (Centro de Estudos de História e Filosofia da Ciência, Terceiro Encontro Nacional de História das Ciências e da Tecnologia, Évora, September 26–28, 2012).

MERCEDES PASCUAL ARTIAGA received her PhD in the history of science and scientific documentation at the University of Alicante in Spain, and her field of research is the history of public health in contemporary Alicante. In addition to various articles and book chapters, she has also published the monograph *Fam, malaltia i mort: La societat alacantina front a l'epidèmia de febra groga de 1804* (Simat de la Valldigna, Spain: La Xara, 1999) and more recently *El desarrollo del municipio liberal y el reto de la alimentación en el Alicante de la primera mitad del siglo XIX* (Alicante: Universidad de Alicante, 2013).

MARÍA-ISABEL PORRAS-GALLO is a professor of the history of science in the Medical Sciences Department and Medical Faculty of Ciudad Real at the University of Castilla–La Mancha, Spain. She has both her MD and PhD in medicine (Complutense University of Madrid, Spain). From 1996 to 1998 she was a Spanish Ministry of Education and Science postdoctoral fellow at the Historical Research Centre-Laboratory, École des Hautes Études en Sciences Sociales, Centre National de la Recherche Scientifique in Paris, France. Her main research field is the history of diseases, especially the 1918–19 influenza pandemic and, more recently, poliomyelitis in Spain. In addition to having published numerous articles and book chapters, she is the author of *Un reto para la sociedad madrileña: La epidemia de gripe de 1918–1919* (Madrid: Complutense / Comunidad Autónoma de Madrid, 1997) and the coeditor of *De la responsabilidad individual a la culpabilización de la víctima: El papel del paciente en la prevención de la enfermedad* (Aranjuez: Doce Calles, 1998) and of *El drama de la polio: Un problema social y familiar en la España franquista* (Madrid: Los Libros de la Catarata, 2013). She is also the principal researcher of the project "The Eradication of the Poliomyelitis in an International Context and Related to Other Diseases by Viruses (Smallpox and Influenza): The Role of the Laboratory, the Epidemiological Research and Socioeconomic Factors," funded by the Ministerio de Economía y Competitividad of Spain (2013–15).

ANNY JACKELINE TORRES SILVEIRA is an associate professor in history at the Universidade Federal de Minas Gerais in Belo Horizonte, Brazil. She received her PhD in history from the Universidade Federal Fluminense in Rio de Janeiro. Her main research fields include the history of health sciences and history of public health in Brazil. She is currently coordinating research on the history of hospitals and hospital assistance in Minas Gerais in the nineteenth century and has researched the history of health and the history of smallpox in Minas Gerais in the nineteenth century, funded by Brazilian research agencies—CNPq (Conselho Nacional de Pesquisa) and FAPEMIG (Fundação de Amparo à Pesquisa do Estado de Minas Gerais). She is also a member of the Grupo Scientia—Diretório de Grupos de Pesquisa, CNPq. She has published *A influenza espanhola numa capital planejada: Belo Horizonte, 1918* (Belo Horizonte: Argvmentvm, 2007) and coedited *História da saúde em minas: História e patrimônio arquietônico, 1808–1950* (Campinas: Minha, 2011) and *História da ciência no cinema 3* (Belo Horizonte: Argvmentvm, 2010). She has authored book chapters and articles in the journals *Dynamis, Ciencia e Saúde Coletiva; Tempo: Revista do Departamento de História da UFF; História, Ciência, Saúde: Manguinhos; Luso-Brazilian Review; Revista de História;* and *Varia História,* of which she has been a coeditor since 2012.

PAULO SILVEIRA E SOUSA is an assistant in the Centro de Estudos de Sociologia da Universidade *Nova* in Lisbon, Portugal. He is a coauthor with Pedro Tavares de Almeida of *Ruling the Portuguese Empire, 1820–1926: The Colonial Office and Its leadership* (Baden-Baden: Nomos, 2006) and coeditor of *A pandemia esquecida: Olhares comparados sobre a pneumónica, 1918–1919* (Lisbon: Imprensa de Ciências Sociais, 2009). His work has also been published in journals such as the *Revista de História das Ideias* and *Análise Social.*

JOSÉ MANUEL SOBRAL is an anthropologist and historian and a senior research fellow at the Instituto de Ciências Sociais, University of Lisbon. He is a former president of the Portuguese Anthropological Association. His research interests include epidemics, Portuguese rural society, family and kinship, social memory, heritage, nationalism, food, and cuisine, and he is the author of several essays and books on these subjects. Recently, he authored *Portugal, Portugueses: Uma identidade nacional* (Lisbon: FFMS, 2012), and coedited *A pandemia esquecida: Olhares comparados sobre a pneumónica, 1918–1919* (Lisbon: Imprensa de Ciências Sociais, 2009) and *Food between the Country and the City: Ethnographies of a Changing Global Foodscape* (Oxford: Berg, 2014).

CHRISTIANE MARIA CRUZ DE SOUZA received her PhD in the history of science from the Casa de Oswaldo Cruz, Fundação Oswaldo Cruz (Rio de Janeiro, Brazil). She is currently a researcher and teacher at the Instituto Federal de Educação, Ciência e Tecnologia da Bahia, IFBA in Salvador, Brazil, and a member of the Núcleo de Tecnologia em Saúde, IFBA. She is the author of *A gripe espanhola na Bahia: Saúde, política e medicina em tempos de epidemia* (Salvador: Editora da Universidade Federal da Bahia / Fundação Oswaldo Cruz, 2009), as well as of several articles on the Spanish flu epidemic in Bahia, Brazil, published in specialized periodicals.

Index

aetiology. *See* etiology
Africa, 5, 26, 32, 39, 41–44, 79; culture,
139; Dakar, 39, 41–44, 113, 114;
Mozambique, 79
aftermath of pandemic, 5, 9;
improvement of health care, 63, 66;
social disruption, 135, 144; support
for mutual benefit societies, 165
agriculture, 75, 119
AIDS, HIV, 4, 5, 26, 28, 35
Alaska, 34
Alicante, 1918–19 pandemic, 10, 183,
215–25; areas most affected, 217;
Arrabal Roig, 220, 224; cleaning
brigades, 221; control mechanisms,
216; demographic impact, 215, 217;
deportation of beggars and vagrants,
220; evacuation and demolition,
222, 226; home visits, 220, 241; Las
Provincias, 217, 219, 221–23, 226;
major inequalities, 222; measures
applied, 221; Permanent Commission
on Health, 219; plague, 223; port
at virtual standstill, 217; San Antón
and the Ensanche, 217; sanitary
conditions, 222; social isolation, 215
Alicante, yellow fever epidemic of 1804,
218
Almería, 182–83
alternative therapies: 122; miracle cures,
139; religion-based healing practices,
132
anthrax, 1, 77
Archives, Portugal, 64; Pamplona, 154,
156, 164; Montreal, 231
Archives of Internal Medicine, 49, 50
Argentina/Argentine, 1918–19
pandemic, 6, 7, 10, 194–210;

alcohol, 207; amulets, 209–10;
citizens, 209; closing of schools,
195, 201; Congress, 194; criticism
of public health authorities, 202,
204–5; disinfection measures, 195,
205; extermination of flies, 208;
plague, 199, 209; press, 194–96, 200;
preventative measures, 199, 204, 206;
Yrigoyen, Hipólito, 7, 194
Argentina, press: *Caras y Caretas*, 198,
206–9; *El Hogar*, 195, 198–99, 202–3;
La Nación, 195–200, 203–5, 208; *La
Prensa*, 201–6
autobiographical accounts, 249, 250

bacteriology, 8, 82, 98, 117
Badajoz, 77, 185
Bahia, 9, 130–44; alcohol, 140; Bonfim,
138–39; effects on daily life, 135–38,
144; *O Imparcial*, 133, 135, 136, 137,
142; personal hygiene, 142; political
and economic context, 133; press,
131, 137; public places disinfected,
142
Barcelona, 101, 176, 181, 183–85, 195,
201
Belo Horizonte, 1918–19 pandemic, 9,
47, 111–24; alcohol, 122; amulets,
121; effects on daily life, 118; first
death, 118; new city, 112, 124;
mobilization of society, 124; society,
113, 124
Bilbao, 183
blame, Great War, 43; fear, 115;
government, 131; people's behavior,
117; Portuguese laborers, 175–76;
psychological need for, 175; SS
Demarara, 130

Board of Public Health, 177, 180–81
bodily fluids, 40, 45–48, 132
body: bodily events, 252; body-mind
    division, 259; role of, body stands in
    for the body politic, 178
border(s), 62–64, 77–78, 175–76, 178,
    181, 184, 209
Boston, 1918–19 pandemic, 4, 248, 252,
    256–57, 260
Brazil, 1918–19 pandemic, 6, 7, 9;
    antisepsis of the mouth and nose,
    43; army, 39; autohemotherapy, 48;
    demographic impact, 40; disinfection
    measures, 39, 118; healing practices,
    10, 121, 130–32, 138, 139, 144;
    isolation of sick, 39, 43–44, 118–19;
    plague, 112–13, 117, 119–21, 124,
    133, 137–38; Recife, 39; Red Cross,
    44, 120; research, 39–51; Rio de
    Janeiro, 6, 8, 39–41, 43–47, 49, 50,
    114–15, 117–18, 123, 130, 144, 195–
    96. See also Bahia, Minas Gerais, Belo
    Horizonte
Brazil, press: A Tarde, 141; Diário de
    Notícias, 130, 141; Jornal de Notícias,
    141
Brazilian Academy of Medicine, 43, 50
British Medical Journal, 50, 252
bubonic plague, 56, 58–59, 120
Buenos Aires, 200–201, 205–6, 208, 210
Butantã Institute, 7, 40, 41, 46
Byerly, Carol R., 94–95

Canada, 11, 230–42, 250; disinfection
    measures, 230; Toronto, 237. See also
    Montreal
Carabanchel, 99
caregiving, 11, 231, 237–40, 242
Cartagena, 183, 223
censorship, 7, 83, 115, 179
Chagas, Dr. Carlos, 45
Chile, 200–201
cholera, 1, 11, 56, 58–59, 63, 85, 98,
    112–13, 116–17, 119, 124, 134, 139,
    175, 215–16, 218–21, 225, 252
Ciudad Real, 180, 181
Civilian Public Health Service, 93

climate, 9, 27, 43, 115, 198
closing of schools, 4, 81, 184, 195, 201
closure of public spaces, 81
Coimbra, 56, 61
Commonwealth, 257–59
conspiracy theories, 63; Germans, 122;
    Judeo-Soviet conspiracy, 210
contagion: airborne, 34, 117; animal
    sources, 27, 28, 31, 32; Argentina,
    199–202; Bahia, 129–30, 132, 136,
    138, 142, 144; demographic, 27;
    ecological, 27; of fear (see fear); in
    literature, 255; Minas Gerais, 112–16,
    118–19, 122; Portugal, 77–83;
    poverty, 27; Spain, 175, 180, 221,
    225; travel, 27
contagion, vectors of: discharge of
    soldiers, 95, 101–3; migrant workers,
    6, 77, 78; travel, 6, 27, 31, 181, 223;
    World War I troops, 6, 34, 39, 42, 43,
    44, 45, 95, 78
contemporary views of pandemic, 42,
    43, 221, 238; as joke, 10, 117, 194,
    195, 200, 201
cordon sanitaire, 63, 64, 81, 258
Crosby, Alfred, 4, 94, 261
Crowell, Bowman C., 45, 46
cultural impact, 9, 10, 59, 93, 112, 122,
    131, 139, 144, 182, 226, 248, 250
cyanosis, 252–53

da Cunha Motta, Dr Ludgero, 41, 42
da Fonseca, Olimpio, 41, 47–50
Dakar, 39, 41–44, 113, 114
death toll. See mortality
Demerara, 39, 130
demographic impact, 4, 5, 40, 27, 55,
    215, 217
dengue, 41, 42, 98, 113, 132, 198
DiLouie, Craig, 249–51
diphtheria, 77, 100
diplococcus, 45
Directorate General of Public Health:
    Brazil, 43, 44, 45, 130, 133, 135, 136,
    141–42; Portugal, 56, 61
disinfection: Argentina, 195, 205; Brazil,
    39, 118, 142; brigades, 156, 184, 221;

Canada, 230; Portugal, 82, 84; Spain, 99, 100, 101, 156, 175, 176, 181, 182, 184, 220, 221, 225

DNA-based biosphere, 22

doctors, 9–11, 39–51; debate over diagnosis/ treatment, 40–42, 44–48, 82, 97–98, 100, 113, 131–32, 141–42; contagion of fear, 115, 137; as functionaries, 185–86; gender, 11, 238, 240, 242; home calls, 158, 184, 201, 220, 233; military, 42, 81, 95–103; modern, 51; mortality among, 58, 196, 201, 231, 238–40; mutual benefit societies, 10, 152–55, 157–59, 162, 165; payment, 182, 185, 186; and politicians, 199, 185, 186; prevention, 77, 96, 99, 103; professional defeat, 86, 94, 95, 99, 103, 240, 242; response to pandemic, 130, 131–32, 195–96; retired, 81; rural, 182; shortage, 39, 76, 81, 82, 233, 234; tensions, 94, 95, 101, 103; and traditional medicine, 139; treatment, 100, 142, 143, 157, 158, 200

domestic medicine, 10, 122, 131, 139, 140, 144. *See also* traditional medicine

dysentery, 175

etiology of 1918–19 influenza pandemic: 2, 40, 41–47, 49, 50, 96–99, 112, 113, 132, 175; bacillus, 1, 40, 44–47, 132; bacterial infections, 35; causative agent, 8, 22, 45; diplococcus, 45; epidemiology, 2, 4, 9, 10, 32, 46, 56, 63, 64, 81, 173, 200, 204, 205, 209; filterable virus/ agents, 8, 40, 45–50, 82, 98; identification of the influenza "germ," 7; influenza bacillus, 50; miasmatic theories of disease, 221; pathogen(ic), 1, 8, 25, 26, 28, 31, 32, 34, 35, 130, 132, 175, 186, 257; pneumococcus, 46; streptococcus, 46; supernatural origin, 84, 144

Europe, 5, 6, 11, 26, 32, 39, 41–44, 57, 63–65, 78, 95, 103, 114, 124, 152, 196, 198, 199, 215, 239

evolution of viruses, 21–35; antibodies, 25, 26; antigenic variation, 25; antigens, 23, 25, 26, 33, 48; cytokine storm, 34; copathogenesis, 35; emergence, 3, 24, 26, 30, 33; fading away of an epidemic, 28; fitness, 22, 28, 30; H subtypes, 25; H1N1, 3, 25, 32, 33, 34, 251; H2N2, 32, 33; H3N2, 25, 32, 33; H5N1, 2, 31, 32, 251; pathogen transmission, 28; reassortment, 22, 23, 25, 26, 31, 32

explanatory framework, 8, 132

famine, 6, 27, 121

financial aid, 81, 155

First World War. *See* World War I

fear, fear of, 9, 210; contagion of, 10, 112, 114–16, 119, 120–21, 123–24, 135, 137, 144, 175, 195, 197, 203–5, 209, 236, 255; of further pandemics, 32, 49; influenzaphobia, 115, 137; ritual as palliative, 138

filterable virus/ agents, 8, 40, 45–50, 82, 98

Foote, Horton, 249–52, 259

Fonseca, Olympio da, 41, 47, 48, 49, 50

France, 8, 42, 43, 51, 60, 63, 79, 95, 97, 103, 113, 122, 175, 198

gender and 1918–19 pandemic, 230–42; caregivers: 11, 230–31, 235, 237–38, 240–42; gender history, 230; healthcare workers, 237; mortality, 230

genetic sequencing, 1, 3, 22

genome, 22–25, 28, 30, 32–33; genetic change, 28, 35; genetic material, 21, 32; role of Viral Genome Variation, 30

germ theory, 1, 8, 123

German, 40, 56, 63, 122

Goldberg, Myla, 3, 248, 250, 257, 259–62

Great Britain, 81; Liverpool, 39

Great War. *See* World War I

grippe, 39, 157, 197, 237

Haemophilus influenza. See Pfeiffer's bacillus

healing practices
historiography, 5, 6, 55, 124
HIV. *See* AIDS
Hospital de Isolamento, 39, 118
Hospital of Isolation, 39, 44, 118
housing, effects of poor, 79, 80, 116,
205, 217, 221, 225

immunity, 2, 48, 96, 117, 209; immune
response, 8, 22, 26; immune system,
25, 35
immunization, 45, 132, 206
influenza pandemics (other than 1918–
19): Asian influenza of 1957, 32;
Hong Kong influenza, 25, 33; major
recorded influenza epidemics, 29;
1957 H2N2, 32; 1997 Hong Kong/
avian flu, 2, 3; Russian influenza, 33;
2009 human influenza pandemic, 24
influenza, 1918–19 pandemic: Alicante,
217, 218, 222; antipyretics, 165;
antisepsis of the mouth and nose,
43; autohemotherapy, 48; Bahia,
130, 144; Belo Horizonte, 112, 115;
benignity of, 39, 42–43, 49, 77, 80,
96, 114, 118, 131–32, 134, 137, 144,
200–201; Brazil, Rio de Janeiro,
São Paulo, 49; Canada, 230; causes,
34–35; characteristics, 3, 32, 41–43,
50, 77, 80, 251; circulation of people
and goods, 60; cleaning brigades,
156, 184, 221; clinical characteristics,
96, 251, 253; closing of public spaces,
81; closing of schools, 4, 81, 184,
195, 201; control mechanisms, 10,
216; cordon sanitaire, 63, 64, 81,
258; daily life, 118, 119, 123–24, 131,
134–38, 144, 154, 201; demographic
impact, 4, 5, 40, 27, 55, 215, 217;
disinfection, 39, 82, 84, 99, 100,
101, 118, 142, 156, 175, 176, 181,
182, 184, 195, 205, 220, 221, 225,
230; egalitarian character, 137–38;
epidemiology, 2, 4, 9, 10, 32, 46,
56, 63, 64, 81, 173, 200, 204–5,
209; estimates (by age sectors), 79;
estimates (by gender), 79; estimates

(by social class), 79; estimates (total),
78; evacuation and demolition, 222,
226; extermination of flies, 208;
gender difference, 230; H1N1, 3,
25, 32–34, 251; historiography, 5,
6, 55, 124; home visits, 158, 220,
241; hygiene, 57, 77, 100, 101,
142; inequality, 103, 176; isolation
(social), 215; isolation of pathogen,
1, 4, 5, 8, 10, 46, 47, 175; isolation
of sick, 4, 39, 43–44, 60–61, 63,
82–83, 96, 99, 101–2, 118–19, 156,
215, 216, 257; kissing, 60; literary
representations, 3, 5, 11, 248–62;
medical-pharmaceutical care, 154;
medication, 143; Montreal, 230–42;
mortality, 2, 3, 11; narrative, 2, 8, 10,
112, 124, 174, 186, 201, 210, 249,
252, 255, 260; origin of, 2, 33, 94,
121, 122, 221, 225; Pamplona, 155,
156; Portugal, 77–78; preventative
measures, 95, 99, 101, 199, 204,
206, 233; quarantine, 4, 81, 82, 117,
201, 205, 258, 259; Quebec, 231;
reconstructed 1918 influenza virus,
3, 34; Salvador, 137; samples for
study, 33–34; sanitary conditions, 81;
serum, 100, 101, 240; shaking hands,
122, 208; shortage of basic goods,
100; Spanish army, 96; spread, 5, 6,
9, 28, 31, 41–44, 46, 60–62, 76–78,
80, 95, 99, 101–3, 113–14, 117–18,
124, 130, 133–35, 137, 144, 156–57,
174, 194, 195, 200, 203, 261, 218,
221, 224, 232; suspension of public
activities, 136, 181, 182, 184, 203,
205; treatment: 44, 84, 122, 132,
140–41, 143, 157, 165, 176; virulence
of, 2, 22, 28, 33–35, 41–44, 48, 78,
94, 113, 130–32, 203, 217, 223; virus,
2–5, 34, 256; virus type A, 23, 25. *See
also* domestic medicine, etiology,
remedies, traditional medicine
influenza virus(es): antibodies, 25,
26; antigenic variation, 23–26, 33;
avian / birds, 2, 25, 27, 31, 32, 33,
34; contagion from animal sources,

27; evolution, 21–22, 35; genetic change, 28, 35; genetic material, 21, 32; genome, 22–25, 28, 30, 32, 33; H1N1, 3, 25, 32, 33, 34, 251; H2N2, 32, 33; H3N2, 25, 32, 33; H5N1, 2, 31, 32, 251; influenza virus type A, 8, 22, 25, 31; mutation, 2, 8, 22, 23, 25, 26, 27, 28, 30, 31, 32, 50; quasispecies dynamics, 22, 28; reassortment, 22, 23, 25, 26, 31, 32; recombination, 8, 22–23, 25, 26, 30, 31, 34; reconstructed 1918 influenza virus, 3, 34; role of viral genome variation, 30; swine, 3, 5, 24, 25, 31, 32, 33, 34, 251

Institut Pasteur, Paris, 50; Tunis, 98
isolation of sick, 4, 39, 43–44, 60–61, 63, 82–83, 96, 99, 101–2, 118–19, 156, 215, 216, 257

Jorge, Ricardo, 7, 9, 55, 59, 62, 64, 65, 76, 79–81; pseudonym, Dr. Mirandela, 62, 63

laborers: migration, 6, 78; Portuguese, 77, 176; professional, 237; public service, 201; Spanish, 95, 103, 176. *See also* workers
Laidlaw, Patrick, 1, 4, 50
Las Provincias, 217, 219, 221–23, 226
Last Town on Earth, The, 3, 250, 252–53, 257–59
Lazcano, Sergio, 154, 158, 159, 165
Leiria, 55, 81
League of Nations, 9, 57, 62–65
Lisbon, 39, 55–56, 58, 60–62, 75, 77, 79–81, 85

Madrid, 79, 94, 95, 97, 99, 100, 177, 181–85
Magalhães, Octavio de, 41, 47–50
malaria, 56, 58, 59, 77, 120, 134, 137, 196
Malthus, Thomas, 94
Marques da Cunha, Aristides, 41, 47, 49, 50
Martín Salazar, Manuel, 64, 97–99, 185
McIntosh, James, 50

measles, 46, 98
medical science, 59, 143, 240
medicine, confidence, 94–95
memory, 55, 58, 134, 144, 250, 254, 255, 258, 261
Mexico, 32, 33
miasmatic theories of disease, 221
Minas Gerais, 9, 47, 111–24. *See also* Belo Horizonte
Ministry of Public Health, 185
Montreal, 1918–19 pandemic, 11, 230–42; archives, 231; blow to doctors' confidence, 240; *La Bonne Parole*, 236; caregivers, 238; Collège du Sacré-Cœur, 232; Conseil d'Hygiène de la Province de Québec, 233; *Le Devoir*, 234; federal Department of Health, 232; Gardes-Malades de Ville-Marie, 234; gender history, 230; gendered, 11, 230–31, 235, 237–38, 240–42; gender-neutral, 230, 238; globally, more men than women died of influenza, 230; Gray Nuns, 231, 234, 239; healthcare workers, gendered, 237; helplessness of medical professionals, 242; heroism, 238, 239, 240, 242; Idola Saint-Jean, 234, 241; immigrants, 232, 236; Lady Lacoste, 237, 238; linguistic and religious configuration, 232; members of the clergy, 235, 237; Municipal authorities, 232; New England, 232; nuns, 11, 231, 234, 236–40, 242; *La Patrie*, 237; plague, 231; preventative measures, 233; priests, 11, 139, 231, 235–36, 238–40, 242; Red Cross, 235; Regalia, 231, 233; rhetoric of heroism, 238–40, 242; Sœurs Grises (Gray Nuns), 231, 234; social responses, 231, 234–36; soldiers, 232
Mullen, Thomas, 3, 250, 252–53, 257–60
mutation, 2, 8, 22–23, 25–28, 30–32, 50
Mutual Benefit Societies. *See* Pamplona

Nabuco de Gouvêa, Dr. José Thomaz, 42, 44
names. *See* terms

national identity, 7, 11, 176
Navarre, 154, 155. *See* Pamplona
newspapers. *See* press
1918 (play), 250–52

O Imparcial, 133, 135, 136, 137, 142
Office Internationale de Hygiène
    Publique, 59
"On Being Ill" (Woolf), 253
Oporto. *See* Porto
Oswaldo Cruz Institute, 7, 40–41, 45,
    47, 49

Pais, Sidónio, 60–63, 76, 83, 85–86
Pale Horse, Pale Rider, 249, 254–57
Palma de Mallorca, 185
Pamplona, 1918–19 pandemic, 10,
    152–59, 164–66; antipyretics, 165;
    archives, 154, 156, 164; cleaning
    brigades, 156; City Council, 164–65;
    Diario de Navarra, 159; home visits,
    158; Instituto Nacional de Previsión,
    153; social protection, 153
Pamplona, 1918–19 pandemic, mutual
    benefit societies, 7, 10, 152–66;
    educational role, 152; financial aid, 155,
    156, 160–64; income and expenses, 160;
    La Conciliación, 154–66; reactions, 156;
    role during influenza, 154; role of their
    doctors, 154
pappataci fever, 41, 42, 132
Paris, 42, 50, 56, 58, 59, 116, 117, 200
Pasteur, Louis, 56, 65
peste pneumónica, 55, 58, 59, 61, 63, 64
Pfeiffer, Richard, 1, 40, 45, 46, 50, 132
Pfeiffer's bacillus, 40, 46, 47, 49, 50, 97,
    98
pharmacies, 76, 81, 119, 141–42, 165,
    195, 200
pharmacists, 44, 120, 143, 208, 209
physical contact: shaking hands, 122,
    208; kissing, 60
physicians. *See* doctors
Pires, Accacio, 143, 144
plague, 56–59, 62, 64, 80, 84–85, 98,
    112–13, 117, 119–21, 124, 133, 137–
    38, 199, 209, 223, 231, 257–58

pneumónica (*also* peste pneumónica),
    55, 57–59, 60–64, 77, 131; influenza
    pneumónica, 57, 80
Pontevedra, 185
popular imagination, 2, 57, 112, 113,
    197, 205
Porter, Katherine Anne, 249, 254–57
Portugal, 1918–19 pandemic, 6, 7,
    9, 55–65, 75–86; age groups, 79;
    Alentejo, 77; Algarve, 55, 78;
    archives, 64; Azores, 78; church
    claimed a key role, 84; Coimbra, 56,
    61; Conselho de Saúde Pública, 60;
    demographic impact, 55; failings of
    authorities, 81; Leiria, 55, 81; Lisbon,
    39, 56, 58, 60–62, 75, 77, 79–81,
    85; medical and nursing services,
    77; mortality, 77–81; mortality by
    socioeconomic group/ class, 79–80;
    movement of soldiers, 95, 103;
    (peste) pneumónica, 55, 57–59,
    60–64; plague, 56–59, 62, 64, 80,
    84–85; Porto, 56, 58–59, 64, 75, 77,
    80; politicization of pandemic, 9,
    77; propagation by migration, 78;
    religious explanation, 85; Red Cross,
    44; Virgin of Fátima, 55, 85–86
Portugal, 1918–19 pandemic, measures
    taken, 79–85; bureaucracy, 82;
    closing of schools, 81; closure of
    public spaces, 81; cordon sanitaire,
    63–64, 81; criticism of Spain's
    measures, 62, 63; daily hygiene,
    57; disinfection measures, 82, 84;
    impeding the circulation of people
    and goods, 60; personal hygiene, 77;
    prohibition of export of drugs, 80;
    social structure, 75, 76
Portuguese press: *Diário de Notícias,* 59,
    60; *O Mundo,* 83; *O Século,* 59–62
Portuguese Republic, 56, 60, 75–86;
    Estado Novo, 56; poverty, 6, 27, 58,
    79, 216, 218, 220–25, 241; separation
    between church and state, 60; social
    unrest, 61
press, 9, 10, 39, 43, 44, 55, 61–63, 80,
    94–96, 98, 101, 112–20, 122–23, 130–

33, 138–39, 141, 156, 158–59, 176, 178, 181, 194–95, 198, 201, 204, 210, 216, 234, 236, 239, 258. *See also under individual countries*

prophylactic/ prophylaxis, 3, 43, 60–63, 64, 96, 98, 99, 100, 102, 118, 122, 131, 134, 139, 142, 195, 198, 205–6, 208, 210; etymology, 208

psychiatric sequelae, 144, 256

psychological closure, 2, 3

purple death, 131

public health: brigades, 184; challenges for, 35, 86; criticism of, 62, 63, 133, 177, 196, 202, 204, 208; improvements, 153, 216, 241; and military doctors, 99, 103; Portugal, 55–65, 83; public health zones, 141; resistance to, 9, 131; responses to, 11, 80, 112, 114, 116, 120, 130, 131, 133, 135, 136, 141, 142, 153, 156, 162, 176, 182, 184–86, 199, 221, 222, 231, 237; shortcomings of, 27, 65, 77, 80, 86, 93, 99, 103, 124, 174, 202, 232

quarantine, 4, 81, 82, 117, 201, 205, 258, 259

quasispecies, 22, 23, 28, 30

quinine, 43, 81, 119, 143, 196, 200, 201, 206

Real Academia Nacional de Medicina (Spain), 98–100

recombination, 8, 22, 23, 25, 26, 30, 31, 34

reconstruction of influenza virus, 3, 34

Red Cross, 44, 62, 120, 235

religion and 1918–19 pandemic, 5, 7, 10, 11; *Bonfim*, 138–39; Christians: Catholic, 9, 75–77, 83–85, 121, 153, 232; church claimed a key role, 84; disruption of rituals, 182; expiation, 121; festivals and rituals, 136, 137, 138, 182, 183, 254; Gray Nuns, 231, 234, 239; healing practices, 10, 121, 130–32, 138; Leiria, 55, 81; linguistic and religious configuration, 232; liturgy, 61, 137; masses, 138, 144,

184; members of the clergy, 235, 237; nuns, 11, 231, 234, 236–40, 242; priests, 11, 139, 231, 235–36, 238–40, 242; Protestants, 85, 232; religious communities, 232, 234; repentance, 85; Virgin of Fátima, 55, 85–86

remedies, 2, 81, 100, 122, 139, 140, 207, 209

Rio de Janeiro, 6, 8, 39–41, 43–47, 49, 50, 114–15, 117–18, 123, 130, 144, 195–96

RNA, viruses, 21–23, 28, 30; (or DNA) polymerases, 21; biosphere, 22

Salvador, 9, 39, 130, 131, 133, 136, 137, 140, 141, 144

sandfly fever, 131, 132

São Paulo, 6, 8, 40, 41, 42, 44, 45, 46, 49, 50, 144

segregation, 220, 226

sequelae, 178, 260; psychiatric, 144, 256

Sisters of Charity, 102

slums, 217, 225, 241

smallpox, 77, 82, 98, 133, 252

social control, 7, 11, 226

social hygiene, 10, 59, 152

social impact, 9, 34, 64, 94, 119–20, 123, 124, 134, 181, 182, 249. *See also* 1918–19 pandemic, effects on daily life

social mobilization, 44, 82, 93, 119, 120, 124, 185

socioeconomic status and mortality, 77, 79, 93, 103, 153, 216, 217

sociosanitary policy, 7, 10, 216

solidarity, 44, 120, 185

Spain, 1918–19 pandemic, 1–11, 32, 46, 56, 63, 93–103, 152–66, 173–86, 215–26; Board of Public Health, 177, 180–81; Cartagena, 183, 223; chronic shortage of basic goods, 100; civilian health service, 9, 93, 94, 96, 100–103; civilian medicine, 7, 11; cleaning brigades, 156, 184, 221; closing of schools, 184; Córdoba, 183, 199; disinfection measures, 99, 100, 101, 156, 175, 176, 181, 184, 220, 221, 225; "epidemic Spain," 10, 174, 181,

Spain—(cont'd)
184, 186; Guipúzcoa, 155, 182;
  La Coruña, 182; Málaga, 184;
  measures against Portugal, 62–64;
  neutrality during WWI, 6, 63, 94,
  173; Pontevedra, 185; sanitary
  dictatorship, 174, 178–81, 184–6;
  "sanitary Spain," 10, 174, 178, 181,
  184–86; Toledo, 180, 182, 183;
  turnismo system, 180; two Spains,
  173, 174; "Wall of China," 63. See also
  Alicante, Pamplona
Spanish army, 93–103; Civilian Public
  Health Service, 93; conflicts with
  Civil Health Service, 9, 94; doctors'
  professional disaster, 94, 103; hygienic
  conditions of barracks, 93, 96, 99,
  101; infrastructure deficiencies, 101,
  103; military medicine, 7, 9, 93, 94,
  99; morbidity rates for soldiers, 96,
  97; personal hygiene, 101; plague,
  98; preventative measures, 95, 99,
  101; proper cleaning of the skin, 100;
  Manuel Martín Salazar, 64, 97–99,
  185; speed of spread of influenza, 101;
  unequal treatment, 101
Spanish flu. See influenza 1918–19
  pandemic
"Spanish Lady," 130, 132–37
Spanish military press: La
  Correspondencia Militar, 95, 98, 102; El
  Heraldo Militar, 95; Revista de Sanidad
  Militar, 95, 98
Spanish press: ABC, 175–78, 180, 182–
  83; El Correo, 223; Diario de Navarra,
  159; Heraldo de Madrid, 182; El Liberal,
  174, 179, 180, 183, 184; El Socialista,
  102; El Sol, 102, 181; El Tiempo, 223;
  La Vanguardia, 176, 183, 196–97, 199,
  201, 206, 208–9
supernatural, interpretation, 84, 85;
  remedies, 144
suspension of public activities, 136, 181,
  182, 184, 203, 205
symptoms, 34, 42, 45, 49–50, 95, 113,
  115, 132, 139, 140–41, 143–44, 177,
  179, 197, 251–52

Taubenberger, Jeffery, 1, 2, 3, 22
terms: nickname, 7, 95; origin of
  nickname, 174; other names, 41, 42,
  131, 132, 197, 198
Thin White Line, The, 250, 252
three-day fever, 42, 131, 132. See
  pappataci fever
Toledo, 180, 182, 183
traditional medicine, 121, 144,
  209–10; alcohol, 122, 140, 207;
  healing practices, 10, 121, 130–32,
  138, 139; herbal teas, 139; sinapism,
  140
tuberculosis, 1, 77, 79, 138
typhoid, 77, 98
typhus, 77, 98, 113, 175, 177

unanswered questions, 2–4, 11, 33, 35
USA: 4, 5, 26, 32, 50, 64, 79, 81, 82, 85,
  232, 240; army, 94; Boston, 1918–19
  pandemic, 4, 248, 252, 256–57, 260;
  Colorado, 257; New England, 232;
  New York, 26, 256
urban areas, 7, 28, 75, 111, 217, 218

vaccine, 2, 4, 33, 48, 64, 82, 99, 100, 185
Virgin of Fátima, 55, 85–86

welfare state, 10, 59, 65, 76
Wickett's Remedy, 3, 248, 250, 257,
  259–61
workers: migration, 6, 78; insurance
  protection, 152–54, 157, 159–65;
  Portuguese, 77, 176; public service,
  201; professional, 237; Spanish,
  95, 103, 176; Workers' Obligatory
  Retirement, 153
Woolf, Virginia, 253–54
World War I, 6, 7, 11, 42, 43, 59–64, 76,
  93–95, 103, 122, 134, 157, 173, 194,
  230–34, 239, 242, 249

yellow fever, 11, 112, 117, 120, 132–34,
  137, 215–16, 220–21, 225
Yrigoyen, Hipólito, 7, 194

Zamora, 101–2

Lightning Source UK Ltd.
Milton Keynes UK
UKHW011846251121
394539UK00002B/85